Confessions
of a
Prolife Missionary

Confessions
of a
Prolife Missionary

The Journeys of Fr. Paul Marx

Fr. Paul Marx, OSB, PhD

With a Foreword by Fr. Joseph Fessio, SJ

Human Life International
Gaithersburg, Maryland

To my long-time collaborators:
Mrs. Virginia Gager
Mrs. Bonnie Manion
Frau Elisabeth Backhaus
Mrs. Elizabeth Trollope

© 1988 by Human Life International
7845-E Airpark Road
Gaithersburg, Maryland 20879 USA
301/670-7884

Printed in the United States of America

ISBN 1-55922-020-1
ISBN 1-55922-021-x pbk.

CONTENTS

FOREWORD

One thing this book does not need is a long foreword, by me or anyone else. This is battlefront reporting from someone who is not just a war correspondent but one of the greatest fighters for the cause of the unborn in this century.

God has his ways of letting his sovereignty be shown. For example, there is one state in the modern world which has made an all-out attempt to eradicate the worship of God—tiny, isolationist Albania. And so God, who will not be mocked, at the very moment that this state was exterminating every last vestige of Christianity that it could find, inspired a young Albanian woman named Agnes Bohaxiu to be the apostle of that very charity that her country had tried to obliterate. Of course, she is better known as Mother Teresa of Calcutta. And what roars of celestial joy there must be for all those around the world who have come to know and love God and his Son Jesus through the labors of this Albanian woman.

So we should not be too surprised by other marks of God's work. A century after a man named Marx infected the whole planet with a deadly ideology, killing tens if not hundreds of millions of people by execution or forced starvation, a century after the beginning of that promethean atheist system which is the principal symbol of a loss of faith in God, a loss which has inevitably led to a loss of faith in man and in man's dignity—and which led in particular to a hatred of the unborn—God responded. He raised up another Marx, and gave him the name of the indefatigable warrior-missionary Paul.

Here is a man with the intrepidity and organizational skills of his distant cousin Karl and the tireless zeal of his patron Paul. And as if to make it inescapably clear that this is God's work and not man's, the Father chose—no doubt amid a cataract of celestial laughter—a man with a vow of *stability*!

Just as St. Benedict became the father of Europe by the enormous spread of his monastic ideal in thousands of monasteries in the ages when the glories of civilization were almost completely disintegrated, so now a disciple of

St. Benedict has become, if not the father, certainly the godfather of prolife activism around the world.

To some extent the *Special Reports* in this book are autobiographical. They tell us about Fr. Marx, his travels and his experiences on the front lines. But they are really a story about the war itself. There is no better way of seeing precisely what is happening and just what spiritual powers and forces of man are in play than by following these reports of the last seven years. They read like a novel, because they are in fact eyewitness accounts of the unfolding great battle of our time, the struggle for life and human dignity.

But this is not just armchair reading for bystanders. It is my hope that every reader will be inspired by the work of Fr. Paul Marx and his Human Life International to take part in the struggle. Because the story has not ended, and it is up to us—with the help of Almighty God— to make this saga the story of heroic victory and not of tragic defeat.

Fr. Joseph Fessio, SJ
Founder, Ignatius Institute
and Ignatius Press

PREFACE

In 1959 the American Law Institute issued the first model abortion bill for states to enact. I was teaching family sociology at Minnesota's St. John's University and the nearby college of St. Benedict, and my flags went up when this threat to the most vulnerable member of the family appeared. How could I, as a citizen, a sociologist, a priest and a man, possibly remain uninvolved? I began writing articles against abortion immediately.

In 1967 Colorado became the first state to adopt the proposed bill, which allowed the killing of preborn babies in certain cases. After only one year, Representative (now Governor) Richard Lamm, who engineered the bill's passage, told Planned Parenthood of Minneapolis, "It was a noble experiment that failed; we must have abortion on demand."

In January 1971 I attended and recorded the whole of a large, semi-secret meeting at the International Hotel in Los Angeles (now the Hyatt at Los Angeles Airport). The purpose of the meeting was to discuss how to bring down all abortion laws, how to justify this legally, how legally to abort teenagers, how to prepare American society for baby-killing and many other unbelievables. I was shocked to the core, but even more astounded at who attended: noted gynecologists, heads of famous medical departments and schools, Planned Parenthood propagandists, pro-abortion Sen. Robert Packwood of Oregon (who spoke by phone from Washington for more than half an hour) and many others.

To attend, you had to have written permission; to record, you had to have a second, special permission slip, signed by an official. Calling myself "Dr. Marx" (I have a doctorate in sociology), I received these documents from a careless secretary who assumed I was an abortionist.

Out of this gathering came my book *The Death Peddlers: War on the Unborn*, which sold 140,000 copies (and transformed my life into an impossibly hectic battle). After the Los Angeles meeting I was convinced that the USA was on its way to abortion on demand, but few believed me. How to awaken bishops, priests, academics, doctors and other leaders to this gigantic threat became a painful ordeal and a preoccupation.

By 1972, 18 states had liberalized their abortion laws, but in the state legislatures the abortion movement as such had been stopped. The abortion promoters then turned to state referenda to advance their ignoble cause. They were defeated both times they tried, by 79 percent of the vote in North Dakota and by 62 percent in Michigan. Despite these signals that the people did not want the slaughter of the unborn, on 22 January 1973 the U.S. Supreme Court imposed upon the nation abortion on demand any time during the nine months of pregnancy.

I was in London at the time, and my first thoughts were: (1) the United States of America has seen its best days, and (2) from now on, the nation will slide back culturally and morally. Any open-minded observer who examines subsequent events must admit that since 1973 the USA has been doing nothing but "going downhill."

On 26 January 1973, four days after the Court's "Black Monday" decision, I spoke for several minutes with Pope Paul VI, who had been briefed. Indeed, he knew about the Court's decision and its consequences. He told me, "Never give up; you are a courageous fighter."

By the time of the Supreme Court's infamous decision, I had already been active in speaking and writing against the baby-killers for more than a decade. I was not surprised that the Supreme Court decreed abortion on demand, given the machinations of the abortion zealots, the decline of the American judiciary, and the weakening of spiritual, moral, and religious forces throughout Western society.

In 1972, after much opposition, I founded the Human Life Center at St. John's University to combat this horrendous new evil nationally and internationally. As a group, intellectuals have a poor record when it comes to fighting the evil of abortion. It was no different at St. John's University. But the Human Life Center flourished despite the hostile environment and, at one time, employed 24 people.

I also founded *Love-Life-Death Issues*, a newsletter now published monthly as *Human Life Issues* by the Human Life Center at Ohio's University of Steubenville, to which HLC escaped for a more favorable environment. Later I founded a monthly prolife newspaper, *Life and Family News*, now edited by my former HLC colleague, Andrew

Scholberg. Today it is published by Joe Scheidler's Pro-Life Action League in Chicago.

Since my ordination in 1947, I have had an abiding interest in modern natural family planning (NFP). I have organized ten international symposia on that subject. In 1976 I founded the *International Review of Natural Family Planning*, still published by the Human Life Center today.

In 1981, I received permission from my Abbot to establish Human Life International in Washington, D.C., the political capital of the world. Long before this, I realized that abortion was the modern world's primary evil; as the Germans say, "Die Abtreibung macht Alles kaput"—"Abortion destroys everything." And indeed it does!

Abortion kills babies, damages women, harms families, degrades the medical profession, weakens nations and destroys Churches. That is why the "common sense of history" has always condemned it: in law, 2,000 years before Christ, in the oldest major law code we know, the Sumerian Code; in medicine, 400 years before Christ in the Hippocratic Oath; and, of course, in Christian teaching about the year 70 AD in the *Didache*, the first non-biblical Christian document that we possess.

Thanks to God's obvious and manifold blessings, HLI is flourishing today. We have 22 international branches on five continents, plus six U.S. chapters. We employ 38 people around the world. HLI is undoubtedly the largest prolife/family organization in the world; surely, it is also the best informed one and the one most in touch with international prolife/family realities. We are a unique missionary effort: you cannot baptize and catechize the child who has already been murdered in the womb—which, by the way, has become the most dangerous place on earth to live today. (What a sad commentary on our times!)

There is a saying that "an organization without a newsletter or publication does not exist." Hence, we founded *HLI Reports*, edited by John Cavanaugh-O'Keefe. This 12-page international prolife/family publication reports prolife activist news and important events and developments from all over the world. It contains news that you cannot find in any other publication.

Seeing how Planned Parenthood preyed on Hispanics, we also founded *Escoge la Vida*, edited by the incomparable Cuban-born Magaly Llaguno; this excellent newsletter for the Spanish-speaking people of the world appears quarterly from our branch office in Miami. From this office, too, Mrs. Llaguno and Fr. Albert Salmon coordinate HLI's prolife activities throughout Latin America.

Because so many people are so interested in our work and so many give it their gracious financial support, I have been sending them a monthly insider's report on what I do and see around the world. This monthly accounting, known as *Special Reports*, has proven fascinating to many, who are shocked by what is happening all over the globe. Some find it hard to believe that abortion, with its accompanying evils, has now spread through three-quarters of mankind. Some also express shock at my prediction that abortion will be legalized in virtually all countries eventually.

The "true blue" prolifer, however, was not surprised to see abortion's twin, the euthanasia monster, rear its ugly head. As early as 1971, I published *The Mercy Killers*, which sold more than half a million copies. It sounded the warning that "mercy" killing was coming. I have updated this publication three times, and it will be available as *Doorways to Death* in the spring of 1989. Currently there are four euthanasia societies in the USA and more than 50 throughout the world. In April 1988 the International Federation of Right-to-Die Societies held its seventh international conference on euthanasia in San Francisco, drawing hundreds of participants from 17 countries.

Along the way, I was enormously encouraged by a 10-minute conversation I had with Pope John Paul II on 17 November 1979. He said he knew me from my talks and writings in the German-speaking countries, where I began to work in 1972. (He was then the Cardinal Archbishop of Krakow in Poland.) Incidentally, the Pope asked me impishly, "Is there a little bit of Karl [Marx] in you?" I responded, "Your Holiness, only through Adam and Eve."

At that point I had made prolife missionary journeys to 48 countries (now 75); I thanked him for condemning contraception in every country he had visited, because I had found that inevitably, without exception, contraception pushes nations into abortion.

Once contraception is widespread, no society has ever been able to keep it within marriage. Then, as surely as morning follows night, liberalized abortion follows, so that people can "remedy" their contraceptive failures. Abortion then becomes a primary means of birth control. And yet even today, so many people still do not know (or will not admit) that foresight contraception leads to hindsight abortion. When I explained to the Pope the social evolution from contraception to abortion to euthanasia in every country I had visited, he said to me in his Polish-English, "That is why the Church, Christianity, condemned contraception from the beginning." (All Protestant denominations did so until 1930.)

Later he remarked, "You have lots of experience. You are doing the most important work on earth." He urged me to bring the prolife/pro-family ministry to the whole world, particularly to the developing countries where, he implied, humanity and the Church have their future. Today nine out of every 10 babies are born in the developing countries, while the over*cop*ulating West is dying from non-reproductive birthrates. After conversing with the Holy Father, I went home with renewed energy, only to learn that I had been relieved as head of HLC—for reasons I might understand in eternity. At that time, HLC had a staff of 24 and was heading toward a million-dollar budget.

An estimated 200,000 people read HLI's *Special Reports*. Readers have urged me to publish the best of these *Reports* in one volume so that more people will learn about HLI's prolife missionary work and perhaps be motivated to join HLI's fight against the mystical body of Satan. My dear prolife friends tell me that this volume will cause HLI to grow even faster.

There are hundreds of thousands more who would read and support us if they learned the true extent of our worldwide pro-family apostolic work. Our *HLI Reports* and *Special Reports* reach 90 countries regularly, and we have shipped prolife literature and audiovisual aids to, or produced them in, 105 countries. Anyone who reads our monthly publications will tap an international reservoir of prolife/family information and experience that exists nowhere else.

John Cavanaugh-O'Keefe, Director of Publications for HLI, has expertly edited the very best from these *Special Reports* into this book, giving you vital information and a priceless, worldwide perspective. I must also acknowledge the contributions of Mike Engler, who skilfully edited nearly all of the *Special Reports* from my rough manuscripts in the first place, making many valuable additions.

We beg you to spread this book far and wide so that more and more people join our battle for life. The situation is truly desperate: of all the developed countries in the world, only Ireland, Poland and little Malta are reproducing themselves. In other words, contraception/sterilization/-abortion is killing the developed nations. Indeed, abortion is the point of no return for any country. As a German cardinal told me, "Abortion is a moral earthquake, undermining the whole structure of law, culture and civilization."

Meanwhile, the euthanasia juggernaut is now upon us. As Pope Leo XIII once said, "We must look at the world as it really exists, and then look elsewhere for the solace of its troubles." He was implying clearly that we cannot be good Christians, good clergymen or good bishops unless we truly understand our cultural environment and the *Zeitgeist*. The basic moral law never changes, but the moral tasks change for each generation. We must take pains not to live in the past, but to confront the present courageously. As Søren Kierkegaard observed, we know life backward but must live it forward.

May this modest effort, then, awaken and inspire many more to oppose contraception, sterilization, abortion and euthanasia intelligently in these unique times; may it lead all to promote an understanding of and reverence for God's great gifts of human sexuality, true love and healthy, happy, holy marriage.

Finally, I wish to thank the many souls across the world who have helped HLI with their prayers, their finances, and their words of encouragement. Only in Heaven will you know how many young people you educated in chastity; how many couples you schooled in NFP; and how many babies you saved from murder in the greatest war of all time, the war on the unborn—an orgy of medical violence rapidly spreading to the elderly and those whom Hitler called "useless eaters."

One day you will defeat the death peddlers, because you truly *do* have God on your side. As Pope Paul VI said to me, never give up, for you are a courageous fighter.

Fr. Paul Marx, OSB, PhD
2 October 1988
7845-E Airpark Road
Human Life International
Gaithersburg, Maryland 20879 USA
301/670-7884

H.L.I.'S BIRTH

(No. 1—October, 1981)

Abbot Jerome Theisen, OSB, my superior, has graciously given me a five-year leave of absence from St. John's Abbey so that I can pursue to the utmost the prolife/pro-family apostolate.

Accordingly, I have founded HUMAN LIFE INTERNATIONAL (HLI), with headquarters on Capitol Hill in Washington, DC. Already my head is filled with ideas for urgent prolife projects.

Why another center? Because HLI will do what *no one else* is doing. From the hub of the political world I shall launch forth to devote two or three months a year to spreading the prolife/pro-family gospel, mostly in the underdeveloped areas that I know so well from having visited 51 countries.

This spring I spent five weeks lecturing in Japan, South Korea and the Philippines. Nuns, interns, nurses, intellectuals, Knights of Columbus, and youth groups gave me their eager attention. In the Philippines I could have talked ten times a day! Its largest religious order begged me to return.

By calling myself Dr. Marx, I obtained much valuable information from the Population Commission, an American-funded antilife base for Southeast Asia. It has trained some 80,000 Filipinos to carry its deadly message to 110 islands. There is evidence that it coaches midwives to induce abortion by massaging the pregnant woman.

In Asia, Africa and Latin America, I shall introduce prolife/pro-family literature and audiovisual aids, planting or nourishing the natural family planning (NFP) movement. Wherever possible I shall help to organize prolife groups, as I did in 1971 in South Australia, Latin America and other regions.

Will I abandon the United States? Never! This country must be saved. We are imitated widely, both in our good deeds and in the evil we propagate internationally. We *are* relentless purveyors of contraception, sterilization and abortion, but our right-to-life movement is incomparable. I shall continue to study and write, to lecture and advise, to help existing groups and organize others. I shall address our nuns, priests, seminarians and college and high-school students.

Day after day, Planned Parenthood, with taxpayers' money, contaminates more of this country's youth with its vicious sex education program. To combat this blight effectively, we must work up positive, truly Christian programs on sexuality. Here is an area to which HLI must devote much time and effort.

Another such area is the U.S. seminaries, which are not adequately preparing future priests to promote positive alternatives to the antilife movement, to build up an intelligent resistance to the destroyers of the family, to teach and foster the priceless virtue of chastity.

Thanks to generous grants in the past, including two from the Propagation of the Faith in Rome, we have distributed more than $200,000 worth of literature and other aids to foreign seminaries, Catholic colleges, high schools, hospitals, dispensaries and mission stations. Through my voluminous correspondence, much of it foreign, I have consulted, advised and encouraged the leaders and workers in this marvelous apostolate.

Right now I am completing plans for a weekend seminar (October 23-25) designed to advise chosen Irish leaders how to pass a constitutional amendment protecting all human life from fertilization onward, thus heading off the abortionists. HLI's first big project in the United States will be to conduct an international NFP symposium in Washington, DC, November 5–8.

More than ever before, I need your prayers and your spiritual sacrifices.

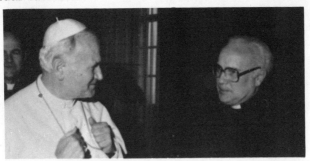

'You are doing the most important work on earth.' —
17 November 1979

IMPENDING BATTLES
ON TWO CONTINENTS

(No. 2—December 1981)

The International Symposium on Natural Family Planning, November 5-8, sponsored by Human Life International (HLI), was the best of ten such international symposia organized so far. Seventy-nine leaders from 13 countries attended. One, a medical student from Stockholm, is starting a natural family planning unit (NFP) at the notorious Karolinska Hospital, where the hideous fetal experiments are done, many financed by American money. A Medical Missionary from Ireland came to promote NFP in that order's vast missionary empire in Africa.

On March 19-21 we will be part of an American delegation organized by HLI and Americans United for Life (AUL) which is to discuss with 50 Irish leaders in a closed, weekend seminar the best way to pass an amendment to the Irish Constitution which could not be challenged, leaving the Catholic Irish with the same antilife mess we have in our country.

I shall leave January 2 for one month in the Philippines, where I expect to be lecturing several times a day on many of the 110 islands that the Filipinos occupy out of a total of 7,000! I have already sent ahead prolife films and slides, and much prolife/pro-family literature. There are opportunities galore in this nation of 50 million, where all speak English and where American money perhaps has done more harm than in any other developing country.

In the early 1970s American authorities prevailed on President Marcos to make a presidential proclamation mandating population control programs at every level of Filipino education. A massive American-financed program of contraception was introduced, with assurances that there would be no sterilization and no abortion. Even in 1974, when I addressed the Filipino population controllers twice, they assured me that there would be no sterilization and no abortion. But in my three-week lecture tour in the Philippines (May 1981), I learned that sterilization had become the chief means of birth control, with programs sponsored by Planned Parenthood (PP) and the United States Agency for International Development (USAID) and other population controllers. Many of these sterilizations are done without informed consent. More than one million illegal abortions are committed each year without government prosecution. There are persistent reports that American money is being used to coach the untrained midwives to massage a pregnant woman so that she miscarries. The evil that American tax money does in these developing nations staggers the imagination.

Pope John Paul II told the Filipinos that, as the only Catholic nation in Asia, they were the Christian hope of Asia, and so they are. I shall introduce the American prolife/pro-family movement, literature, films, and slides there. I know from the response I got last May that this will do much good, because the Filipinos are Catholic in their very bones even if not always in their Sunday Mass attendance.

In visiting 51 countries, I have learned of the prolife/pro-family opportunities in the developing nations. Here is where the future of the Church lies; here parents are still having many children; here vocations are many; the dying West will be or already is in a post-Christian stage; to it will come in the future missionaries from countries where I hope to organize a prolife/pro-family movement. Financial help for international prolife work is most important and will do more for the Lord than any money spent for any cause anywhere else.

HLI not only tries to save the unborn—the least and so the dearest—but also works to build up family life, to spread NFP, to prepare people for marriage, and to save the developing nations from the antilife incursions of the pagan West (or at least to *minimize* Western paganism).

A September lecture tour in Ireland and England and then visiting prolife leaders in Belgium, Switzerland, and Austria, convinces me how right Solzhenitsyn was when he said, "The West has lost its will to live." That is perhaps no more true than in Europe, where conditions are much worse than in the USA, where at least we have a flourishing prolife resistance, much lacking in the old country. In Belgium and Austria, prolifers told me flatly that "the Church is dead."

This fall in Belgium, there will another effort to legalize abortion. In interviews with two large Catholic papers, I tried to describe for the Belgians what they would be in for if they introduced massive abortion. Of course, in many ways, they already have it. There is a Belgian doctor who claims to have committed 2,000 abortions and has dared the state to prosecute him.

In Holland an abortion law was passed last spring after being defeated for years. The deciding vote in the Senate was cast by a priest! And a second priest delivered a key vote on behalf of abortion!

The battle is now raging in six small Catholic countries of Europe: Malta, Luxembourg, Spain, Portugal, Belgium and Ireland. These countries are being told by the abortionists that they are backward, that they must be fashionable and up-to-date like the rest of Europe—in short, that they too must relax the law and allow "post-conceptive family planning."

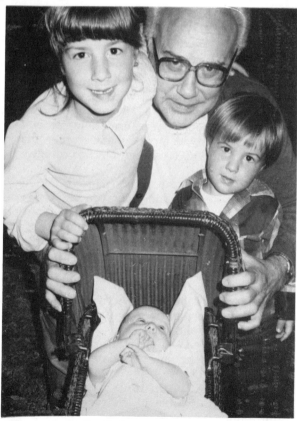

Three reasons for fighting on.

PROLIFE MISSIONARIES TO ASIA

(No. 3—March 1982)

Loaded down with 17 films, 50 slides, and as much prolife/pro-family literature as could be carried, I invaded the Philippines on 4 January 1982. I spoke three or four times a day for almost a month—sometimes all day—using films and slides. In the audiences were bishops, priests, nuns, doctors, medical students, midwives, government population controllers, parents, students of all kinds, and spies of Marcos. The response was truly total. These people have virtually no prolife literature or audiovisual aids. Imagine yourself seeing for the first time a multitude of the slides and films we Americans have.

Sponsoring me were the Sisters of St. Paul of Chartres, French-founded but now entirely Filipina, the largest religious order in this nation of 7,200 islands and 47 million people. Among the many good works these nuns carry out are running 15 colleges and 11 hospitals (I spoke at most of them) including their Sister Formation Center outside of Manila. I always prayed for a religious order that wanted to be totally prolife and carried on accordingly. Now I have found it!

By tolerating illegal abortion (more than one million annually) and by encouraging abortifacient Pills and devices, massive sterilization, "menstrual extraction" and every form of contraception, the government has been able, in just 10 years, to bring down the annual population growth rate from 3.2 to 2.4 percent. Thanks to fierce American pressure (from Planned Parenthood, United States Agency for International Development, United Nations Fund for Population Activities, the Pathfinder Fund, and others), population control "education" is mandated in all the public schools. By government order, purely physical sex education starts in the fourth grade. To reach Catholics, the law mandates that before people can get a marriage license, they must attend a three-hour government-sponsored birth control session, where they learn how to use all manner of contraception, abortifacients and sterilization.

To discourage births, government policy is that maternity leave is granted only for the first three pregnancies; for a fourth pregnancy, no maternity leave is given. From the first pregnancy on, but especially during the third, sterilization is pushed strongly. Poor and illiterate women are often sterilized without their knowledge or informed consent. Courageous nuns watch like hawks to prevent sterilization by irresponsible doctors. On one occasion, these so-called Catholic doctors told the nuns, "We'll go to hell; you won't have to." Equal to the occasion, a nun-administrator shot back, "I for one don't care to go with you."

Nearly 100,000 "motivators" have been trained by the government to find "acceptors" of a vicious, use-any-means-to-reduce-the-population program.

Remember, the American taxpayer pays for nearly all of this. Is there a worse imperialism than to destroy the family and corrupt the young of another nation? The irony of it all, when you think that the average American completed family size is 1.8 children, and we need 2.2 for reproduction!

(Ireland is among the few developed countries in the world that have a reproductive birthrate, but the Irish are acting as stupidly as their neighbors, now taking massive amounts of contraceptives. Their so-called Catholic doctors give the abortifacient Pill to some 75,000 Irish women, telling them they are "merely regulating the cycle," and the plea for abortion to remedy failed contraception is already loud, while each year some 4,000 girls go to England to kill their Irish children.)

NFP is making headway, especially in Mindanao, where they have the best programs. Everywhere, I found the young intensely interested in NFP, gobbling up every piece of literature that I had— which was, of course, never enough. One perceptive female doctor who fights the government's population-control program told me, after seeing my films, that all I had to do was to show my films on abortion to Filipina girls, and "they will never have an abortion." She confirmed what I sensed all along, that many young women in the Philippines have the notion that an abortion only involves a little blood-letting and the removal of a little meaningless tissue. That is why films are so important. We have to educate the whole world about intrauterine life!

With NFP, we must teach people thoroughly and clearly about the unique human reproductive system, because the enemy trades on ignorance. I have always maintained that one reason priests promote NFP so little is that they have such a poor concept of the magnificent human reproductive system, not realizing how specific fertility is, how well the Lord has provided!

I am sure that is why the present pope in 1980 had four world-famous medical experts explain the human reproductive system to 216 bishops assembled in Rome for the Synod on the Family. He wanted them to understand NFP. They were totally attentive, and someone remarked to me, "This may be the first time that the bishops are learning where babies come from!" But alas, the bishops are not alone in this! As every NFP teacher knows, most adults know virtually nothing about the fine points of human reproduction. That is why so many do not see the common sense in *Humanae Vitae*, do not see in it the best solution to the fertility problem. Is there anything more important in this world than to educate our young against abortion and for chastity, to teach those getting married about NFP, to build beautiful families out of which will come the vocations we are so lacking?

The Filipinos are shy but lovely people. They are happy, generous, gentle, kind, and very eager to learn and to improve themselves. Their patience seems infinite. What an example for impatient me, who have too often prayed through the years, "Oh God, give me patience, and do it fast."

Many educated and trained Filipinos leave the country. Ten thousand Filipino doctors and many more nurses are in the USA, and many more will come. The brain drain of educated and skilled people is great. In five years, there may be two million Filipinos in the Moslem Near East, a strange counterpart to Moslems just now taking over Western Europe.

I left half my films in the hands of prolife leaders, and I have begun to ship as much as I can afford. At the nation's second largest city, Cebu, the doctors of their prestigious hospital invited me to a special meeting. They proposed becoming a branch of Human Life International fighting the antilifers all over the Philippines, with programs of all kinds that I would help them to engender. I am not an emotional man, but I almost wept at this obvious sign of Divine Providence, because I myself had not thought of founding branches of Human Life International all over the developing countries to carry on what Pope John Paul II called "the most important work on earth." This is one more example—and true prolifers will know what I am talking about—of how those who really fight the antilife devil, despite all their suffering and contradiction, are in the hands of God! How often I have observed this or been told this as I meet these selfless leaders in the 54 countries I have now visited! It is at such moments that one wishes (though frustrated in the wish) that all those who have ever contributed a dollar could be present to see the obvious workings of God. Let me risk misunderstanding and perhaps even ridicule to tell you that I am convinced that Human Life International is doing the most important work on earth. Without life and good families, society and the Church and mankind collapse. There is a massive collapse in many parts of the world. Europe is already beyond the point of no return, says the greatest prolifer in Europe, the Lutheran Dr. Siegfried Ernst—and I agree.

In this island nation, the Church is hampered by a shortage of priests (fewer than 10,000), religious (fewer than 20,000) and catechists. It came home to me forcefully as never before what the Christian decline in the West has done to the Church in the developing countries. The flow of missionaries from the West has all but dried up. Parishes of 100,000 people served by two or three old priests are not uncommon. I spoke for hours at two 100-bed hospitals where 20 nuns worked all day; none of them were younger than 50. A number of them were over 70, still doing a full day's work. In one instance, they were running a boarding school for 250 poor girls.

One bishop told me that the vast majority of Filipinos grow up without any organized religious education whatsoever. They lack priestly and religious personnel and the money to train an adequate number of catechists. In the light of this, Church attendance and the religious spirit of the people are surprisingly good. I once offered Mass and preached to 1,600 high-school students who almost sang off the church roof. The Philippines are the only Catholic country in Asia; that is why the Pope told the Filipinos they were the hope of Asia.

The number of vocations is considerably higher than in the USA. The larger religious orders are sending missionaries to neighboring countries, responding to the will of

the Pope.   But the enemies of the Church are great, including the government—which is beholden to the antilife
American government for needed loans, loans which are
given only if the needy recipients bow to the antilife
imperialists—the media, and the increasing flood of pornographic films and magazines from the USA.

I spoke on many islands.   What a sight to fly over
these islands, some covered with beautiful coconut trees,
with a few houses along the edge!   Only 105 islands are
inhabited.   You make acts of faith in God as you take off
from a lawn or a lonely pasture—after the goats are
shooed away!

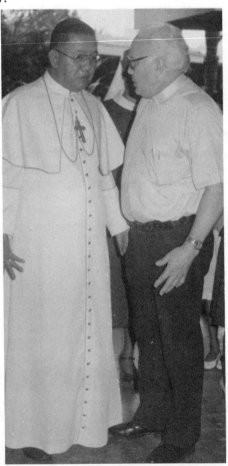

Jaime Cardinal Sin of Manila was an early supporter of HLI.

PROLIFE NEEDED IN SOUTH AFRICA

On the last day of January, I flew (18 hours) to Cape Town, South Africa. Between Hong Kong and Mauritius, I thought the plane would never land! On these long air trips when you know there is only water below, it is easy to pray!

How does one describe the crazy country called the Republic of South Africa—with its many tribes, languages, cultures, injustices and apartheid! The country is huge and wealthy. It is 2,000 miles wide and 1,600 miles long. Four and one-half million whites, whose ancestors migrated there beginning in 1650 to raise vegetables and furnish fresh water for Dutch traders going to the Far East, are mostly Dutch Reformed Calvinist Protestants, enslaving 15 million blacks, 2.5 million "Coloreds" (of mixed race) and 800,000 Asiatics, mostly Indians. Twenty-two thousand educated and skilled whites have entered from collapsed Rhodesia (now known as Zimbabwe), leaving Zimbabwe in a mess.

The parliament of white Calvinist South Africans (one Catholic) runs a vicious police state, the likes of which exists nowhere else in the world. Blacks, Coloreds, and Asiatics have no vote. They can live only in specified areas known as federal homelands. Arbitrarily, a section of the city is declared white, and the Blacks are moved forcibly out to a country area with virtually no facilities for human life. Here, I saw some of the worst slums in the world.

The government, coached by Planned Parenthood, has a strong, inhuman population-control program, but only the whites follow it. Completed family size for whites is 2.12 children; no one knows the average number of children the Blacks and Coloreds have. The Blacks tell you openly that children are their weapons—and indeed they are!

In 1975, the government passed a loose abortion law. At dinner in the government house one evening, a parliamentarian tried to tell me it was a tight law. That would have been funny, except that thousands of lives were at stake.

The government claims there are only 500 legal abortions, but one would have to be utterly stupid to believe that. Now they want to open more loopholes in the law. One amendment called for aborting children conceived after a botched sterilization!

There is no law against sterilization. This barnyard approach to birth control is available virtually on request, with many women returning later for "repairs."

As is common amongst the poor and developing countries, illegal abortion is rampant. Women are often sterilized without their knowledge or consent. In fact, every form of fertility control is used on the Blacks, among whom abortion *must* be common. At age 14, girls are given the Pill at government expense, and Depo-Provera is freely injected in the Blacks. They were surprised to learn that this drug is forbidden to Americans.

One strictly controlled boarding school for girls injected Depo-Provera in the students before they left for vacations at home, on the assumption that they cannot, will not or should not control themselves. At our conference, a young lady, a freshman medical-school student, related that they were told in their first year of orientation to use the Pill because abortion was a messy business. No wonder VD is rampant in this colossal, isolated country, where the handwriting for the whites is clearly on the wall.

But how do you get affluent people to see the handwriting on the wall these days? I discussed that with a Catholic doctor. He confessed that he thought about the situation in realistic terms. "But then at a certain point I drop the shade in front of me." The pervasive fear and hatred that the whites feel towards the Blacks (and the future) is terrible to behold.

In 54 countries I have visited, I have never seen the Church so weak, the priests so "Pill-happy" and so opposed to *Humanae Vitae*. I was warned that most Catholics have hardly heard of that prophetic encyclical, perhaps because of an incredible dissenting statement from the bishops on *Humanae Vitae* (delayed until 1974).

Most of the 1.5 million Catholics are black. There are comparatively few vocations. Incoming missionaries are down to a trickle, in part due to government screening because the bishops have so frequently spoken out against the apartheid. Unfortunately, according to Catholic leaders, the bishops seem to see only one problem, apartheid. Archbishop Lefebvre has no small hold on the leading active Catholics, who complain bitterly about their bishops. Their chief complaints are that the bishops do not uphold orthodoxy and are not supplying chaplains to the armies at the border where their sons are in danger.

NFP is spotty, but there is a real potential for expanding the program, with a number of impressive leaders. Here as everywhere, prolife literature and audiovisual aids are lacking.

I gave four addresses to the First National Pro-Life Conference, attended by 70 people. After the conference, I spoke several times every day to all kinds of groups, including medical students in both Cape Town and Johannesburg. These students were surprisingly subdued, shocked by the filmed reality of abortion. But one medical student attacked me boldly as "too emotional for bright medical students." I assured him that cameras had no emotions, that the aborted babies and the abortion techniques displayed were indeed real, and asked, "Shouldn't medical students face reality?" The crowd roared. He tried again, "You mean to tell me that an unborn baby can kill the mother but the mother can't kill the baby?" I shot back, "Unborn babies are not known to kill their mothers." His fellow medical students clapped uproariously.

I gave eight sermons at the cathedrals of Cape Town and Johannesburg. The people were shocked by my description of the prolife situation around the world, and they listened carefully to the remedies.

The opportunities to promote life and family in the developing countries are mind-boggling. South Africa has a flourishing prolife group, but it is little supported by the hierarchy, which has yet to awaken to the antilife threat, as is so often the case around the world. But as in every country, there are those stalwart and alert Catholics and Christians who are heroic in their concern, work, and sacrifice. I met with such heroes for many hours, often far into the night. They had no idea what prolife literature and audiovisual aids were available to them. I promised to help them in every possible way, especially with the literature and films they lack. I told them that my good prolife friends in the States would help me with money to help them.

DEPOPULATION CRISIS IN EUROPE

(No. 4—May 1982)

March 5, I left for Scotland to lecture for a week. The Scots have a country all their own; to this day it is good to distinguish them from the English and the Welsh. There are four million Scots, most of them Calvinist Presbyterians, living with 850,000 Catholics, most of them concentrated in Glasgow. Scotland's Catholic Church has its own hierarchy. I spoke in all the large cities, including Dundee, Aberdeen, Glasgow and Edinburgh. In Glasgow, I spoke to the Society for the Protection of Unborn Children (SPUC), the British national right to life organization. I also spoke at the seminary in Glasgow. They have a wonderful bishop in Glasgow, who has sponsored two NFP seminars.

The last figure on abortion in Scotland was 8,000 per year.

Only two percent of the Scots go to Church on Sunday. For England and Wales, attendance is only one percent. There are 4.5 million Catholics in Britain; of these an estimated 2.5 million practice their faith. It is said that the number of Catholics going to Church on Sunday in the UK is larger than the number of Anglicans and Protestants combined. In light of this and given the lack of any agreement on basic morality, you wonder whether all the fuss about ecumenism is so much unrealistic sweet-talk.

IRELAND: PILL 'EM OR KILL 'EM

Ireland is the only major developed country in the free world that has a good and reproductive birthrate, 21.9 per 1,000 (USA: 15.2). Unfortunately, in 1979, the government passed a Health Family Planning Bill (note the propaganda: it promoted neither health nor family life) which unleashed the Family Planning Association (as Planned Parenthood calls its national affiliates).

The FPA had been softening up Ireland since 1969 by passing out contraceptives. To circumvent the law against selling contraceptives, they gave them out free and then asked for a donation. The "family planning" bill was passed with virtually no opposition from the bishops, although Pope John Paul II condemned contraception twice when he was in Ireland. The Irish foolishly hoped that conscientious doctors and pharmacists would control the distribution of contraception and abortifacients. But the law was a disaster. For conscience reasons, many pharmacists refuse to handle contraceptives and abortifacient pills and IUDs, and some doctors refuse to prescribe them. But a disappointing number of doctors are giving out the abortifacient Pill.

Two years before the "family planning" bill was passed, doctors were courted by Pill companies; often, they received large amounts of these contraceptives (really abortifacients) free. I have observed over and over that when a country begins with contraception, it moves on to abortion and ends with infanticide and euthanasia. Thus, in 1979, the Irish government imitated the ugly Americans and squeezed out of their Constitution a phony "right to privacy," interpreted to include the right to contraception. Now, if someone challenges the Irish Constitution (as in this country), the courts could issue a destructive decision, and the Irish would have the same situation Americans have.

To halt the trend of events, an American team (consisting of Carl Anderson, Dr. Herbert Ratner, Pat Trueman, Fr. Charles Corcoran and myself) offered a weekend seminar for 60 leaders, chosen by Irish prolife leaders. The seminar was co-sponsored by Human Life International and Americans United for Life. We discussed an immediate amendment to the Constitution by referendum. An all-inclusive amendment passed by referendum is the only way the Irish are going to stop legalized abortion. The amendment must leave no exceptions, must protect all life from fertilization on. But for this, the Irish are going to have to be educated, persuaded to go out to vote and to push their parliament.

Many Irish have the naive idea that they are Catholic and therefore are not in danger, forgetting that already almost 4,000 girls go to England for abortions every year.

Before this seminar we did a prolife weekend at Knock, the famous shrine where Mary is said to have appeared in the 19th century.

I shall never forget an evening at Maynooth, the liberal national seminary, attached to a college. We were stunned by how little the students learned about sexual morality, how fixated they were on contraception, having no suspicion whatsoever that contraception is the gateway to abortion. After the session there, conducted by Dr. Ratner and myself, we met with about 25 prolife students, including a few seminarians. They told us they had never heard anything convincing on sexual morality from their teachers. They had heard no promotion of *Humanae Vitae.* The students assured us that some professors on the seminary faculty were in favor of contraception, and taught their views.

Pro-abortionists, of course, have been very active in Ireland for some time, especially on the university level. In years past, I have lectured to students and have armed the prolife students with literature, slides, films and other aids, but they are still outgunned. A large pro-abortion "information" meeting was conducted recently in Dublin. Pro-abortion money pours in from other countries to bring down this Catholic country, the source in the past of so many vocations and of such beautiful family life.

In a recent report from Ireland's chief prolifer (an engineer), I learned that the passage of an amendment is a real possibility.

SWEDEN, THE SEX PARADISE

I flew to Sweden for four days. Sweden has often been proclaimed the sex paradise. In 1956, they initiated sex education from kindergarten on. In their view, sexual intercourse is as natural as eating, drinking, urinating and defecating—just another bodily function. VD, alcoholism, and suicide are rampant among the young. Contraception is seen as an essential part of sex education; abortion is explained openly as necessary to remedy failed birth control. Homosexuality is widely accepted, as are living together and frequent divorce among those who do bother to marry.

PP is a big part of the mess. The Swedes see they have gone too far, but because religion is more or less dead, do not know the way back. The chaplain to Swedish Catholic youth insisted that *chastity* is a word neither understood nor taught. "We have to begin all over," he emphasized.

The Swedes are a nation of eight million people with one million foreigners from 30 countries. I talked to three parliamentarians who were prolife; they told me that the government now has to import people to keep the country going.

There are 100,000 Catholics, mostly foreigners, with only 12,000 native Catholic Swedes. The Lutheran Church, of course, is the state church, and the ministers are functionaries of the State.

As a wonderful Lutheran editor told me, religion there is not so much taught as taught about, and *anyone* can teach *about* religion, even atheists. In short, the doctrines of the Christian faith are no longer really taught and therefore are not lived.

Sweden has an enormous number of young people living together; the distinction between legitimacy and illegitimacy has been wiped out. There were about 92,000 babies born and 32,000 abortions in 1981. The average family size, including foreigners, is 1.6 children.

I stayed with Karl and Theres Degen, who have nine children. Theres learned about NFP attending one of my early NFP symposia in Minnesota. The Degens are a magnificent Catholic family, proving once more that you can raise a beautifully Catholic family in a horrible environment. Theres teaches NFP and has 12 teachers. One of her sons is a priest (the head of the Catholic youth in Sweden).

Karl has driven trucks into Poland, and it was interesting to get his comments on Polish life before martial law, how the Poles would stand in line for hours to buy a cup of powdered soap for washing clothes.

IN DYING DENMARK

I spent five days in Denmark, staying with the Oblates of Mary Immaculate in Copenhagen. My nephew, who bears the same name I do, is pastor of a parish; he is also a former missionary in Greenland, where the teachers actually lead girls out of the high schools over to abortion mills. Among five million Danes are 30,000 Catholics with some 100 priests (mostly foreign), two Catholic hospitals, and two Catholic high schools. As in Sweden, Lutherans constitute the state church, and the ministers are the functionaries of the State, with grave consequences. They are required to baptize, for example, whether they want to or not. There are 57,000 births and 25,000 abortions annually.

The birthrate is low. What a delight to speak to Dr. and Mrs. Jensen, another couple who have raised a magnificent family in so much moral muck and who teach NFP and fight abortion without the Church's help! I had been

in contact with Dr. Jensen for years. One way of remaining Catholic and raising children in the faith successfully
is to fight the Church's battles even when bishops, priests
and nuns do not.

I was surprised that the lay editor of the only Catholic
paper interviewing me was unfamiliar with *Humanae Vitae*
and was really pro-contraception (as a matter of "conscience"). It is in countries like Sweden and Denmark that
one sees how right the Church is and how bad sex education in the schools is. There is more than something
rotten in Denmark!

HOLLAND: BISHOP vs. BISHOP

I carried my prolife apostolate to Holland, a sad country in almost total disarray from a Catholic point of view.
At one time, the Dutch produced the highest number of
missionaries; no more. Holland has seven dioceses, five
against the Pope and two for the Pope. The situation is
truly incredible. The special synod of Dutch bishops with
the Pope seems only to have aggravated the situation.

I had flown to Brussels, where another truly Catholic
stalwart, Dr. Philippe Schepens, came to meet me. He
edits the newsletter of the World Federation of Doctors
Who Respect Human Life, a group I helped to found. I
have been collaborating with Dr. Schepens for years. He
took me to Rolduc, where is the only traditional (orthodox)
seminary in Holland, in the southwest, a stone's throw
from Belgium and Germany. About 10 years ago Pope
Paul VI appointed Fr. Jylsen bishop of Roermond and
asked him to clean up the mess. The primate of Holland,
Cardinal Alfrink, refused to install him. Fr. Jylsen called
Pope Paul VI, who invited him to Rome for installation.

Bishop Jylsen then started the only traditional seminary in Holland. All other seminaries have been abandoned. Theological students live like other students in
residential houses of universities. That has not worked.

The orthodox seminary is built out of the enormous
ruins of an Augustinian monastery dating back to 1106.
During its eight years of existence, it has produced more
priests than the rest of Holland put together. The seminary has also educated priests for Rotterdam, the other
loyal diocese.

Currently there are 80 very mature seminarians with a
sophisticated faculty of 40, some teaching only one course
or institute. The seminarians at Rolduc tend to be older; I

met a young doctor and several young lawyers studying for the priesthood.

The seminary is sponsored by the dioceses of Roermond and Rotterdam, where Bishop Simonis is the other orthodox bishop. Both Jylsen and Simonis spoke out fiercely against abortion last year when Holland passed a law permitting abortion in the first three months of pregnancy. It passed by one vote, the one vote cast by a priest—a Dutch Drinan! The liberal bishops hardly spoke out against the proposed killing. In fact, the Primate of Holland, Cardinal Willebrands, was pathetically weak in his stance and even excused the abortion-voting priest. During the abortion battle, Willebrands said something like, "We must allow the State to do its best in a difficult, disputed question." The Health Minister said he "took comfort" in the Cardinal's observation. It is said that St. Alphonse once remarked that one side of hell was lined with bishops.

I addressed the seminarians twice. It was a great experience. The intellectual climate is excellent and the standards are high. Eager and sensible seminarians come from many parts of Europe. Once ordained, they may function only in these two dioceses, not in the other five! The rector, a shrewd Jesuit, wants to start a family center (at the suggestion of the bishop) which will cover the whole of marriage, including marriage-preparation courses and NFP in the two dioceses.

A large part of the huge old monastery was being renovated for training permanent deacons. The Dutch bishops have refused to foster the permanent diaconate up to now because they still hope to have a married clergy!

I told the rector of the seminary that the future of Holland is in that seminary. There is no seminary like it in the USA, with a faculty highly competent and having a proven publishing record and thoroughly orthodox. Until we reform American seminaries—most of them—little is going to change. Disloyal theologians flirting with heresy pollute the whole instructional process of the future priest, nun and catechist.

There are 40,000 abortions each year in Holland. Busloads of women come from Belgium and France and Germany; they come to hide the killings. Of the 40,000 abortions, only 13,000 are Dutch babies.

The Protestant church is virtually dead. A euthanasia society has organized. The young doctor now studying for the priesthood at Rolduc told me that in Rotterdam medical professionals routinely give the Pill to 14-year-old girls!

I am pouring books into the 40,000-book library at this seminary, for their family-life center, for training priests for this apostolate. They are eager to start teaching NFP everywhere, because they are as convinced as I am that contraception means abortion and euthanasia, the breakdown of the family, low birthrates, divorce and all the rest.

The Pope invited all the seminarians and faculty to Rome on Easter Monday, gave them a special private interview, and offered Mass for them. This was his way of showing his support in their struggle. Already Rolduc has produced more priests in eight years than the rest of Holland combined; 14 are to be ordained this June, while the rest of Holland has only three.

SWITZERLAND: SEX, YES; BABIES, NO

I visited the Bonaventur Meyer family; they have a large catechetical center with which I have been in contact and where I lectured as early as 1973. I also had a great visit with the most knowledgeable Granges family in Bern. I had met them years ago and had sent them much literature. They are the heart of the battle for life in Switzerland. The Swiss prolife forces collected 270,000 signatures for the protection of all human life from conception on, which means that the government is now forced within the next four years to have the nation vote on that issue. The Swiss could be the one European nation that will turn back the abortionists. But then, the Swiss can cross four borders and be aborted.

Actually there still are many abortions in Switzerland even though abortions are allowed for strictly medical reasons only. Like the Germans, the Swiss have more coffins than cradles.

In a nation of 6.3 million people, they have almost one million foreign workers! Archbishop Lefebvre has more seminarians in Switzerland at his seminary at Econe than all other seminaries combined!

I was shocked when Meyer showed me a TV broadcast from Germany about sex education. The broadcast openly showed a 17-year-old girl having an abortion. The German law requires that, before abortion, a doctor and social worker must counsel the woman (or couple) who comes in to have her (their) baby killed. The female counselor/social worker was a member of Pro-Familia, Germany's equiva-

lent of PP. The "counseling" of the couple was unbelievable:

> *You are students; you do not want to interrupt*
> *your education to have a baby?*
> *No.*
> *As students, you have little money -- right?*
> *Right, we have little money.*
> *You are not ready to be parents now, are you?*
> *No, we are not at all ready.*
> *Then you have a social indication for abortion.*
> *I'll process the papers.*

What shocked me even more was the young abortionist
talking to the couple. He described the possible consequences of abortion graphically. Then he said, "Now after the
abortion you can take no tub bath for a week, no swim-
ming for 10 days, and no intercourse for one month." So
he spoke to a fornicating couple ready to kill their baby.

In Germany as in other countries, extramarital intercourse is taken for granted, while chastity is unknown.
That is why the Germans have the lowest birthrate in the
world—lots of sex but few babies.

This program of sex education was broadcast over
German TV, which also covers Switzerland. The previous
week, this official course in sex education had dealt entirely with contraception. All types of contraceptives and
abortifacients were shown clinically—how they work, how
they fit, everything! Sterilization was recommended for
some people and circumstances. One cannot say that no
values were presented: the *worst* were presented ever so
subtly, the values of PP, with no call for chastity, self-
control and responsibility. These values have evaporated
in a Europe which is "down the drain," says the great
German abortion opponent, Dr. Siegfried Ernst.

I went to see Dr. Ernst for a day. He is convinced
that the Russians will move west, that Europe is beyond
salvaging, that the Church (both Lutherans and Catholics)
has much to answer for. He proposes that we set up a
university in Paraguay to train Christians who will fight
back. He maintains that such a training project can no
longer be done in Europe because the environment is so
pagan. This Paraguayan center would aim to save the
best of the German Christian culture, train prolifers on a
wide scale, publish prolife and pro-family literature, and be

a worldwide base for training and research. He suggested
we could appeal to the many Germans in South America
for support.

What a great family Dr. Ernst has! He is a Lutheran
and wonderfully Christian. Of his children, four are doctors or in medical school. Two have become Catholics.
They all fight abortion.

IN JAPAN WITH MOTHER TERESA

April 21-27 I participated with Mother Teresa and
others in an international symposium on NFP in Tokyo. I
had great chats with this saintly nun. She was invited by
the Health Minister, who is prolife, to speak to as many
parliamentarians as wished to hear her at a breakfast at
the Tokyo Hilton. More than 200 came. She was superb.
She did not prepare, but appealed to God to speak through
her—and He did! Only a saint could say what she said to
them about poverty, materialism and abortion, and get by
with it! In the end, she wheedled a collection out of them
to which virtually all contributed amply.

She also spoke magnificently to the youth on chastity,
and to adults on other subjects. Everywhere, she was
mobbed. Then she did the same in other Japanese cities.
At Nagasaki she knelt at the spot where the first atomic
bomb had exploded, to pray for peace and sanity, that
mankind be spared the ultimate insanity of a nuclear
holocaust.

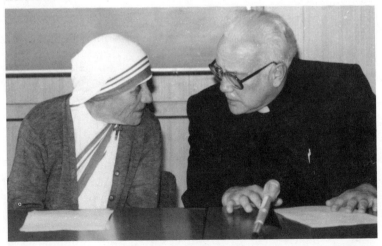

Tokyo, 1982.

IRELAND: ABORTION ON DEMAND?

(No. 5—October 1982)

We are working desperately to save the Irish from abortion-on-demand. Briefly, the Irish constitution, like the American, does not mention the unborn. In 1973, the Irish Supreme Court "discovered" a right to privacy in the constitution wide enough to include contraception. The sale and advertising of contraception had been forbidden in this country, 95 percent Catholic. In 1979, the Irish Dail (Parliament) passed a horrendous Health and Family Planning Bill which aimed to contain contraception within marriage by making a doctor's prescription necessary for all contraceptives and abortifacients and by stipulating that these could be secured only from certified pharmacists. Truly Catholic doctors and pharmacists refused to be involved in immorality. But the law, unenforced, only unleashed Planned Parenthood, which had begun its deadly work in 1969 when they set up contraceptive clinics, gave out Pills, fitted IUDs, and began to refer for abortion. They got by the law by asking for "donations"! The whole effort was orchestrated from the world's center of contraception/abortionism, International Planned Parenthood Federation (IPPF) of London, 40 percent of whose budget is paid by the American taxpayer.

After *Humanae Vitae* appeared in 1968, wild Irish theologians, some teaching at the national seminary in Maynooth, dissented publicly. They were not disciplined by the bishops, and the media picked up their propaganda. Today, the Irish are deep into contraception, on which the Irish bishops have repeatedly waffled, despite the fact that the Pope twice condemned contraception in that country when there.

Now the only way the Irish can avoid a bad decision from their Supreme Court, which could easily extend the "right to privacy" to abortion, is by passing an amendment to the Constitution through a national referendum, which may take place in early 1983. This amendment must say that all human life is protected under the law from fertilization on.

Irish legislators—misled by the antilife media, the woolly theologians, and many Planned Parenthood-type influences—are haggling over the wording. Even though 4,000 Irish girls already go annually to England to kill Irish babies, the Irish have no experience in fighting abortion. They believe too easily that because they are Irish and Catholic, this war on the unborn will not engulf them! The bishops have done virtually nothing, saying they will speak out only when they see the wording of the amendment. But by then it may be too late!

In 1973, I came to Ireland to warn them about what was happening. I spoke to a well-known bishop for half an hour, gave him the documentation, and explained to him how the Planned Parenthooders start with contraception but end with abortion. The bishop was most polite, but he refused the documentation and obviously did not take me very seriously. If he remembers that encounter, he knows now that I predicted exactly what has happened since then, what is happening today, and what may happen tomorrow!

It would be the tragedy of tragedies if the Irish went down to abortionism. Remember that 35 percent of American priests are of Irish extraction, and even more of the nuns. The clergy in countries such as Australia and New Zealand are primarily Irish. Go where you may in this world (and I have been in 55 countries) and you will find the Irish missionary priest, nun, brother—and not least, the Irish Catholic doctor—manning the mission stations. (Ireland has five major medical schools, but only three million people.)

Planned Parenthood abortionists know exactly what they are doing in Ireland. They laid their plans well, and want to move in for the kill, which amounts to preventing a referendum. They are arguing now that it is an unnecessary expenditure, since abortion is already forbidden.

Prolifers, on the other hand, are desperately trying to educate the Irish about the dangers they face, urging them to vote correctly.

On September 23 I began my fourth lecture tour in Ireland. On October 4 I spoke to all the priests of the Archdiocese of Glasgow, to the prolife groups in that and neighboring cities in the days following. Then I moved on to Austria, where I keynoted the International Symposium on *Humanae Vitae* and *Familiaris Consortio*. The bishops of the Western world have virtually buried this latter document, which is the Pope's response to the Synod of Bishops in Rome on the family. It contains the Church's latest teaching on responsible family planning and on sexual morality.

Then I invaded my 56th country, Portugal, where the battle is raging, as in Spain. In Portugal, during the recent revolution, a Planned Parenthood doctor (who calls himself a Catholic, by the way) became head of the health services. He introduced contraception, which always includes the abortifacient Pill and IUD, into the health services, paid for by the government.

SWITZERLAND AND AUSTRIA

Speaking in Zurich to prolifers from several countries, I saw once again that the greatest Christians on earth are the prolifers. I tried to give them an overall picture of the worldwide prolife/pro-family situation and what we need to do. They were shocked by conditions worldwide. It is so easy to think that only your own country, and perhaps neighboring countries, have the bad situation. But the devil is everywhere and never sleeps. That is why we must work internationally!

After the Zurich meeting I went to Austria, a country I know very well. Supposedly Catholic, among seven million people there are 115,000 abortions and approximately 85,000 births! In 10 years the number of vocations has dropped by half! Again, the Cardinal Archbishop of Vienna and the bishops seem to be sleeping. NFP is only getting on its feet. Again, you meet the few good and heroic priests, the dedicated prolife lay people, who are at wits' end over what more to do and how to maximize their resources.

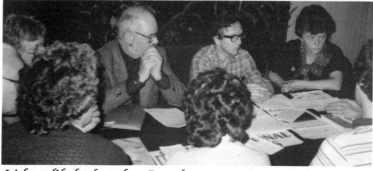

Irish prolife leaders plan Amendment campaign.

SPIRITUAL CRISIS IN THE WEST

(No. 6—December 1982)

Our Ninth International Symposium on Sexuality, Chastity, and NFP was our best yet. Participating were 230 people from 20 countries and 22 states. It was largely a leadership crowd. All those who came from overseas are leaders in their own countries, doing great things to fight abortion, promote NFP, and promote family life. A number of Protestants from other countries were with us. With the exception of one, all talks were excellent, and any number of them super.

Pat Driscoll, the creator of Womanity, an organization promoting chastity and virginity, drew the largest seminar among four. Until recently, she worked out of the Family Life Office in Oakland, California. This good woman, promoting chastity with her creative literature in this country and abroad, was dismissed, with dishonest reasons given. Briefly, she is too orthodox. But Pat is too much like me and will not quit!

She has often told me how some priests laugh at her promotion of chastity and virginity. Alas, another sign of our corrupt times when the nation is rotting from within— like the whole Western world, which, as Solzhenitsyn has said, "has lost its will to live."

IRELAND vs. THE ABORTIONISTS

The Irish government has passed a bill paving the way for an amendment to the constitution explicitly protecting the unborn. The Irish constitution, written in 1937, does not even mention them. But the government has fallen on a no-confidence vote; November 24th will see another election in Ireland. The battle is on, and the opposition could win, thus making it all the harder to save Ireland from abortion. The opposition leader who would be the prime minister was pressured in the previous election campaign into saying that, if elected, he would propose an amendment. We suspect that he does not mean it. He instigated a vote in the last session of the parliament on a resolution saying that an amendment was not necessary. If the resolution were not overwhelmingly defeated (and it was not), he could renege on his promise.

Frankly, I am not optimistic. PP and their collaborators (perhaps unwitting), the wild theologians dissenting from *Humanae Vitae*, are seeing the results of the process of moral erosion they began after that prophetic encyclical. The bishops have not promoted NFP and have been more or less impotent. We are pouring as much literature and audiovisual aids as we can afford into Ireland, the kind that will work in Ireland, and into the hands of those who truly know how to fight the battle. But we never have enough financing.

I urged the Irish prolife leaders to bring Dr. Bernard Nathanson to their country. We debated the issue for days, because Nathanson allows the rarest exception for abortion, and any exception in Ireland would defeat the whole amendment drive. Nathanson gave two lectures to two huge audiences after being completely briefed on the Irish situation. He performed magnificently. He was scheduled to appear on the Gay Byrne show, the equivalent of Johnny Carson's show in the USA; but the night before he was to appear the producers backed out. This shows that the abortionists have the media on their side and they can use them as they wish.

The tactics of the abortionists are devilishly subtle. Because of the high Irish birthrates over the last decades, some 60 percent of the Irish are under 25 years of age. Naturally, the abortionists concentrate their propaganda on winning the young, especially the university students. Usually, because these students stand for nothing, they fall for anything, like so many of their professors. I do not expect salvation from scholarship! Meanwhile, more than 4,000 Irish girls will be going to England for abortions this year.

Back in the United States, I had a great evening in Wheeling, West Virginia, talking to the right-to-lifers there and to the students of Wheeling College, perhaps the most sensible of all Jesuit colleges in this country. I was delighted to meet young orthodox teaching Jesuits who have taken the measure of the Jesuit McCormicks. Yes, there is hope, even for the Jesuits.

A day-long prolife seminar for the students at Mt. St. Mary's Seminary in Emmitsburg, Maryland, one of the few totally orthodox seminaries in the country, went superbly. We had an excellent faculty, and all the talks dovetailed

beautifully. Twenty of these seminarians came to the
seminar. It is an encouraging experience to move among
devoted and devout future priests, although they make
your hair stand on end when they tell you what is going
on in other seminaries from which they escaped.

Mt. St. Mary's turns out some 60 seminarians a year.
It struck me that the good bishops in this country have
their men there. The situation in the seminaries in this
country is pathetic.

PORTUGAL AND THE CRISIS OF THE WEST

The Portuguese are lovely people, but they are not
reproducing. They are the only country in the West apart
from France to throw the Communists out (after a seven-
month rule), and very recently they defeated the abortionists in parliament. The pro-abortion bill was entered by
the Communists, of course.

Portugal is the poorest country in Europe, and the best
guess is that for 10 million people there are perhaps
50,000 abortions. I heard that the Portuguese have suffered from a century of Freemasonry, with roots stemming
back to the French Revolution.

An informed and delightful prolifer told me that Por-
tugal will never have legalized abortion for two reasons: (1)
The parliament will not pass such a law, and (2) "Our
Lady of Fatima will not stand for it."

I spent a day traveling to and from Fatima, about 70
miles from Lisbon, in the middle of nowhere, high in the
mountains. The facts of Our Lady's appearances present
an enormous challenge to the disbelieving modern pagan.
The crowds build up every Saturday.

We were there on a Wednesday, with several hundred
people. Religious houses and hotels are building up
around this shrine.

Pope John Paul II drew 600,000 people here. When he
knelt at the site of Our Lady's appearances, there was a
noise in the crowd, until someone asked over the loud-
speaker system that the crowd be silent to allow the Pope
to pray. For one hour, so they told me, 600,000 people
were totally silent.

Of the three children to whom Mary appeared, two
died quite early and are buried at Fatima. Sister Lucia is
still living; the Pope had a long chat with her. She slips
from convent to convent to escape the crowds and
publicity.

The children to whom the Mother of God appeared did not even know the Hail Mary and said only, "Hail Mary, Holy Mary." She taught them the whole prayer.

Unfortunately I did not have time to offer Mass there, at this sacred shrine that so contradicts the machinations of proud worldlings and teaches us once more that it is the little people through whom God works.

The more I travel, the more I see the total spiritual crisis facing Christianity in the West, including the USA. The Hatch Amendment was an unmitigated disaster. We would not have lost the prolife bill sponsored by Sen. Jesse Helms by one vote if the bishops had consulted the best legal prolife experts who have fought the battle for a decade. Sen. Hatch almost lost his shirt in the last election in Utah, because the Mormons felt he was too soft on abortion! Yet the bishops embrace him.

I continue to think that the bishops should stay with the moral and spiritual aspects of the abortion tragedy and let the experienced legal and political minds of the movement plot the political course against abortion! In short, I wish the bishops would promote basic morality, clean up the catechetical mess because the young are not learning their Faith even in Catholic schools, arrange creative programs on chastity, and work up serious and comprehensive marriage-preparation programs containing substantial emphasis on NFP. Thus they would save many more babies than by dabbling in politics, in which they have neither expertise nor role and which seems to be only a distraction from what they should really be doing.

Approximately 75 percent of abortions in this country, as in all countries of the decadent West, come from sinful sex. Why does not that fact help the bishops and their wilder advising theologians to see that *Humanae Vitae* was right, that chastity and virginity need to be promoted, and that if we are going to clean up the abortion holocaust—as the early Christians did, over a long period of time—we must, like them, teach people to live chastely and maturely? More than that, people must see marriage as a very special vocation and see the gift of human sexuality as the source of life which, as Pope John Paul II said in Washington, "lasts forever."

As I view the international antilife mess which now has engulfed more than two-thirds of mankind, I keep asking myself what a different world it would be if our bishops had followed the lead of Pope Pius XII in 1951—

31 years ago! Twice, that far-seeing Pope pleaded for NFP. How I wish that every American bishop would visit the Diocese of Chun Cheon in South Korea, where Bishop Thomas Stewart has more than 95 percent of all couples who need to practice fertility control using NFP. The Archdiocese of Calcutta still has the only seminary in the world that I know of that gives decent training in NFP to future priests.

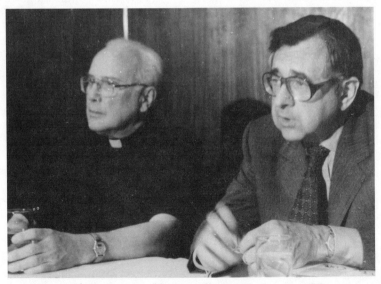

Dr. Bernard Nathanson—former abortionist, now prolife activist —fought to protect Irish babies.

THE GLOBAL THREAT TO LIFE

(No. 7—June 1983)

We have poured more than $100,000 worth of prolife audiovisual aids and literature into Eire, the only major developed country in the free world still welcoming enough babies to stay in existence. On September 7, the Irish will vote on a referendum designed to prevent both their supreme court and their parliament from ever legalizing abortion. Planned Parenthood and other antilife forces are frantically spreading their devilish propaganda everywhere. We could still lose, even though the consequences are too horrible to contemplate—for the babies, for Ireland, and for the whole Church.

In 1973, I went to Ireland to organize prolife forces while there was still time. In the late 1960s, PP had set up contraception centers in Irish cities. In country after country, I had already seen the inexorable march of the antilife movement from contraception to abortion-infanticide-euthanasia. So, in five national lecture tours, I warned every Irish bishop, priest, sister and lay person who would listen, about what was coming.

St. Paul once boasted of his successes, even while admitting he was talking foolishly. Allow me the same privilege: I honestly believe that except for my constant prayers, urgings, national lecture tours, lavish distribution of prolife materials, stateside publicity and a 1982 weekend seminar for 60 Irish leaders on how to write a tight amendment, Ireland would *already* have legal baby-killing.

Even after winning the referendum—assuming that they do—the Irish will have to step up their prolife work: contraception is spreading fast, and almost 100,000 Irish women now use the Pill. The government proposes free contraceptives for everyone and threatens to withdraw even the 60,000 pounds for teaching NFP it gave as a sop when introducing contraception in 1979.

[Prolifers won the referendum, by a 2–1 margin. The Irish constitution protects unborn children from conception, setting an example for the world.]

CANADA: SAYING THE "C" WORDS

Recently I made two extended lecture tours in this country. For the first time in my 36 years as a priest, I was boycotted by some priests and nuns. Nuns running one school for girls said they did not want "that priest" giving their girls "the old hang-ups." Later I learned that PP and speakers from the Welfare Department showed contraceptives to the girls there.

The situation in Canada is worse than in the United States, because the Canadian bishops dissented, in effect, to *Humanae Vitae*. The priests seem very sympathetic to contraception and generally unaware of the abortifacient character of Pills and IUDs. They know little or nothing about NFP. The seminaries are emptying, as in the United States. Many women told me they had been sterilized by Catholic doctors who claimed to have had permission from bishops. Several people quoted their priests as saying that today Catholics obey the bishops, not the pope.

Recently, His Holiness told 18 bishops of Ontario to denounce divorce and contraception "so long as God gives you breath to preach." One bishop later told his people that the Pope had told them to "work with broken families"! Forty percent of Canadian marriages end in divorce. Abortion is rampant; the average family has 1.7 children (United States: 1.8).

Thanks to prolife friends, I spoke in several Canadian churches and high schools. Preaching about contraception and chastity made news in every parish! In the hundreds of Catholic high schools where I have spoken during 20 years of fighting the antilife devil, I have never before met such resistance to my defense of Christian chastity, nor did the students seem to know the elementary truths of their faith. For the first time, I heard of high-school students "living together."

In several provinces, the private schools are fully supported by the Canadian government. Formerly these schools were staffed by orthodox religious and priests; today they are run by laymen, most of whom contracept or are sterilized. A Catholic high school run by contracepting laymen cannot be a truly Catholic high school.

In one city I was asked to evaluate a "Catholic" family life course (sex education) in which contraception was taken for granted, NFP was not even mentioned, a totally false view of conscience was given, and each couple were encouraged to decide what form of fertility control was best

for them. As always, the course was far too biological,
with virtually nothing said about chastity, self-control or
personal responsibility. The weak and vacillating bishop,
wanting to please everyone, finally allowed the truly Catholic parents to withdraw their children from the course—
but how is that a solution when so-called sex education
pervades the whole curriculum?

Thank God, I spent one evening with eight NFP teaching couples. They were great, as these couples always
are—truly loving their families and their Church. But
they were never even consulted about the "Catholic family
life" course. They say their work receives no support
whatsoever from either their bishop or any priest. They
spend their own money to advance this crucial apostolate,
so dear to the Pope.

In Yellowknife, an isolated Canadian community of
10,000 people, I met an apostolic couple who, in years past,
had taught NFP to 212 couples in another city. In just
one year, this couple had started a right to life group,
Birthright and NFP in Yellowknife! I asked them the
origin of their apostolate. They replied, "Paul Marx." I
had forgotten!

There is friction between the French- and English-
speaking hierarchies in Canada. Amidst this squabble, the
combined hierarchies did not insist that the new constitution fully protect unborn babies from conception onward.
Once again bishops fiddle while babies burn. In Canada—
as, indeed, all over the world—informed Catholics ask me
why their bishops do not speak out like the Pope.

UPDATE ON SPAIN AND PORTUGAL

Despite 500,000 prolife protesters who took to the
streets of Madrid, the Socialist government in Spain has
completed the first step in the process of legalizing abortion for rape up to three months, for a defective baby up to
22 weeks, and for "the health and life" of the mother up to
the day of birth. Twenty thousand Spanish women get
abortions in London annually. You know the rest: the
propaganda is always the same.

Prolifers won a temporary victory in Portugal when the
leader of the autonomous government of the Azores, which
belong to Portugal, made it clear he will never cooperate
with any party that sanctions baby-killing.

Portuguese and Spanish Catholic leaders say the bishops are weak, sometimes providing more hindrance than help.

Most priests and bishops of the Western world seem utterly befuddled by the deadly challenge of sex obsession propagated by the international monster PP and fueled with massive government money. They do not know how to deal with the situation, with their seminaries floundering, their teenagers fornicating in increasing numbers, with VD flourishing and abortion raging. The whole Western world is collapsing from within through the same moral-spiritual rot that brought down the great nations of the past.

WEST GERMANY DISAPPEARING

In this country, which has the lowest birthrate in the world, the average German wife rarely has more than one child. One-half of all married women have only one child or none at all. The 4.7 million foreign workers, one-third of them Moslem, have more children in the schools of the large German cities than the Germans do! Germany is losing half a million people every year   If this trend continues, there will be fewer than 20,000 Germans in the year 2100.

. . . ALONG WITH ITALY

Last year 204,000 abortions were reported. The Italians have contracepted and aborted themselves into the world's second-lowest birthrate. There is little evidence of any improvement.

WILL FRANCE BE MOSLEM?

With 300,000 babies aborted annually, a birthrate higher than Germany's but still below the replacement level, and hundreds of thousands of Moslem foreign workers with large families, this "eldest daughter of the Catholic Church" will be a Moslem country by the year 2035. As in Germany, seminaries are emptying and parishes are closing. In the Archdiocese of Paris, a city of six million, 400 of 800 secular priests are 70 or older. Few bishops and priests say anything about the causes of this tragic situation: a loss of faith, sex obsession, and the resultant contraception-sterilization-abortion.

SCANDINAVIA'S PROBLEMS

Of the eight million people in Sweden, one million are now foreigners. The average family has 1.6 children. There are endless abortions, much divorce, the world's highest teen suicide and alcoholic rates, and an increasing number of couples living together without marriage. "Sex education" has destroyed millions of lives. Denmark, Norway and Finland have similar conditions. Thank God, NFP is off to a good start in Sweden.

AUSTRIA ON THE CRITICAL LIST

Last year there were 85,000 births and 120,000 estimated abortions among seven million so-called Catholics and the now-usual army of foreign workers, many of them Moslems. Austria has the world's third-lowest birthrate.

SWITZERLAND: BABIES NOT WELCOME

Since 1955, as many babies have been aborted as have been born. One million foreigners now live in this nation of 6.3 million. Switzerland, which boasts the world's highest standard of living, evidently cannot afford to let its own babies live.

HOLLAND'S ABORTIONS

Abortion was legalized in 1981 by one vote, that of a Drinan-type Catholic priest. An estimated 40,000 babies are killed before birth each year in a nation of 14 million.

BELGIUM SLIPPING

The law forbidding abortion is hardly observed, and killing babies will soon be legalized.

SOUTH AFRICA DEPOPULATION

The government recently prevented further relaxation of the already-permissive law. The 4.5 million whites, enslaving 24 million blacks and "Coloreds," are barely achieving a replacement birthrate. The Church is weak.

HLI has opened a branch headquarters there.

BEHIND THE IRON CURTAIN

One of the USSR's greatest problems is abortion. The average married woman has eight to ten abortions. The average Soviet family has 1.9 surviving children, but most babies now are born to the 90 million Moslems, who will soon outnumber the White Russians.

All of the Iron Curtain nations legalized abortion in the 1950s. All of them have since tried to restrict abortion because of its bad effects on both maternal health and the birthrate. *Romania* forbade abortion in 1966, but it continues illegally. No East European country has a replacement birthrate. To prop up the birthrate, the Communists in *East Germany* offer the most lavish family allowances in the world. *Poland* currently records as many abortions as births (though the statistics may be manipulated by the government, to discredit the Church). The government promotes and pays for abortions, and the shortage of food and housing tempts even Catholics to resort to it. Grace abounds, however; last year Poland ordained 688 priests, 200 of whom went to the foreign missions.

JAPAN AND ABORTION

Eighty percent of the women in the 50-54 age group admit to having aborted at least one baby. Abortion in Japan has really become just another means of birth control—two to four million abortions every year in a nation of 117 million, with an average family size of 1.6 children.

An authentic prolife movement seeks to limit abortions in Japan because of their horrendous social effects. But the Catholic bishops of Japan have never condemned abortion in a national statement. Nor have they fostered NFP in the nation that gave it birth, where some 24 percent of all couples still practice the old calendar rhythm.

UNITED STATES: WHERE ARE THE BISHOPS?

One could appreciate the bishops' statement on the war and peace movement if they were also properly fighting the greatest war of all time, Satan's war against the unborn, which has already engulfed two-thirds of the world's countries and slaughters an estimated 60-100 million babies each year. The bishops-sponsored Hatch Amendment divided, and thereby destroyed the effectiveness of, the prolife movement, and the National Right to Life Committee has become the bishops' tool.

The final version of the nuclear "freeze" statement is not so bad. But again, one could take the bishops more seriously if they had spoken out when the Soviets brutally raped Afghanistan, when the Communists inflicted genocide on Cambodia, when Castro's Soviet-directed soldiers invaded Africa, and when the Soviets used chemical-biological warfare against helpless Laotians and Yemenis.

My close friends in Central America tell me what
Solzhenitsyn also says: Soviet Communists are inspiring
terrorism and revolution in Latin America even as they
support and promote the "peace" movement in Europe.
They make war while we make "peace"—through surrender. The big goal: the red flag over the United States of
America. "It can't happen here"? That is what some
people said about abortion.

Again, the bishops should have upheld unwaveringly
the principle that abortion—because it takes innocent,
defenseless human life—can *never* be allowed. They should
have let competent laymen plot the battle in the political
area. They should have ordered prayers said against
abortion at every Mass in every church. They should have
led public prayers of reparation to God like those offered at
Los Angeles' Procession and Mass of Reparation for Abortion, held every year at Christmastime. They should have
taught NFP vigorously.

And they should have preached in every manner possible the Church's wise social doctrine and encouraged our
government to help the poor countries, to avoid falling to
Communism. Instead, the bishops seem almost as unaware of the gigantic threat of world Communism as they
are of the moral-spiritual collapse under their very noses.

Do our bishops know that at least 75 percent of all
abortions are performed on unmarried mothers whose lack
of chastity was caused in part by "organ recital" and contraceptive "sex education" programs? When will the bishops *really* start promoting chastity and NFP?

Stated negatively, "prolife" must imply no contraception, no sterilization, no purely secular sex education, no
abortion, no infanticide, no euthanasia. Positively, "prolife"
must imply parent-guided education in Christian sexuality,
rather than humanistic education in physical sex. Needed
in every diocese immediately: an intensive preparation for
marriage with serious emphasis on NFP and parent-train-
ing courses in the light of *Humanae Vitae* and *Familiaris
Consortio*.

We were not baptized in order to finance bishops who
will not join the Pope in combatting the Satanic evils now
destroying the Church and society. Therefore, bishops who
do not resist abortion to the maximum, who do nothing to
foster chastity, who do not work to clean up the catechetical mess in their own seminaries, who do not actively
promote NFP, and who on the contrary set up "sex educa-

tion" courses (as in New Jersey) that resemble Planned
Parenthood's, do not deserve financial support.

With millions of abortion-murders, with infanticide
spreading, with seminaries emptying, with fornicating
teenagers making future healthy marriages virtually impossible, with VD out of control, with a birthrate below
replacement level, with mushrooming divorce and easy
annulments, with homosexuality tolerated, with shrinking
Catholic-school enrollments, with the Mormons now raising
the largest families in this country, with so-called Catholic
colleges sponsoring the Drinans and Currans and McCormicks and Kosniks—who needs bishops who are unfaithful
to the Holy Father?

When the majority of Catholic teachers contracept or
have been sterilized, with some having had abortions (as I
know from Minnesota's Saint John's University), what can
so many bishops, priests and nuns be thinking about?
Certainly not Catholicism!   DO NOT SUPPORT THEM.
SUPPORT THOSE WHO STAND WITH CHRIST AND
HIS VICAR.

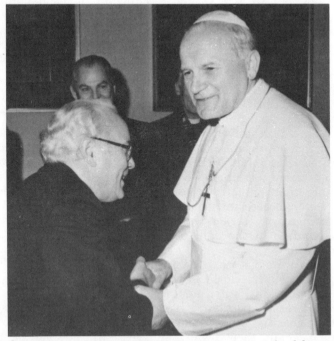

Throughout the century, the popes have pleaded for life.

RED CHINA AND 10 OTHER BATTLEFRONTS

(No. 8—December 1983)

SPAIN: POPE vs. ABORTION

Godless Socialists and Communists now run this nation, control its media, and are fast snuffing out Catholic education—and the right to life.

The Chamber of Deputies has passed a virtual abortion-on-demand law that surely will pass in the Senate. The law will be challenged in the Supreme Court, because the new constitution claims to protect all Spanish citizens. Like the Irish constitution, it says nothing about the first nine months of life, but unlike the Irish, it makes a prolife amendment via national referendum impossible.

Although sterilization is illegal, its existence is winked at. The government would like to pay for all contraception and give contraceptives to teens, but it cannot afford to. The Catholic bishops and religious leaders have wasted the years they had to prepare the nation against the inevitable onslaught of the antilife movement. Soon, thanks to legalized abortion, the current birthrate of 2.3 children per family will fall below replacement level.

There are still laws against prostitution and pornography, but they are "honored more in the breach than in the observance." NFP is virtually unknown. Spain was the first country in the world to legalize marijuana and cocaine.

Vocations are few. Opus Dei is strong. About 15 percent of the people in the cities go to Mass regularly, compared with some 30 percent in the country areas.

In Madrid the Pope's Mass and sermon drew his largest crowd ever: 2.1 million. He begged the Spanish bishops to speak out against contraception, abortion and divorce (divorce has already been legalized). He pleaded with them to stand up and be counted. They did speak out against abortion, comparing it to war crimes and blatant terrorism—but alas, years too late! Even Mother Teresa came to do her part, drawing a record crowd.

FRANCE IN EXTREMIS

The French hierarchy was one of 12 national hierarchies that dissented to *Humanae Vitae*. All twelve of those nations are now dying of contraception-sterilization-abortion. This "eldest daughter of the Catholic Church" legalized contraception in 1975 under Gen. Charles DeGaulle; there went his nationalistic dream of 100 million Frenchmen! Despite the highest family allowances in the Western world, intended to induce French couples to have children, they are not replacing themselves. The average family now has only 1.9 children, and that is *including* the children of the four million foreign workers, more than a third of whom are Moslems with large families.

A French scientist has calculated that France will be a Moslem country by the year 2035. Planned Barrenhood played a big part in bringing contraception and abortion to France. The bishops are exceedingly weak, parishes are closing and vocations are few. Attendance at Mass is pitifully low. *La Belle France* is rotting from within.

According to a study in the *Augsburger Zeitung* for Easter 1983, 90 percent of the French people no longer believe in sin, and only four percent still use the word "sin" in its traditional sense. Sixty-nine percent say they do not go to Confession; 13 percent say they go at least once a year.

Meanwhile, a dehumanizing sex education program, sponsored by the government, amounting to the open promotion of permissiveness, has taken over France. Good Catholic French parents complain that their children no longer learn the Faith in so-called Catholic schools, but do learn all about sex. Thus, a vicious physical sex education course replaces religion to explain the mysteries of life. Some French priests argue that for children in the early grades it is too early to teach the doctrines of the Church. But it never seems too early for dehumanizing sex education!

The millionaire Socialist President Francois Mitterrand will almost certainly nationalize the Catholic schools.

WEST GERMANY: PILLS, PORN AND P.P.

This country has the worst theologians, the worst seminaries, the worst bishops, and the worst antilife conditions of any country in the world! With almost a million surgical abortions for 59 million people, paid for by the government, and with 57 percent of all couples having only one or no children, Pill-happy Germany has the lowest birthrate in the world—1.2 children per couple.

There are now 4.7 million foreign workers, one-third of whom are the mosque-building Moslems. Having founded a euthanasia society, the Germans have begun edging their way back to Hitlerian "mercy" killing, for which they are as theologically programmed as they were for the Pill. Germany's prolife movement is weak and divided. Prostitution, pornography and the horrible "sex shops" are legal; in fact, the largest sex shop in the world flourishes at the Frankfurt airport. The German bishops still dissent to *Humanae Vitae*. One of them told me the encyclical was "not a dogma." I said that the content *was* infallible, that is, unchangeable, having been taught for so many centuries under the guidance of the Holy Spirit.

Our new pamphlet, *The Betrayal of the Theologians*, will help you and your friends understand the moral and theological situation not only in Germany but also in the United States.

In Germany, Planned Parenthood is known as "Pro Familia," which is like calling the Nazi Party "Pro Juden." Since 1952, PP has gone unopposed. Today, the federal government gives it 20 million deutschemarks each year to conduct the country's sex education program, which is perhaps even worse than Sweden's. Church attendance has dropped drastically. The youth are out of control, symbolized in part by the idiotic, pro-abortion, "peace" (surrender) movement, undoubtedly financed by the Soviet KGB.

Once they were users of "die Anti-Baby-Pille" on a massive scale, but now German women are moving to sterilization and abortion because of bad reports on the Pill. In Germany, it has been known since 1967 that the Pill is an abortifacient. This was admitted by the gigantic Schering pharmaceutical company in Berlin. Well-known German theologians have justified the Pill by asserting that *implantation* is the beginning of human life.

Germany's worst theologians (in touch with one of America's worst, the Jesuit Richard McCormick at the Kennedy Institute in Washington, DC) are advisers to the bishops. Josef Cardinal Höffner has admitted that when it comes to NFP, Germany is an undeveloped country. What a shame that such a talented and powerful and "Christian" nation may have gone beyond the point of no return, while the wild theologians go almost unopposed by their colleagues and the weak, cowardly bishops!

AUSTRIAN DEBACLE

In 1972 and 1975, I gave some 50 anti-abortion talks in Austria, fighting the murderous tide. The Socialist government passed an abortion-on-demand law in 1975. Today this beautiful country of seven million so-called Catholics has the highest ratio of abortions to births in Western Europe: 120,000 estimated abortions to 85,000 births.

There are almost 400,000 foreign workers in Austria. Again, many of them Moslems.

Vienna's Francis Cardinal König and the bishops do virtually nothing to stop the moral decline. The Benedictine archbishop of Linz has been warned by the Holy See. The sabotaging of the Church by theologians and religious "educators" is sad to behold—a far cry from 30 years ago, when 700,000 Catholics drove the Soviet Army of Occupation out of Austria by pledging to pray the Rosary for that purpose!

H.L.I. BATTLES DEATH IN ITALY

Italy has the second-lowest birthrate in the world. Estimates of legal abortions vary between 500,000 and 750,000, prolifers having lost the abortion referendum. The Moslems are building a mosque in Rome, and the Mormons a temple. The atheistic Socialists and Communists are murdering both the body and the soul of this nation that does not know how to establish a viable government. The prolife movement is limping.

Last September HLI and PLAN (Protect Life in All Nations) sponsored the first international prolife meeting, with a view of organizing a worldwide network of prolife/pro-family collaboration. Our meeting in Rome drew 100 delegates from 34 countries.

MEXICO THREATENED, H.L.I. RESPONDS

For the second time since 1977, Mexico's government had hinted that it was considering the legalization of abortion. A vote was to come in early September. Then a prolife Mexican businessman who asked for our guidance and with whom we are still working, published *The American Holocaust* in a metropolitan Mexico City newspaper. This publication, with its horrifying abortion photos, aroused an enormous furor; the newspaper was only too glad to print thousands of additional copies that sold for 25 pesos each!

We also instigated a letter-writing campaign directed to the parliament. A small group of doctors and lawyers gave out individual statements exposing the tragedy of legal abortion. A delegation went to lobby the Catholic, Opus Dei wife of the president. She said she obviously could not do anything publicly but would do all she could privately. The president is a Freemason and may well be a crypto-communist.

In any case, the government pulled in its horns, and no vote took place in September. After we threatened huge demonstrations, the president said in December that he considered abortion inappropriate for Mexico. We do not believe him, of course, but now we have time to educate the nation, thank God. In the early 1970s, PP laid the usual groundwork for legalizing abortion by promoting contraceptives and abortifacients, including the hideous abortifacient Depo-Provera, judged too dangerous for *Yanqui* women but good enough for poor Mexicans. I saw a woman buy that stuff over the counter!

PP operates very secretively. In every large government hospital there is a "family planning" center where anyone, married or not, can get free contraceptives, abortifacients, and sterilization. I am trying to prove that this is paid for by the U.S. taxpayer with laundered money. Abortions are also committed in these hospitals.

As in every underdeveloped country, illegal abortion is widespread in Mexico. The killings are done mostly by the *coma drona*, untrained midwives. At a news conference, a Communist woman told me that 144,000 women were dying every year from illegal abortions in Mexico. It was hard not to laugh in her face, because this kind of wild exaggeration is a lie used in every country to legalize abortion.

Thanks to prolife connections in the media, I was able to do a long nationwide radio program. I also spoke here and there in Mexico, but spent most of my time meeting with the various prolife leaders to plot our counteroffensive.

HLI was a major factor in saving Ireland, and with the grace of God and your magnificent help we can save Mexico, a most important nation of 75 million people, whose example is widely imitated in Latin America.

We have begun to pour Spanish-language literature into Mexico; we are producing as much of it as possible in Mexico because printing and transportation costs are low

there, especially since the big decline of the peso. With
our battery of English-dubbed films and literature, we are
going into the high schools and universities as fast as we
can.

UNITED STATES: TENDING THE GRASSROOTS

After Mexico I worked two weeks on the West Coast,
preaching at 22 Masses, lecturing to nine groups, and
consulting and fact-finding with key organizations and
individuals.

It seems some people get discouraged more easily than
I do; it was music to my vain ears to hear them say I re-
charged their batteries for continuing the fight in California, where more than 250,000 surgical abortions are committed each year.

WE BRING PROLIFE TO SINGAPORE

The government of this fascinating, wealthy country is
a benign dictatorship (also called a "guided democracy").
Archbishop Gregory Yong said I worked a miracle by getting $10,000 worth of prolife films and literature through
customs. This island nation has 80,000 Catholics among
2.5 million people living in a land area of 240 square
miles. There is no organized prolife movement; the government would not stand for it. So I started a clandestine
one! For five days I spoke every day, and sometimes all
day, to all kinds of groups, including seminarians, priests,
nuns and archdiocesan staffs. The reaction was absolutely
enthusiastic, because my prolife films were like manna
fallen from heaven. The Catholic Church here still has
missionary status.

In Singapore, couples are allowed two children, severe
penalties being imposed for having more. You are under
the worst propaganda disincentives to have children, all
brought here in the 1960s by—you guessed it—PP. There
are some 30 NFP teachers, with too much work and insuf-
ficient resources. I met the finest Catholics, including four
young and active Catholic doctors. The nuns are the devoted kind we remember so fondly. Although short on
priests, Singapore has many young nuns.

Politically, the people fear Red Vietnam puppeted by
the Soviets more than they fear Red China.

Between 50 and 60 abortions every day are reported in
this country; that represents a great underenumeration. I

was amazed at the wide use of prostaglandin pessaries and "menstrual extraction."

KOREAN CHURCH EXPLODES

Nowhere is the Catholic Church growing faster than in South Korea, whose 1.7 million Catholics make more converts each year than the USA's 52 million Catholics! South Korea has 50 times more seminarians and 70 times more religious novices proportionately than the United States; there are three major seminaries, and a fourth one is being built. There are 3,450 nuns, 1,000 native priests and 200 foreign priests. Already Korea is sending missionaries into foreign countries! When will they come to the United States? Metropolitan Seoul has 130 parishes, offering an average of six or seven Masses on Saturday and Sunday. The churches are filled for all of them.

Thanks to PP, which invaded Korea in 1962, there is a great deal of contraception/sterilization/abortion. In a nation of 40 million people, one million babies are born and 1.5 million are surgically slaughtered annually. About 20 percent of Korean couples have been sterilized. The good news is that Korea has perhaps more NFP couples than any other country, proportionately speaking; in one diocese, 95 percent of the couples practice NFP! The reason? The bishops, priests and sisters promote it. So it *can* be done. (When will the bishops, priests and nuns of North America and Europe learn that *Humanae Vitae* was a most wise, prophetic and *practical* document?)

One doctor maintains that the flourishing of Catholicism is due to the great suffering of the Korean people during the civil war of 30 years ago and the cruel Japanese occupation that preceded it. Many Koreans have family members in the North about whom they know nothing; there is no communication whatsoever. Some 18 million North Koreans have as their chief industry the manufacturing of weapons that go to Communist countries and terrorists around the world, including Red guerrillas in Africa and Central America.

What a sight, though, to see so many young religious priests, seminarians, nuns—and babies on the backs of their mothers, totally content with the world! When the Angelus rings on Sunday, Korean Catholics stop to pray in public. And at Mass the singing makes your spine tingle. Next May the Koreans will give the Pope a welcome such as he has never received anywhere! The Pope will feel at home in this land of martyrs, 103 of whom he will canonize.

RED CHINA: PLUSSES AND MINUSES

I spent a fascinating week in this Communist colossus, a nation of one billion people. Only one child per couple is allowed; you suffer severe penalties if you have more, including forced abortion even in the seventh or eight month of pregnancy. Marriage licenses are issued at ages 25 and 27. Female infanticide is common, because firstborn boys are preferred. The number of abortions and sterilizations boggles the mind. But there is virtually no fornication, prostitution, pornography, homosexuality or immodesty. Divorce is frowned on, and great efforts at reconciliation are made, because "divorce is hard on women and children." The annual income is about $300 per capita. Three TV channels, two national and one local, are used to educate/propagandize; the whole nation seems to be going to school. I have never before seen so much construction going on in any country, or so many bicycles.

There is a strong but small underground Catholic Church; an official "Patriotic Catholic Church" and seminaries exist for propaganda purposes, and the regime persecutes priests and bishops who will not collaborate. Protestants seem to be flourishing in Red China. There are about 20 million Christians in all.

PROLIFERS IN THE PHILIPPINES

This nation of 51 million is in total turmoil and depression, with a $25 billion debt! Caught in one of several daily demonstrations, I was scared to see thousands of angry students march. There is more and more hatred of Americans for backing the dictator Marcos, who may be finished.

I visited HLI's promising sub-center in Cebu City. I also did a seminar in Tacloban and met with the Board of Directors of the Filipino Pro-Life Society, which I founded in 1974; they gave me a very special gift, a unique carved wood sculpture. Parishes are huge; priests and nuns are too few, but vocations are picking up in this nation which is 95 percent Catholic and has a high birthrate. The Filipinos refuse to buckle under the gigantic USA-financed population control Program.

GOODBYE, HONG KONG

I attended the second meeting of the International Federation for Family Life Promotion, mostly an NFP group. In this island nation of 5.5 million people, there are 279,000 Chinese Catholics, mostly converts. The singing of an English-Chinese Mass at the cathedral made my spine tingle. But Hong Kong is doomed: in 1997 the British contract with the Communists will run out, and the Red Chinese will swallow Hong Kong, as a lion a mouse. Priests in Hong Kong are telling their people to move out of the country—and the people are. The sum total of suffering in the world never ceases to amaze me.

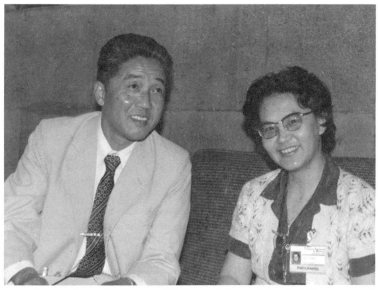

At the U.N. conference, a Chinese minister defended his country's coercive policies genially.

A WORLDWIDE PLAGUE

(No. 9—April 1984)

Contraception-sterilization-abortion is a worldwide
plague that has already engulfed more than two-thirds of
mankind, and I am convinced it will spread through the
rest. What will be left, I do not know.

H.L.I. COMES TO CANADA

In March I spent 10 days in the Montreal area of
French Canada, preaching at all the Masses in two parishes and lecturing to various groups, including several
high schools.

Thanks to the Canadian bishops' dissent to *Humanae
Vitae*, Canada is now a dying nation. Quebec has the
lowest birthrate of all the provinces, 1.3 children per completed family. The prolife movement is very weak, and
there is little NFP.

Quebec is the only Canadian province to have set up
abortion centers. Approximately 100,000 abortions are
reported per year, but in fact there are many, many more,
including those done over the border in the United States,
in places such as Grand Forks, North Dakota, and Buffalo,
New York.

Sex reigns supreme, as I learned from discussions with
high school students who seem never to have heard of the
crucial virtue of chastity. The government still subsidizes
the Catholic schools, now taught almost entirely by lay
people. I was told again and again that teachers who
neither believe in nor practice their Faith are pushed into
conducting religion classes! Religion courses have been
almost completely emptied of essential Christian doctrines.
Twenty-five years ago, 95 percent of French Canadians
went to Sunday Mass weekly; today barely 15 percent do.

I had not realized the enormous political disarray
caused by French Canadian people's desire to break away
from Canada. The government of Quebec is riddled with
fallen-away Catholics (most Socialists, some Communists),
and plenty of Freemasons.

Oh, yes, there are those worried laymen and their
too-few good priests who bemoan the cookie Masses, the

girl altar-servers, the blatant disregard of liturgical rules, and the ignorance of basic morality and the essential teachings of the Church. But harbingers of a heretical national church (Gallicanism) are even more pronounced in Canada than in the United States. I did meet a magnificent, apostolic prolife nun with whom we have just founded a Canadian branch of Human Life International. (This is an addition to our branches in the Philippines, South Africa and Mexico.)

How sad it was to have truly informed Catholics present evidence that a certain important auxiliary bishop has lost his faith! An important Catholic churchman in Europe has observed that the crisis of the Catholic Church is the crisis of the bishops and priests. The more I travel, the more I see that. In no other city or country have I heard more complaints about the Pope's coming than I did in Canada. Misled and half-practicing Catholics do not like to hear the truth.

YUGOSLAVIA: H.L.I. BOOSTS PROLIFERS

I spent two cold, rainy, difficult and rewarding weeks in beautiful but economically troubled Yugoslavia.

Some socioeconomic and other facts: A nation of 22 million people, Yugoslavia is described as one nation with two alphabets, three religions, four main languages, five principal nationalities, six republics and seven borders! The size of Oregon, Yugoslavia counts almost seven million Catholics (Croatians mostly, plus Slovenians and some Hungarians and Albanians), two million unemployed, one and a half million citizens working in foreign countries (including 700,000 in dying West Germany), 17 percent inflation, and 23 dioceses. There are four million indigenous Moslems (as leftovers from the Ottoman Turkish conquest); the rest are Greek Orthodox of weak faith and weaker practice. All three bishops whom I spoke to threw up their hands when I asked about the future of the Catholic Church.

One Catholic archbishop claims there are 800,000 abortions every year in Yugoslavia, including 40,000 to 80,000 among the five million Catholic Croatians. The government is now urgently warning people that abortion is a barbaric means of birth control because it is hard on women's health. Contraceptives and abortifacients (including Depo-Provera—"the Shot") are being introduced as fast as possible. Yes, Planned Parenthood is there too—as a division of governmental health service! Medicine is entirely socialized; Catholic doctors who do not commit abortions are penalized subtly and denied promotions. Thus, new Catholic doctors tend to avoid gynecology, while others abort as few as possible by talking women out of abortion. It is strange and eerie to discuss the issue with them, knowing that they kill!

In all my lectures and conversations, I did not meet a single priest who favored contraception, and virtually all of them agonized over how to help their people. NFP has barely begun, but there is great interest and I will be going back in October to conduct a number of workshops to train NFP teachers.

I met a magnificent young doctor whom I am coaching and whose training I am guiding with European NFP specialists; he wants to spend his life serving the Church, above all teaching NFP and fighting abortion. Given my work, I know a great many Catholic doctors, but I do not think I have ever met another one who seems so clearly to have been chosen by God. If I could find $3,000 for him, he could go around the country doing prolife work, teaching NFP and helping the bishops, priests and nuns, all of whom impressed me.

Catholicism in Yugoslavia dates back to the seventh century, when Benedictine missionary monks converted the Slavs. At one time they had 150 monasteries in Yugoslavia, only to give way to the Franciscans in the 13th century when St. Francis of Assisi charmed the Moslem conqueror. Today the Franciscans have five provinces. The vocation situation is fairly good, except in the diocese with the most tourism, which is a curse everywhere. (The nude sunbathers on Yugoslavian beaches are mostly Germans.) There are 10 minor seminaries and eight major seminaries. Some parishes have begun to run kindergartens, which saves the government money.

In rural areas and small towns, Moslem families average eight children; in cities, five or six children. Catholics, however, are barely replacing themselves. Moslems in Yugoslavia say to conquer Europe they will not need the sword—only children! One priest started an interesting movement called "One More Child" to fight abortion and boost the Catholic birthrate. It has worked: within two years he increased baptisms by 40 percent in his parish! The Church has only the parish with which to educate, its other institutions being nonexistent. The many religious are, however, devout and wear their habits. There are countless young Catholic families who do their best despite difficult circumstances.

For three years we at HLI have been in touch with prolife Yugoslavs and have shipped them much literature. They are now trying to find $20,000 to publish a million more copies of a pamphlet showing aborted babies and having good commentary, including the government quotation that abortion is barbaric. This project has been very successful in saving babies. The new edition will be published in several languages for the benefit of the many tourists who come to Yugoslavia from other Socialist countries.

While in Yugoslavia I made it a point to go to the village of Medjugorje (near Dubrovnik), where the Blessed Virgin Mary reportedly has appeared daily to six teenagers since 24 June 1981, first on a hillside and now in a room in the local church.

More than three million people have come to Medjugorje from all parts of the world. Besides the visions, there have been some 150 miraculous healings, thousands of spiritual healings and conversions, and a repetition of the 1917 Miracle of the Sun of Fatima. I was right next to the teenagers (or visionaries, as they are called) during the reported 1,000th apparition, on April 1.

I talked to four of them before and after, through an interpreter, and found them to be sincere, unaffected, normal and very likeable young people. Some 4,000 people attended Mass immediately after the apparition, most of them standing outside the packed church. I was most impressed.

Mary's messages warn of an impending world catastrophe in punishment for sin. She begs for penance, fasting, prayer, faith, reconciliation, and loyalty to Church and Pope. She is also giving the teenagers 10 secrets, and says she will leave a permanent visible miracle near the village when she leaves. The consistency of the reports and above all their theological soundness are what impress me most about this whole astounding phenomenon.

I was told that several American Catholic bishops have blocked the showing of Fr. John Bertolucci's video documentary on Medjugorje, for reasons unknown to me. While I naturally leave the final judgment to the Church, which is investigating the appearances, they seem to me to be

authentic, as they do to the priests I talked to who are
familiar with the whole story.

GERMANY'S THEOLOGICAL THICKETS

The Church faces many problems in Yugoslavia, but
my distinct impression is that Catholicism there is health-
ier than in Western Europe. Hence, the great contrast I
saw in going straight from Yugoslavia to a dying Germany
to do research and writing.

Germany, in the heart of Europe, is a very important
country and has always boasted the most important and
influential theologians and theological schools. When these
theologians, imitated so much by others, go bad, the disease soon infects many other countries. Münster alone has
4,000 students of theology!

When I asked jokingly whether these students were all
in the seminary, I got a quick reaction, because vocations
in continental Europe are exceedingly few and the Church
in many ways is in dire straits. Poland, for example,
produces more priests in one year than Germany, France
and England combined. As for the Church's "strength" in
the rest of Western Europe: Portugal recently passed a
virtual abortion-on-demand law, Spain's law is before the
Supreme Court to test its constitutionality, and Belgium is
now the only European country forbidding abortion, although the law is widely ignored.

Germany is one of 12 countries whose Catholic hierarchy dissented to *Humanae Vitae*. All 12 countries are
now dying, with Germany having the lowest birthrate in
the world, 1.2 children per completed family! Here Pro
Familia, our Planned Parenthood, has functioned freely
and unopposed since 1952! In 1976 one of the world's
worst abortion-on-demand laws was passed, setting up a
cumbersome typically German legal apparatus (with the
aid of some Catholic theologians and Catholic legal authorities). The law requires a pre-abortion counseling session
with a social worker. One doctor fabricates an "indication"
for abortion and another does the killing.

The moral theologian Fr. Franz Gründel, together with
other theologians in the democratized German diocesan
bureaucracy, advised the bishops to support this chain of
"Catholic" counseling centers to be set up mostly at government expense. In these centers, the counseling must by
law be "nondirective"; no pressure may be put upon the
woman not to abort; her "conscience" must be fully res-

pected. In pertinent German literature I read that the counselor *must* accept the woman's decision to abort, and state in writing that she has been counseled—thus creating a dishonest and rationalized justification for abortion! Some theologians call this "remote, justifiable, material cooperation," but it is anything but that. In short, the German Catholic Church is immediately involved in the promotion and execution of abortion!

When asked repeatedly for an explanation, informed Catholics told me that it is money, and that the bishops do not have the moral strength to stand up to the government, to the pro-abortion, Socialist-controlled media, or to the notoriously pro-abortion national magazines *Der Spiegl* and *Der Stern*. It is unbelievable, but true, that there is only one private counseling center in Germany like our Birthright. It is run by a nun in disguise, Hedi Lebert, who has saved 700 babies in 2,000 counseling sessions, but who is incredibly persecuted by *Der Stern*, by the leaders of the German Catholic counseling centers, and by her own order.

As recently as 1979, the late theologian Fr. Karl Rahner, SJ, published the biological fairy tale that human beings after conception go through stages of animality. He even questioned whether babies are human at birth! These false notions of the biologist Haeckl, I was assured, still appear in many German biology books. Another notable theologian who has betrayed Germany is Father Bernard Häring, who once published an article (without evidence) asserting that couples who practice NFP have more miscarriages and defective children.

Then there is Father (Professor, Doctor) Franz Böckle, head of the university at Bonn, who has been told by Cardinal Josef Höffner himself that he does not speak for the Church in prolife matters. Asked why the German bishops tolerate him in so high a position and accept him as an advisor, my German prolife colleagues gestured in despair. Other theologians who have done tremendous damage are Fr. Alfons Auer and legal scholar Albin Eser, who has a high station in the German Catholic bureaucracy and who—in rationalizing abortions—has re-opened the door for Hitlerian euthanasia. About five years ago the Germans started a euthanasia society.

What makes Germany's theological situation unique is that when big German moral theologians speak foolishly and heretically, there is virtually no one of similar stature to counter them. It is different in the United States, which has several good, prominent Catholic theologians to point out the fallacies and heresies of the likes of Jesuit Fr. Richard McCormick and Catholic University's moral theology professor Fr. Charles E. Curran. The writings of even the latter, however, are mild compared with what the German theologians have written. No doubt the Fellowship of Catholic Scholars and their peers act as counterweights in the United States.

In Germany the prolife movement is weak, small and much opposed. Prostitution and pornography (the world's worst) are legal. The suicide rate, especially among the young, is high (40,000 last year for 59 million people). Pro Familia, which does most of the pro-abortion counseling and killing, has gone unhindered, but will soon be exposed by dogged prolifers. Although they finance NFP in other countries through their considerable charities, the Germans themselves have hardly begun with NFP and are still under the spell of "die Anti-Baby-Pille." Politically, Socialists and Freemasons occupy key places.

Catholic education has been gutted of essential doctrines, as it has been in France, the United States and other Western countries. I was impressed by the nuns I met, still in their habits, although their orders suffer from a lack of vocations. Asked by some bishops to help improve the German Catholic situation, the leader of the Christian Democratic Party, Josef Strauss, bluntly told them "to clean up their own pig sty." (Germans are nothing if not blunt!)

SEX-OBSESSED SWITZERLAND

I spent several days comparing notes with my great friends Dr. and Mrs. Rudolf Vollman, two of the world's top experts on NFP. A good Catholic theologian completely familiar with the Swiss situation thinks that the theological mess there is perhaps even worse than in Germany. Very few go to Confession. While there is still some kind of anti-abortion law, abortions are common. One Swiss lawyer told me he could name 40 abortion centers in Zurich alone, and Geneva has always been wide open for abortion.

Zurich alone has 1,570 registered prostitutes who are examined weekly and who pay high taxes. Some 600 prostitutes walk the streets, among them 30 from foreign countries as far away as Thailand. This city of Calvin supports 312 massage parlors and 22 sex shops, the latter being a sickening sign of the times in Western Europe. (The continent's biggest sex shop is in Frankfurt airport.) The Swiss are wealthy, irreligious, in many ways pagan, and obsessed with sex. There are more than a million foreign workers in this little country of 6.3 million people, who will not be spared in the next war, guilty as they are of sex-run-wild and abortion, the greatest war of all time.

MOSQUES IN "CATHOLIC" AUSTRIA

As in the other German-speaking countries, sex reigns supreme, with more abortions than births in this so-called Catholic country of seven million. *Humanae Vitae* was actively opposed and *Familiaris Consortio* virtually ignored in Austria, as were the last two documents from the Holy See. Here, as elsewhere in Europe, the Moslems, already five million strong, quietly build their mosques and rear their many children. Islam is now the second religion in France.

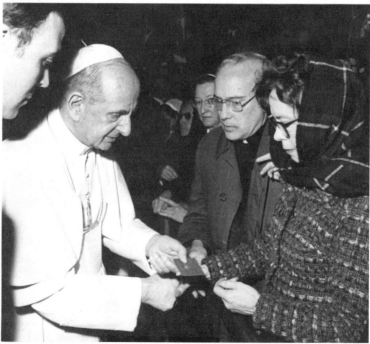

26 January 1973, four days after Black Monday, with Pope Paul VI, who said, 'Never give up, you are a courageous fighter.'

POPULATION CONTROLLERS DESCEND ON MEXICO

(No. 10—September 1984)

I gave prolife seminars in the ancient and beautiful city of Morelia (the capital for vocations in Mexico), in the poor community of Salamanca, and for Mother Teresa's sisters, assembled in Mexico City from her South American convents.

From Mother Teresa's sisters I learned that they have five novitiates worldwide with 525 novices, 325 of these in India. What a powerful force for good are Mother Teresa's 3,500 professed sisters in more than 34 countries! (And what lessons American convents could learn from this holy woman and her devoted followers, who always wear their habits in obedience to the Pope.)

I also lectured to various youth and parish groups. The opportunities in Latin America are overwhelming. Our Spanish-language anti-abortion films are like manna fallen from heaven on these good people, so victimized by their government, by PRO FAM (Planned Parenthood) and by U.S. tax money promoting the death movement.

AT THE SECOND INTERNATIONAL WORLD POPULATION CONFERENCE

A decade ago I was a prolife spy at the first such meeting, in Bucharest. This time I was an official observer at this pre-planned, gigantic act of international deception and manipulation.

An important Mexican official who was in on the planning of this conference told us privately and confidentially that all the important issues were settled, the conclusions written, and the tactics plotted long before the conference began. These antilife/anti-family conclusions were accepted by the president of Mexico before the conference began; he also appointed a committee to advise him on how they can be implemented.

More than that, Mexico's elected dictator signed a contract with the United Nations Fund for Population Activities (UNFPA) to study population "problems" and (final) "solutions" in Mexico. These "solutions" will most likely set a pattern of massive slaughter by abortion and coerced sterilization during the coming decade in Latin America, where up until now only Uruguay has legalized abortion (with the usual tragic results).

Months before the conference began, the fallen-away Catholic, abortionist head of the UNFPA, Rafael Salas (Philippines), admitted that the UN had already spent $80 million for population control on our brothers and sisters south of the border. This is the same Salas who mysteriously visited Pope John Paul II shortly before the conference began. He received a tongue-lashing, in the politest language, from the Pontiff, who condemned contraception-sterilization-abortion and who reminded Salas that it is immoral to bribe nations to reduce their populations.

At the conference, some official observers were allowed to speak for three minutes daily. When my turn came, I was judged not acceptable.

At the daily morning briefings for the non-government organizations (NGO) such as HLI, we heard endless lecturers, virtually all of whom were known abortionists and population controllers. Only one prolife person in nine days was allowed time—five minutes! I was that prolife person.

At these briefings it was made clear that one could not make a statement, only ask questions. After a long harangue on how every country's wishes must be respected, I spoke out on what really happens in the various countries I had visited—giving country, fact and figure. After about five minutes I was shouted down as one making a statement. Did I have a question to ask?

Indeed! At an earlier NGO briefing I revealed, in response to the lies being spoken, that in Mexican Social Security hospitals women who come in pregnant for the second time (or more) must sign a statement agreeing to be sterilized after the birth as a condition for registration in the hospital. I also exposed the fact that simple women are often sterilized there without their consent or even their knowledge.

What is more, I revealed that many babies were being aborted in these hospitals, as I learned from various reliable sources inside, including a chaplain and a social worker who is writing a doctoral dissertation on abortion and asked for my help.

A day later, international pro-abortionist David Poin-
dexter told the briefing audience (in my absence) that Paul
Marx is wrong, that these things do not happen at the
Social Security hospitals. He also said that at the first
International Population Conference at Bucharest in 1974,
Paul Marx showed fetuses in bottles.

Did I have a question? Indeed! After (1) denying
what Poindexter accused me of, (2) offering my evidence
concerning the hospitals and (3) assuring my audience that
I did no such thing at Bucharest but showed only pictures
of aborted and preborn babies (which I now also offered to
anyone outside the door), my question was: Will abortionist Poindexter accept my evidence and sources, make his
own investigation, and then report back to the group?

The highly disturbed lady chairperson could only say
that we can make no such requests of Poindexter. But I
had made my point. Outside the door three-fourths of the
audience accepted *The American Holocaust*, which I was
later forbidden to circulate since it was "not approved."
(Did I quit? No!)

The International Planned Parenthood Federation
(IPPF), with its 114 affiliates throughout the world, was
all over the place. So were its literature and that of its
cohorts. We were not allowed to put prolife literature on
the tables, but we did anyway. We also stuck prolife
stickers everywhere we could, keeping many people busy
removing them (they never caught all of them).

NFP was consistently mocked at the conference. A
report from the Carnegie Foundation proclaimed snidely
that NFP was a good means of birth control—with backup
abortion.

A document from an international women's group
pointed out that not enough women could be sterilized in
any country to solve the mythical overpopulation problem,
and therefore that there must be legalized abortion as well
in every country. Contraception? That is too little, too
late; you must have abortion. (A colleague of ours insisted
that any priest or bishop who still does not believe contraception leads to abortion should be sentenced to spend a
month with Planned Parenthood.)

The Population Institute, with its millions of dollars,
held a six-day seminar attended by all the major abortion
groups in the world. Our man John Cavanaugh-O'Keefe
infiltrated it. The purpose of the seminar was to bring
antilife propaganda to every hamlet on the planet! Among

other techniques, they hired 47 student journalists whose
sole purpose was to write articles and news releases that
were disseminated all over the world. We have reason to
believe that these 47 also helped to put out the daily conference newspaper which purportedly gave the highlights of
the conference proceedings, but was actually loaded with
lies and more lies, distortions and more distortions, such
as only the devil could invent.

For example, former Sen. James Buckley, who headed
the mostly prolife U.S. delegation appointed by President
Reagan, declared that American tax money would never
again be given to private international organizations (e.g.,
IPPF) that in any way engage in abortion-related activities,
and would be given to governments involved with abortion
only if they kept segregated accounts. The official "ob-
jective" conference newspaper headlined his remarks as
"Voodoo Demography"! (The prolife U.S. position, coupled
with the idea that a free market solves more problems
than the antilife Socialist approach, drove the pro-abortionists crazy.)

I attended the large news conference of the U.S. delegation. Among the nine members were three pro-abortionists— first, the head of the U.S. Agency for International
Development (USAID) Peter McPherson; second, the head
of the abortionist Population Crisis Committee, William
Draper; and third, writer Ben Wattenberg.

On a table in a prominent place in the entryway of the
hotel was a single document, that of IPPF, pleading their
innocence of abortion-guilt, boasting of all the good they
had done, and giving the reasons they should not be deprived of the $15 million they get annually from the U.S.
taxpayer just because of Reagan's decree. Strangely, they
admitted in this document that they had always said that
contraception was the "first line of defense" against the
unwanted child, thus implying openly that contraception is
not enough and that abortion is necessary! Buckley defended the American position well, while McPherson tried
to reassure a nervous IPPF. We just found a recent document from IPPF urging its members to bring all abortion
laws down everywhere. One of its authors is Faye Wattleton, president of Planned Parenthood.

At the official meeting, abortion was hardly mentioned;
the word got around that abortion should not be discussed
because it is too emotional a topic. The real goal was to
convince the world that it is overloaded with people and

that therefore every drastic measure must be taken lest we all fall off the earth (depicted graphically on the cover of one of many antilife publications there). At a crucial point, the Holy See presented a resolution saying abortion should never be considered contraception and thus never be promoted. Red China and the USSR immediately sprang to counterattack, but there was enough support for the Vatican's resolution for it to go through.

On another occasion, when a recommendation was made that all adolescents should be "contraceptively educated," the Holy See objected vigorously. Too little support prevented the resolution from passing.

The bishop-chairman of the Vatican delegation gave a magnificent presentation, deploring all the doom and gloom rhetoric, and reminding his audience that life comes from God as a very precious gift to be valued and guarded, and that the Catholic Church, so conscious of God's providence in the world, is much more optimistic.

Fertility control, he proclaimed, should be based on true love, chastity and self-control—not on gadgetry and chemicals, which depersonalize, give bad example to the young, and cause sexual promiscuity. The evidence shows, he stressed, that God had provided for His people through NFP.

Nor, he declared, should birth control ever take the form of mutilation through sterilization. The papal document was so beautifully reasoned and so positively stated that every Catholic or Christian should be proud and happy over it.

We learned from several reliable sources that IPPF and their cohorts did everything possible to have representatives from even Catholic countries be antilife. The evil that infests the environment and circulates at a meeting like this is overwhelming! As at Bucharest 10 years before, every notorious pro-abortionist was in Mexico City.

Truth, logic and reason go overboard when the devil's lying agents speak for bringing down the family, God and His Church. Sexual intercourse is a right, to be performed any time with anyone willing, and if there is an unwanted pregnancy because of failed contraception, there must be legal abortion for every woman in every country for any reason, paid for by the taxpayers—so pleaded an abortionist female delegate from Sweden.

At the Population Institute's seminar, the prize-winning agronomist Norman Borlaug openly admitted that the world could produce food and fiber sufficient for very many more people. Nonetheless, according to him, we need abortion to prevent pollution and overcrowding.

Nothing was ever said about the developed countries, all of which are now dying through depopulation (except for Ireland, which alone has a good, reproductive birthrate). Nothing was said about the low birthrates in resource-rich and empty lands such as Chile, Argentina and Uruguay. Nothing was said about Taiwan, much more crowded than mainland China, but enjoying a vastly higher standard of living, thanks to greater economic freedom.

Nothing was said about there being enough in the world for everyone's need but not for everyone's greed, virtually nothing about social justice, proper distribution, and fair trade laws. Virtually nothing was said about the out-of-control VD, the record number of divorces, the mounting single-parent families, the epidemic of teenage fornication and abortion, the homosexual trend, the increasing illegitimacy, the fast-spreading infanticide, the threatening euthanasia, etc.

Meetings like this convince me that legalized abortion will run through the whole of mankind. There is no stopping it now. The abortionists have the money and the media. They have infiltrated governments all over the world. In the West the Church is weak, decimated by lack of clergy and religious, afflicted with dissenting theologians and too many weak bishops. What will be left? I do not know.

But I do know, as never before, that HLI and our friends are on the right track. Only a serious moral-spiritual revival, the teaching and learning of chastity before marriage and NFP within marriage, inspired and serious preparation for marriage, and cleaning up of the catechetical mess—to say nothing of more prayer and self-denial—can make a real difference. And I know we need to keep working as never before and, with optimism, to leave the future to God, Who will guide and console us.

HLI helped the Mexican Committee for Life to organize a march of 25,000 people against the World Population Conference. We started at the meeting place and for a time drowned out their deliberations! We then marched to the basilica of Our Lady of Guadalupe, whose appearances in 1531 converted then-pagan and antilife Mexico. Once at the basilica, a bishop and concelebrating priests from various countries offered the Holy Sacrifice of the Mass before

the miraculous image of Mary, preserved to this day on the
cactus-fiber cloak of the Indian Juan Diego. HLI gave out
2,000 copies of *The American Holocaust* in Spanish, plus
other good prolife literature, to participants in the march,
who came from all over Mexico.

Despite government persecution of the Church, Mexico
today is a country in many ways far more Catholic than
the United States. Mexicans are Catholic in their bones
and culture, with a hierarchy loyal to the Holy See. In
response to the World Population Conference held in their
midst, the bishops issued an official statement decrying
contraception-sterilization-abortion and the practice of rich
countries, forcing poor countries to adopt antilife programs
as the price of desperately-needed loans.

On TV the Cardinal and Primate of Mexico condemned
contraception-sterilization-abortion for half an hour, despite
the sensitive relations between the godless government and
the Church. He warned his people that they could be
excommunicated for sterilization, because that sin is now
so seriously pushed in Mexico by the government, most
likely with U.S. money, which also pays for the use of the
injectable abortifacient Depo-Provera, considered too dangerous for U.S. women, but good enough for poor Mexican
(Catholic) women.

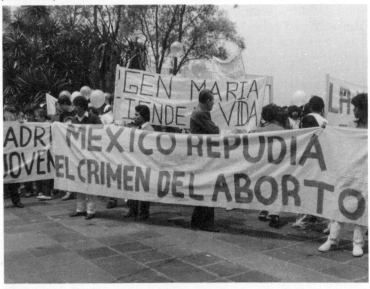

The U.N. conference did not please the Mexican people.

WILL QUEBEC BE EXTINCT?

(No. 11—November 1984)

If you want to know where the contraceptive mentality is taking the United States, all you have to do is visit dying Europe. But I am afraid you can get just as disturbing a glimpse of the future *right next door in Canada.*

And let me tell you, the handwriting is on the wall there, in black and white, for anybody who still thinks the Church's teachings on sexuality can be dispensed with!

THE POPE EVANGELIZES DYING CANADA

I spent 10 days lecturing in Canada and planning our future Canadian prolife programs with the marvelous staff of our new branch headquarters in Laval, Quebec.

My stay overlapped the visit of the Pope, who drew enormous crowds, addressing young and old, Catholics and non-Catholics, French and English, and every ethnic group. One noted psychiatrist said the Pope did more to unite Canada than all the politicians combined. When a saintly, fearless Pope proclaims the truth, even the godless listen and are impressed. There is power in the Word!

In a hospital for sick children, the Pope found an armless, legless little boy who had never smiled. He picked him up and carried him about for more than 10 minutes. I was told the boy smiles readily now.

Totally in touch with God, and therefore His instrument, His Holiness has a way of always saying the right things in the right way for the right people—never mincing words, never being misunderstood, never having to explain what he really meant (unlike some Canadian bishops, my Canadian prolife friends told me).

He roundly and repeatedly condemned contraception and other antilife evils, and praised Catholics loyal to *Humanae Vitae.* The Pontiff addressed himself particularly to the loss of faith by French Catholics when he spoke in Quebec City and Montreal, and to contraception-abortion in the abortion capital of Vancouver.

The Pope's hour-long meeting with 2,500 10- and 11-year-olds in the cathedral in Montreal was phenomenal; they laughed, cried, climbed all over him, and drank in

everything he said. Later he held 65,000 youths spell-
bound with his words on the Church's doctrine as it
applied to them. (Good Catholics in Europe and the U.S.A.
keep asking me why their bishops do not speak like the
Pope.)

John Paul II lamented the French Canadians' plunge
in Mass attendance from 90 percent when he visited Canada 15 years ago to only 15 percent today. He begged and
pleaded and cajoled them to come back to the true fold. In
Quebec City, when he learned that some were actually
taking home the consecrated Host as a souvenir of his
visit, he stopped giving Communion in the hand there.

The French Canadian hierarchy had advised the Pope
to minimize his comments on sexual morality because
people would be "turned off." But the great Polish Pope
followed his own advice (given a few months ago to 30 U.S.
bishops) that the first thing the Church owed the world is
the whole truth.

I spent many hours in Catholic high schools in Ontario.
The students were well behaved but morally confused. A
good Catholic teacher told me some faculty members teach
them that there are no moral absolutes, and said most
teachers in the Catholic high schools are contracepting or
using abortifacients. We wondered out loud how these and
other teachers who do not even attend Mass are capable of
teaching an assigned class in religion—a subject more
"caught" than taught.

A good pastor in Ontario told me that in preparing
people for marriage, it is the Catholic in a mixed marriage
who gives him a hard time—not the non-Catholic, who
"has been standing in the cold for so long that he wel-
comes the warmth of true and full doctrine." The same
pastor deplored the common "living together" made possible
by the acceptance of contraception among Catholics.

Going the rounds in "Catholic" schools in "Catholic"
Quebec province is an unbelievable play called "Children
Have No Sex?" This slick production ever so subtly pushes
the physical side of sex, has no moral values, and suggests
all kinds of sexual activities. A few parents object, but the
vast majority of "Catholics" approve. Many do not know
what is happening.

Thanks to their bishops' dissent to *Humanae Vitae* in
1968, Canadian Catholics are mired much more deeply in
contraception than Catholics in the USA. And far fewer
Canadian Catholics use NFP.

Even worse than American priests and bishops, the Canadian clergy do not speak out on contraception, sterilization, abortion, premarital sex, "living together," overcopulation and underpopulation.

"Catholic" Quebec is the only province in Canada that has set up free-standing abortion centers. It has the lowest birthrate of all the provinces, plus a law designed to destroy parental rights over their children. This Big Brother type legislation, the "Protection [!] of Youth" bill, provides for the government to pay for apartments for liberated 15- and 16-year-olds who cannot cope with their old-fashioned parents!

Meanwhile, Quebecers are now discussing how to raise their dangerously low birthrate. *Bon chance!*

The government of Ontario province has mandated sex education in which ninth graders will be taught contraception as a part of health instruction. Planned Parenthood explained that children have to be taught contraception so the soaring number of teen abortions can be curbed.

They cited a poll—taken by PP, naturally—that "showed" that 94 percent of parents think they should discuss sex and sexual behavior with their children, and that 83 percent want teachers to tell their children about sex, but that only half of the country's schools provide sex education. The president of PP declared that the figures "show a clear gap between what Canadians want and what the educational system is giving them."

PP also "discovered" that only 20 percent of adults were given "the facts of life" when they were growing up, and that 64 percent now say they would have liked more information. With tongue in cheek, PP's president remarked that the parents' lack of sex education could be inhibiting them in teaching their children about sex.

PP warned that "a vocal minority is reported as working to limit sex education.. . . Some of these people believe that if you provide information, you are pushing young people to be sexually active—which is not true."

What a lie—and even they must know it by now! In a pamphlet we have just published, with all facts and sources documented, Valerie Riches of England proves clearly what all careful observers know, or should know: purely biological, value-free sex-education only *increases* the problems it is supposed to solve.

In *every country*, humanistic, "organ recital" sex education has been followed by ever-more sexual irresponsibility

among teens, ever-more teen pregnancies, ever-more illegitimate births, ever-more abortions, ever-more VD, ever-more
"living together" and ever-more ruined future marriages—
plus the frightening increase in divorces, single-parent
families and emotionally crippled children.

As the wise and holy Pope Pius XII said 'way back in
the 1950s, there is no great secret why an increasing number of young people are unchaste; it is not sexual ignorance but spiritual and moral deprivation.

Tragically, PP has much less opposition in Canada
than in the States. They write and do things they would
never get by with in the USA. Thus *Telus*, a Planned
Barrenhood magazine pushing contraception-sterilization-
abortion and unbridled sexual activity (to which "everyone
has a right," they say) was reportedly sent to masses of
Canadian voters at Canadian government expense. Piles of
them were at the Second World Population Conference that
I attended in Mexico City.

Meanwhile, this vast, resource-rich country of 25 million people has a lower birthrate than the dying USA, 1.7
children per completed family. Canada now has to import
people to keep herself going and would be better off in
every way if she had *twice* her present population. The
government reports about 75,000 abortions annually in
Canada, but everyone knows the true figure is much higher—to say nothing of the Canadians who sneak across the
border to have their babies killed.

The Canadian bishops had their great chance to stop
abortion when Canada broke away from Dominion status
with Britain. The Charter of Rights came up for ratifica-
tion. But instead of insisting that the Charter include
protection for all Canadians from conception onward (as
the Irish did in their referendum), the Canadian bishops
made no such major effort. In fact, a cardinal conversed
with Prime Minister Trudeau about the matter, only to
come back to say that all was well, to the consternation of
the right-to-lifers.

It was Trudeau, by the way, who introduced abortion
to Canada in 1969, saying that "the Catholic Church has
no business in the bedroom." As a former law professor,
he surely knew better. O God, deliver us from godless,
cowardly, dishonest, antilife, anti-family politicians who are
"personally opposed, but . . ."!

The anti-family situation in Canada is far worse than
in the developing countries, where HLI has been able to

found seven branch headquarters. For example, in Montreal, a city the size of Chicago, there is only a sprinkling of prolifers and few NFP promoters and teachers. But we have already introduced to Canada all of the best prolife films, a number of them unknown there even in the prolife circles, plus the most effective prolife literature in the world. We are now translating some of this literature into French for the six million should-be Catholics who seem mostly untouched by the right-to-life movement.

What will the Pope find if he comes back to Canada in another 15 years? Perhaps a prolife Christian nation once again.

WHAT I LEARNED IN EUROPE

ROMANIA BANS "CHOICE"!

Astounding news from this Communist country—*they have outlawed abortion!* On March 7, the Central Committee of the Communist Party banned practically all abortions (exceptions: mother over age 42, parents having four or more children, and "juridical" cases).

A fine and prison sentence now await any doctor caught committing an abortion; if he is caught a second time, he gets the death sentence! (It reminds me of what Mother Teresa said in New York City: "Doctors who abort should be put in jail.")

Romania lately has had as many as 1,311 abortions for every 1,000 live births. In 1983, 421,000 babies were killed out of 742,000 conceived. Desperate to keep Romania from disappearing, dictator Ceaucescu has declared that he wants four children from every married woman. Romanian women are now examined medically after each cycle; if they are found pregnant in one cycle but not in the next, they have some explaining to do.

What is more, the Party has also banned the importation of contraceptives. On top of that, they have slapped an extra five percent tax on couples with no children and on people still single at age 25!

How ironic—how insanely ironic!—that an atheist, Communist country should lead the way in banning abortion, while "Christian" nations and theologians in the West are still falling for abortion *en masse!*

(Of course, you did not read any of this in the *New York Times*, just as you did not read in our Catholic press

the Pope's repeated condemnation of contraception in
Canada.)

As for the rest of Europe, I feel like crying when I
recall Belloc's declaration that "The Faith is Europe and
Europe is the Faith." (The whirring noise in the background is poor Hilaire turning over in his grave . . .)

BELGIAN PROLIFERS IN ACTION

In Ostend I attended the 10th Anniversary meeting of
the World Federation of Doctors Who Respect Human Life.
About 250 doctors and other medical personnel from 35
countries took part. The lectures were excellent and the
intellectual exchange was stimulating. Plans for future
growth were discussed. All are awaiting a proposed papal
encyclical on *in vitro* fertilization and related subjects,
which will echo *Humanae Vitae* (Frs. McCormick, Curran,
Kosnik, etc., take note!).

Besides Ireland, Belgium is the only European country
that has not relaxed its abortion law (of course, Ireland is
the only developed country still reproducing itself). Belgians go to neighboring countries for abortions. There is
an annual 100-kilometer march against abortion, but abortions are done even at "Catholic" Louvain University Medical School! There are now thousands of foreign workers in
Belgium; it is another dying country.

DENMARK IN CRISIS

Recently 75,000 Danes marched in protest against
NATO and nuclear weapons. Can they really not see how
they play into the Soviets' hands? It does not matter
much, though, because at the rate Denmark is committing
national suicide, there will not be anyone left for the Red
Army to drive its tanks over.

Very few Danes marry today; they just "live together."
There is massive abortion among the fornicating teens, lots
of VD, pornography everywhere, and great unhappiness.
Foreign workers abound.

Denmark has the highest abortion rate in Western
Europe. (Italy is next with 38 babies murdered for every
100 born.) The Lutheran State Church in Denmark, as in
the rest of Scandinavia, is all but dead—it is little more
than a bookkeeping agent for the State. Less than three
percent in any Scandinavian country still attend church.
Prolifers are only a handful, crying out in the wilderness.

EMPTY NORWAY

This beautiful, empty land of four million people now aborts 29,000 babies each year. The average completed family size is only 1.6, and that *includes* the children of the 400,000 foreigners. The average completed family size for native Norwegians is under one. There are more dogs than babies in Norway. Abortion is simply a means of birth control. But the oil-rich Norwegians do not seem worried.

One wise old Norwegian doctor told me that "it is the attempt at prevention of birth [contraception] that is the real cause of abortion." Why don't most Catholic priests and bishops know this, and do something about it?

CRUCIFIXES REMOVED IN HOLLAND

In some ways, Holland is worse off than any other country I have visited. The Dutch Church makes Canada's seem downright healthy.

A number of priests are openly married, some having children and still functioning as priests. Only about 10 percent of the people and priests still believe. There are horrendous abuses with the Mass, which is often celebrated as if there were no Real Presence.

Fortunately, the Pope has been able to increase the number of good bishops to five out of seven. But they are faced with incredible conditions. For example, nine Catholic churches are for sale in the "Catholic" city of Nijmegen alone! (Archbishop Marcel Lefebvre, who has a large following in Europe, wants to buy one.)

All crucifixes have been removed from the once-Catholic University of Nijmegen. In the diocese of Hertogenbosch, two priest members of the four-member liturgy committee live openly with housekeepers; one has two children. Of course, Catholic students and other young people sleep around in homage to "sexual freedom."

There are 100,000 abortions per year in this prosperous land of 14 million, and no sign of a turnaround.

WEST GERMANY'S WOES

This key to NATO's defense of central Europe is disappearing before our eyes. Wealthy Germany has the lowest birthrate in the world, only 1.2 children per completed family. Next year, the Germans will be unable to supply the 225,000 18-year-old boys needed for the armed forces.

Germany commits some 500,000 abortions annually for
58 million people. The trend now is away from "die Anti-
Baby-Pille" to sterilization. There are more pets than
babies, and the renowned Catholic jurist Albin Eser has
programmed the whole country to accept active euthanasia—the direct killing of patients.

The shocking gains of the Greens and the Reds in a
recent state election prompt some leaders to expect those
parties to be in the next national government coalition.
That would end NATO and thereby invite the Soviets in.

Meanwhile, there are now 4.7 million foreign workers
(and children of same). More than a third of them are
Moslems, who are converting some young Germans disillusioned by what they see in their affluent, dying churches. Nationally, only 17 percent of Catholics go to church;
in Catholic Munich, fewer than 10 percent.

A few bishops are finally waking up to reality and
have spoken out. So have several good theologians who
are bucking the tide with their excellent journal *Theologisches*. Perhaps they will lead the way to better days in
the German Church.

Can Germany be turned around? Can the West be
turned around? Barring a miracle, no. Let us pray (and
work) for that miracle.

ENGLAND: ANGLICANS BLESS FORNICATION

Britain is a nation of educated pagans that is dying
out. PP & Co. now want legal authority to give contraceptives to 10-year-olds, because more and more children are
getting pregnant and being aborted. (After all, they have
a "right" to intercourse.)

Out of 36 million baptized Anglicans, only 750,000 still
go to church on Sunday. An official Anglican document
recently gave its blessing to contraceptive intercourse for
unmarried couples to prove their love (read: lust). The
Anglicans were the first denomination in 20 centuries of
Christianity to give in on contraception (1930). Once you
are on the way down the slippery slope, you reach bottom
fast! The British are there now.

Will there "always be an England"? Maybe so, but do
not expect it to be populated by the English!

IRELAND'S POLITICIANS vs. DECENCY

Evil is the only word to describe the current Irish government, still smarting over losing the constitutional referendum on abortion in 1983.

The politicians now want to rewrite the whole constitution as a secularist manifesto. To make it palatable to the British-ruled North, abortion and divorce would be made legal. (At the moment, another national referendum is being proposed, this time to legalize divorce.) So the abortion battle is far from over in "the land of saints and scholars."

Ireland's prolifers have been unable to close the abortion referral centers run by PP types; in 1983 the latter sent 3,677 girls to England for baby-killings. PP-type doctors are setting up sterilization centers, aimed mainly at women, not men. Ireland's birthrate is falling. NFP is floundering. Pornography is increasing. Yet too many priests are Pill-happy. The bishops seem befuddled and indifferent.

It strikes me that in Europe, as elsewhere in the Western world, most priests and bishops seem unprepared, unwilling and/or incapable of fighting the new paganism—while the Pope, who does know the score, goes unheeded by too many bishops and theologians.

Meanwhile, a state sex ed program is on the Irish horizon. Increasingly, it seems that the laity must save the Church, in Ireland and in the countless lands which Erin's missionaries once converted.

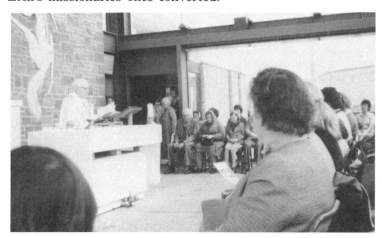

Celebrating Mass at the shrine at Knock in Ireland.

BISHOPS OWE THE WHOLE TRUTH

(No. 12—February 1985)

Ireland today is the only developed country in the world with a good reproductive birthrate.[1] The average family size there is three children (compared with 1.8 in the USA and with 1.4 in the economic community of Europe). But the Irish birthrate is dropping fast because of increasing contraception, and PP-type doctors who are building facilities to sterilize women, and uninformed Pill-happy priests.

Now the coalition government of Prime Minister Garret Fitzgerald is pushing a bill to make non-medical contraceptives available to everyone over 18. (Under current law, only married couples can get them, and then only from a pharmacy, via prescription.)

Thank God, Archbishop Kevin McNamara of Dublin is rallying the forces of decency and sanity to fight back against the feminists and secularists. "Once permissive legislation is passed," he warns, "it is almost impossible to undo it." Unlike so many bishops, he realizes that "the path to moral decline is a one-way street." He told the media that the "choice lies clearly between opting for education in self-control and encouraging self-indulgence in our young people."

This fine bishop was chosen by Pope John Paul II, who was just about the only person who wanted him. In 1974 McNamara had me speak to 600 at Ireland's famous Maynooth Seminary. I still remember how the theologians attacked my orthodox views.

Poor Ireland. It is so hard to survive as an island surrounded by oceans of cynicism, godlessness and the new paganism. Before I first visited Ireland in 1973 to warn them of the coming abortion threat (PP had moved in in 1969), I dreamt that Ireland could be the one, living example of flourishing family life and NFP, proving to the

---

1. Fr. Marx later amended this statement to include Poland and Malta.

world the feasibility and beauty of Catholic teaching in this area.

THE PROBLEM OF THE BISHOPS

A wise man observed, "The problem with the Church is the problem of its priests and bishops." Traveling constantly and being privy to much confidential information, I can only say that there are priests and bishops who no longer believe, judging by their conduct—or should I say, *non*-conduct.

Today the West is dying because of its low birthrates, caused by massive contraception-sterilization-abortion; VD is out of control; and millions of young people fornicate, then abort or give birth to illegitimate babies, thus creating single-parent families in frightening numbers. Seventy-nine percent of all abortions are committed on babies conceived through unmarried sex, while bishops fiddle futilely over the economy and speak vaguely about peace and justice.

This year will bring an estimated 1.6 million divorces in the USA alone. Two million couples "live together" in an "alternative lifestyle" we used to call "shacking up." (PP calls it "being sexually active," and the Bible, "fornicating.") Totally immoral test-tube baby stations continue to be set up. "Mercy" killing is not just around the corner, it is very much with us, especially by way of medical neglect of babies with imperfections.

Young people in Catholic schools seem no longer to learn their Faith; brazen, dissenting theologians, too often invited by bishops to talk to their seminarians, priests and people, continue to pollute the theological streams; our seminaries are practically empty, having suffered a 72 percent student decline since 1967, while most religious orders are dying; the arrogant, asinine, pro-choice-to-kill "Vatican 24" nuns advertise in the *New York Times* and tell Phil Donahue's seven-million-mostly-women audience that there is more than one Catholic view on abortion.

Should anyone be surprised? Most bishops have allowed the theologians to teach that there are no moral absolutes. Hence the nuns say there are multiple Catholic views on abortion. Hence the Church in the West, and humanity itself, is in total crisis.

And the US bishops today—what do they do? Virtually nothing. Most prattle on about peace and justice, or work up partisan statements on economics and the role of wo-

men instead of basic Christian morality—not to mention
the fundamental Catholic social doctrine that should be the
envy of the Western world (in which it is no longer taught,
not even in Catholic schools!).

Have the bishops forgotten that "justice walks on two
legs," that only *just men* can produce a just society and the
peace that is the fruit of a deep and vibrant faith—which
is the bishop's chief duty to nurse and promote?

Again, what a contrast: In South America the Pope
condemned contraception as "gravely illicit" and, unlike our
bishops, criticized both raw capitalist and communist economic systems from a *moral* viewpoint—while acknowledg-
ing that the Church (including the bishops) must seek to
"enlighten consciences and change hearts."

Too many American bishops preoccupy themselves with
"technical solutions" (which they are not qualified in anyway), while neglecting to morally "enlighten consciences
and change hearts."   These bishops are like the captain of
a leaking ship who worries about a distant, barely visible
iceberg, while ignoring the water pouring into his fast-
sinking vessel.

Last summer the Pope told some 30 American bishops
that the first duty the Catholic Church owes the world is
"the whole truth."   He insisted that the compassionate
bishop "will proclaim the doctrine of *Humanae Vitae* and
Familiaris Consortio in its full beauty, not passing over the
unpopular truth that artificial birth control is against
God's law."   Have the bishops as a whole obeyed?   Not
that I have noticed.

These bishops cannot believe with the Pope that abortion comes from the abuse of God's great gift of human
sexuality, that contraception is the gateway to abortion
and other sexual evils, and that the remedies are the
intensive teaching of chastity, a serious preparation for
marriage, and instruction in NFP, especially before marriage. The Pope's Heaven-sent example is lost on them.

As I travel I always get two questions: (1) Why do the
bishops not speak like the Pope? and (2) how can we save
our children from the doctrinal-moral mess in our local
"Catholic" schools?   I am never asked these questions in
the developing countries of the world, where the Church is
flourishing because the bishops and the priests obey the
Pope, carrying out their mandate of teaching and healing,
preaching and catechizing in the true faith. These bishops

will be the Pope's allies at the forthcoming general assembly of bishops in Rome next November.

Meanwhile, we have heard so much about the "seamless garment" concept of prolife issues, a so-called "consistent life ethic," from a certain American cardinal never known for his enthusiasm in promoting *Humanae Vitae.* This same prelate graced the head table at a banquet of a huge secular charity which handed loads of money to the greatest enemy of the unborn (and the Church): Planned Parenthood.

The "seamless garment" theory makes little sense when you remember that suitable armaments may prevent a war and thus may be a positive good; that capital punishment has never been condemned by the Church and has to do with convicted criminals, so at the very least could be a relative good; and that any nation's greatest poverty is to kill its unborn, as Mother Teresa reminds us, and thus liquidate its future.

The "seamless garment" becomes a crazy quilt when you remember that the cardinal in question gave a speech at Georgetown University last fall criticizing Archbishop O'Connor's prolife position (while O'Connor was out of the country, incidentally). The same cardinal stopped a good priest in his diocese (Chicago) from having a Mass and Holy Hour in reparation for the grave sin of contraception. He said, "My concern about the Holy Hour of reparation for the sin of contraception, at least as it was advertised, was that it was too narrow and negatively focused." We wait for the cardinal to come forth with something broader and more positive.

Meanwhile, perhaps he should look into his chancery office, where out of some 60 working priests only four or five are loyal to *Humanae Vitae.* Perhaps he should do something about one of his clergy, Fr. Andrew Greeley, who feeds off the Church while publicly undermining her teaching on sexuality and penning smutty novels. And perhaps said cardinal should have more than one priest and a secretary or two in his low-budget prolife office, since his diocese is the largest in the country.

Before the presidential election, some American bishops put out a statement that there were *14* prolife issues—an obvious ploy to broaden "prolife" so as to make *any* candidate acceptable, even pro-abortion ones. Thanks be to God for the few such as Archbishops O'Connor and Law of New York and Boston, respectively, along with the rem-

nant of our once-solid episcopate. Even so, I am convinced
that this is an age when the laity must save the Church.

MASS PICKETING AND SIT-INS

Our executive director, John Cavanaugh-O'Keefe, is an
originator of and authority on mass picketing and sit-ins to
stop baby-killings. John coaches and courageously leads
effective, *totally peaceful* sit-ins in abortion chambers here
and elsewhere. Perhaps you saw him on TV on January
22, leading the peaceful sit-in on the steps of the Supreme
Court during the huge March for Life.

HONDURAS AND LATIN AMERICA: GOOD NEWS

Just as I was about to tell you the sad news that Honduras had legalized abortion, the Honduran legislature
voted to rescind the law—before it could even go into effect!

The law was a change in the penal code, pushed aggressively by international Planned Parenthood and USA
population control fanatics funded with your tax dollars.
Practically no one in Honduras—right, left or center—
wanted it. It would have allowed abortion in cases of
rape, genetic damage or "health of the mother"—i.e., abortion on demand. Worst of all, it would have allowed husbands, fathers, boyfriends and guardians to force women to
abort if they were judged mentally incompetent or even a
little slow! HLI poured in literature and funds, urged
decisive and immediate action, and organized picketing at
the Honduran embassy in Washington.

This was the first time in Honduran history that the
legislature had repealed one of its laws before it took
effect. What made them do it? A threat by the Church
and the prolifers to paralyze the country with a protest
march in every town, village and parish (accompanied by
work slowdowns, of course) on Ash Wednesday.

Let us give thanks to God for this triumph! But let us
not rest on our laurels, because Satan never sleeps, and
especially not when there is all of Latin America for him
to abort. Honduras would have been only the second Latin
country to fall. (Uruguay was the first, in 1970.)

Right now the Mexican government is keeping quiet
about legalizing abortion; we are convinced it will come up
sooner or later, though. I like to think HLI had a big
hand in forcing the politicians to back off. We believe,
perhaps foolishly, that if we can educate enough Mexican

leaders quickly, we can stave off the war on the unborn in that country, whose 5.2 children per family compares so favorably to the USA's suicidal 1.8.

In Latin America various governments are testing the waters for legalized abortion, as in Costa Rica and Argentina. They only alert us to rush films and literature to their countries' prolife leaders.

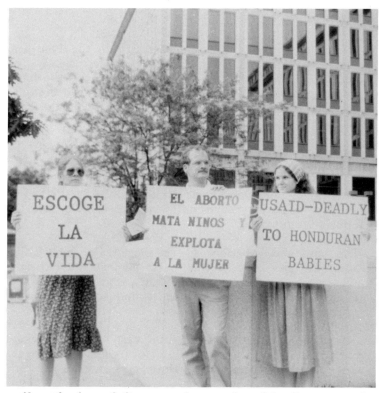

When Honduran babies were threatened, prolifers began to picket the Honduran embassy in Washington.

SYMPOSIUM DRAWS 500 LEADERS

(No. 13—May 1985)

The International Symposium on Human Sexuality in Silver Spring, Maryland, was a huge success—the best I have seen in 10 years of holding international meetings! We had more than 500 participants from 14 countries, including 40 priests and representatives from four of our 13 international branches. Both the Pope and the President sent messages of welcome. Fifteen of the best prolife exhibitors displayed their wares.

A few highlights of the talks:

—Monsignor Diarmuid Martin, secretary to the Pontifical Council for the Family in Rome, explained clearly the teachings of the Church on human sexuality and the family in his excellent keynote address. (He substituted for Archbishop Gagnon, just made a Cardinal, whom the Pope asked to stay in Rome.)

—America's most prolife Senator, Jesse Helms, insightfully and wittily discussed abortion and today's political scene.

—Dr. Wanda Poltawska came all the way from Poland to share her beautiful wisdom on Christian sexuality and the Church's teachings.

—The wise and experienced gynecologist Dr. John Hillabrand, who has been in the courts against the Pill companies more than 100 times, told us of the dirty work of the money-grubbing Pill merchants and the abortifacient workings of *all* Pills and IUDs.

—Jesuit Marc Calegari spoke from vast experience about promoting chastity and fertility awareness among the young, preparing them for NFP in a loving marriage.

—The humorous Dr. José Espinosa gave a devastating talk on how doctors lie about birth control.

—Fr. William Smith, the best moral theologian in the USA, spoke brilliantly on the nature, formation, and function of conscience and its interplay with morality.

—John Cavanaugh-O'Keefe and Joe Scheidler trained scores in peaceful direct-action methods to rescue babies and close abortion mills.

—Robert Marshall and Scotland's Sara Brown gave talks exposing Planned Parenthood's racist, pagan roots as they have never been exposed before.

—Thirty-five symposium participants picketed, prayed and sidewalk-counseled for three hours at an abortion mill two blocks from the hotel. At least two babies were saved, and a priest exorcised the death chamber. Four brave souls were arrested for going inside to stop the butchery.

TEXAS TOUR

I preached at two huge parishes in Houston and got an excellent response. I was astonished at the number of Latin Americans, nearly all of them recently arrived aliens. In one parish they filled the church to overflowing at three Masses, with countless babes-in-arms.

As Bishop Drury of Corpus Christi told me a long time ago, the Mexicans make very fine Catholics; all you have to do is instruct them well. Their many and much-loved children foretell the future of the overcopulating (but underpopulating) USA, whose completed family size is 1.8 versus Mexico's 5.2 (2.2 is needed for national survival).

PROLIFE AND ANTILIFE IN IOWA

In Sioux City, I met informally with doctors, lawyers and other professionals one evening; I showed *The Silent Scream*. I kept a good Catholic high-school audience of 800 boys and girls going from 8:30 to 12:10 with films and talks and dialogue. Thank God, young people still respond to the truth, especially if most of their teachers are still orthodox. This high school has five priests teaching full time; that must be absolutely unique in the USA. (I was shocked, though, to note the influence of Planned Parenthood in this hometown of Ann Landers and Dear Abby.)

Very different was the situation in a 75 percent Catholic town of some 10,000 (better not named) which has two parishes and a Catholic high school. The head of the

"theology department" warned his fellow teachers that they
would get "strange questions after Paul Marx talked to the
students."

I told the priest-principal I was quite prepared to take
on any faculty members who disputed my "strange" (i.e.,
orthodox) theological positions. Only one did, asking me
where I stood on capital punishment. After my response
he lost his courage and wanted no more. (When you stand
up to them, "progressives" are cowards even if they are
priests.)

This "seamless garment" priest, I found out later, did
all he could in subsequent days to destroy what I said.
The same young priest, only recently out of a wild seminary that shall also go unnamed, told people from the
pulpit to vote for pro-abortion Mondale and Ferraro last
fall because Reagan was a warmonger. He has also been
seen in a local go-go joint—trying, perhaps, to convert the
go-go girls?

For the first time ever I was refused the second collection, although it had been promised. Later on, true-blue
prolifers told me why: In neither parish do they ever hear
about chastity, contraception, sterilization, abortion, euthanasia, *Humanae Vitae* or *Familiaris Consortio*. They hear
plenty about "the seamless garment," though.

Girls are referred for abortion from this "Catholic"
town, but only recently was a Birthright center started.
Astonishingly, even in a small Catholic enclave such as
this you find all the evils that you encounter in the large
cities. But then, it is not really surprising: rock and Hol-
lywood have homogenized the culture, and the media are
largely in the hands of the antilife/anti-family devil. All
too many clergy and nuns, seemingly befuddled, stand by
helplessly . . . or simply snooze on.

CANADA

On the way to Canada again I spent a busy day consulting with the authorities of a huge, truly Catholic nursing home run by fully Catholic Carmelite nuns. What a
joy to find the old values and spirit alive and flourishing!

Under the incomparable Josephite Sister Lucille Durocher, HLI's branch in Montreal is thriving, and its success
stands out all the more because there is so little prolife-
pro-family work going on there. Today the Catholic province of Quebec has the lowest birthrate in the world—1.2

per "completed" family! Ironically, the government is more worried about this than the bishops. Our growing prolife gang in Canada has inspired and led lots of healthy picketing against the fanatical abortionist Henry Morgentaler. He defies the Canadian abortion laws by opening mills in the big Canadian cities, in order to challenge the last legal restrictions, as he did in "Catholic" Quebec. He even committed an abortion on television on Mother's Day. Pray for this wretched man, who claims he is a Holocaust survivor but is now waging his own holocaust.

H.L.I. INVADES ARGENTINA
Loaded down with $4,000 worth of films, tapes and literature, I invaded this South American giant April 6-16. It was the most fruitful foreign prolife trip I have ever taken.

In 10 days I addressed nine bishops (two of whom wept when I showed them *The Silent Scream*) and consulted at length with three archbishops; I spoke to doctors, lawyers, law students, seminarians, and university and high school students; I appeared on seven TV programs (one for 35 minutes), had eight radio interviews and confronted news reporters at least 10 times. Two TV stations copied three of my films for multiple future viewings. The serious-minded Argentines, like the Filipinos, must have decided I am tireless, because they flew me from one large city to the next for well-publicized and well-organized appearances.

With runaway inflation and a huge deficit ($30 billion), Argentina's socio-economic and political situation is extremely tense and unstable. The military is ever ready in the wings.

Argentina has two main political parties: the Radical Left, now in power, and the Peronists. There are also many splinter groups. Freemasonry took its toll in the 19th century. A small Communist Party exploits the political and economic turmoil.

The Socialist government of President Raul Alfonsin is anti-clerical, opposed to Catholic education, pro-divorce, and treacherously (although silently) pro-abortion. Ever since Alfonsin took over less than two years ago from the bumbling military, pornography has surfaced increasingly. It is inherent in Socialist policy to lessen the authority of Church and parents, to divide parents and children, to allow or ignore pornography, to foster a humanistic sex education, and to install the leveling state.

When Alfonsin addressed the International Eucharistic Congress last year in "B.A." (Buenos Aires), his theme was the benefits of the pluralistic state, to the visible consternation of bishops and priests, who still are not sure what to expect from him. The speech was written by a seminary theologian, indicating a cancer you and I know all too well.

An interesting spiritual phenomenon has appeared in Argentina: a mini-Medjugorje. The Blessed Virgin is allegedly appearing to a woman who is barely literate but who writes down beautifully the reported messages from Mary. Themes: penance, prayer, faith, reverence, and obedience to the Pope.

Already there are pilgrimages. The Church authorities are trying to keep the whole situation quiet while watching and investigating it. Several miraculous cures have been reported. A young man, full of incurable cancer, was healed. I talked to him; he is going into the seminary. I also spoke with his parents several times. They told me an atheistic Jewish doctor attested to the miracle.

Although poor, the Church wields considerable power through its schools (50 percent of Argentine education) and the trade unions. The seminaries are filled, and several new ones are being built. In this Catholic country there are approximately 2,000 secular priests, 6,000 religious priests and brothers, and 12,000 nuns, all in habit. The hierarchy stood firm on *Humanae Vitae*, except for a wild dissenting theologian here and there. NFP is only in its beginnings, though, and needs our help and coaching.

Although the government kicked Planned Parenthood out of Argentina in the early 1970s, their poison stayed behind in the form of sex education in the public schools. Tragically, some Catholic schools send their students over for this "instruction."

The Penal Code of 1922, still in force, allows abortions for rape and "serious medical reasons." Legally, before an abortion may be committed, it must be cleared with a judge—a requirement long since abandoned in practice.

Estimates of the number of surgical abortions range from 100,000 to 500,000; from consultations with doctors and others, I estimated there are at least 150,000 annually. There is no agreement on whether more abortions are done by doctors or by untrained midwives, or on whether the married have more abortions than the single. Observers maintain, though, that the poor have more abortions than the rich, who use Pills, diaphragms and, increasingly, sterilization. Argentina has a large middle class. Although the birth rate is still reproductive, the infant mortality rate is high; so national growth is minimal. Argentina needs more people. This resources-rich country of one-and-a-half million square miles has fewer than 30 million inhabitants. At the first World Population Conference in Bucharest in 1974, the Argentine delegation was the first to tell the rich nations to stay out of the bedrooms of the poor countries.

A drive to open wide the floodgates of abortion will surely come. But the Argentines have time to build a resistance movement and save their nation—and perhaps all of Latin America. I promised their bishops and lay leaders many more films, a small mountain of Spanish-language literature, and a return trip. The prolife movement here is still in the cradle stage, but it has great possibilities, thanks to Argentina's fierce, orthodox Catholics. (B.A. will soon have HLI's 13th international branch headquarters under an experienced businessman, Victor Taussig, leader of the family life movement.) The Argentines are lovely people, educated, conservative, Catholic and cultured (in the cities).

LATIN AMERICA IN DANGER

As I reported to you from the Second International Population Conference in Mexico City last year, the world abortion movement is now poised to bring down Latin America.

So far only Uruguay has relaxed its abortion law, with the usual effects—150,000 abortions yearly for three million people. Uruguay is truly a dying nation.

In 1972 and again in 1976, I was all over little El Salvador with prolife lectures, literature and films, trying to start the prolife movement I knew they would need. That country is no stranger to me, nor is Nicaragua, which I visited in 1972, for the same reason. Make no mistake, Castro is deeply involved in both countries, helping the Soviets to expand their beachhead. The Communists in Nicaragua are busy feeding weapons to their comrades in El Salvador, while complaining about *Yanqui* interference in *their* internal affairs.

Yes, there are great injustices in Latin America, and the Church must address herself to them fully. But the tragedy of tragedies would be to stand by while Moscow inflicts the greatest of all injustices, namely atheistic Communism, on this Catholic continent.

I worry about nuns and priests and bishops who mouth slogans and ignore history. Allow me to remind them of life today in Vietnam, Cambodia, Afghanistan, etc. Is this what they want for our Latin friends? These clergy will see the light when they themselves go to the Gulag. But by then they will be forgotten in the clamor to "liberate" the next domino.

HLI must concentrate its resources in Latin America, because 40 percent of the Catholic Church is there. By the year 2000, *half* of all Catholics will live on this continent. Brazil is the largest Catholic country in the world. Countless Latin American immigrants are now pouring into the USA, legally and otherwise. These people are Catholics, at least culturally, and properly handled and instructed they could be a great asset to the Catholic Church here. (Have all your children learn Spanish!) Hopefully, the Vatican can nip in the bud the Latin America's loud, false prophets of so-called liberation theology.

PLANNED PARENTHOOD THREATENS LAWSUIT

In February, I really stung Planned Parenthood in Ottawa, Canada, on "Open Line," that city's most popular radio talk show, hosted by abortion sympathizer Lowell Green. Apparently they do not like being exposed as perversion-pushers and child-killers. The Planned Parenthood Federation in Canada has thrown a million-dollar lawsuit for libel against the radio station. At the same time they have told us they intend to sue HLI and me for libel.

Frankly, I have expected this, because I act as a guerrilla against PP all over the world and have sniped away at them for 30 years! At their national meeting in Atlanta in the late 1970s, they called me "Public Enemy Number One of Planned Parenthood."

HLI's lawyers consider the lawsuit threat an attempt to intimidate me and HLI. If PP thinks it can silence us this way, we've got news for them!

The radio station is required to keep tapes of this show for 30 days. PP sued on day 31, thinking the court would have to accept their version as the truth. Fortunately,

HLI has a tape of the whole show (thank you, Guardian Angel!).

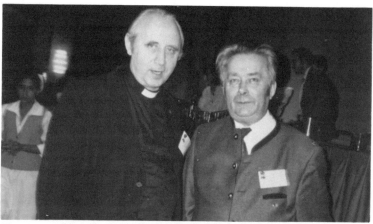

Fr. Otto Maier (Germany) and Martin Humer (Austria).

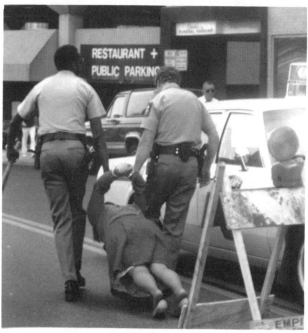

HLI's meetings inspire action. Four people were arrested at a rescue (or 'sit-in') at an abortion clinic near the symposium in Silver Spring.

CATHOLIC COLLEGES: R.I.P.

(No. 14—August 1985)

In the last few months, I have spoken at two secular and two Catholic "institutions of higher learning." The secular campuses were San Jose State University and East Valley College in California; the "Catholic" universities were Santa Clara and Notre Dame. The difference in moral and intellectual climates between "Catholic" and public schools is now practically nil.

At Notre Dame, for example, out of 40 staff theologians, only two accept *Humanae Vitae*; one is an admitted atheist! Contraception seems to be no moral problem here, despite being one for 20 centuries of Catholicism and four centuries of Protestantism (until 1930).

When I asked prolife students whether the faculty points out the abortifacient character of the Pill and IUD, they said contraception is not even discussed, because it is not a problem. People are experimenting on fetal brains at this university named for the Mother of Jesus.

At Jesuit Santa Clara, a new student prolife group, aware of the antilife climate on campus (where signs announcing my talk were torn down), insisted I not show the film *The Silent Scream* because it would be "counterproductive." At both "Catholic" universities, students told me various faculty members were pro-abortion. At St. Mary's College near Notre Dame, the women are very enthusiastic about contraception, and woe to anyone who speaks about NFP.

At San Jose State and East Valley College, recreational sex is simply taken for granted. Contraception is the great blessing; should it fail, there is always Planned Parenthood's "post-conceptive family planning" (abortion). That human life begins at conception was "your opinion"; allow others to have theirs, pontificated a student.

A smart-looking young lady commented brazenly, "Do you really think young people won't do what comes so naturally?" The same girl volunteered, "I use contraception myself." I neglected to ask her whether she charged for her favors or whether she belonged to the 10 percent of female college students in this country who have the latest form of VD, chlamydia.

I held my ground in this sea of ignorance and naivete about religion, history, biology and human realities. The stupidity and arrogance that one encounters among these pseudo-sophisticated students is appalling. But they are to be pitied, because they are only regurgitating what they have been spoon-fed in the classroom by professors whose own lives might appall decent people.

When you enter these dens of iniquity you find out how misled these young people have been, yet how eager they are to learn nonetheless. They have been betrayed by contracepting parents and teachers—and sometimes even by cowardly clergymen who are perhaps little better than the sex-happy sex educators who have turned so many campuses into moral cesspools, destroyed our families, and produced doctrinally ignorant graduates, many of whom are incapable of establishing loving marriages.

I often remember Einstein's famous remark about not expecting so-called intellectuals to defend the best interests of society in times of national crisis. Anyone who supports such so-called Catholic education will have much to answer for in the next life.

I also preached at three parishes. In a California church, five people walked out when I mentioned contraception. The truth will set you free, but it won't make you any friends! These days its demands are too great for too many who do not know their Faith or refuse to live it.

LIFE IN EAST GERMANY

This Communist-enslaved country of 17 million has one million confirmed alcoholics (*vs.* two million for 60 million West Germans). The "German Democratic Republic" has only about 500,000 practicing Catholics, with 1,000 priests, 3,000 nuns and a sprinkling of brothers, supported mostly by West Germany's Catholics. At the end of World War II, East Germany was approximately 50 percent Protestant; today the Protestant Church is all but dead. Apart from alcoholism, there is no drug problem, because such drugs are not available in this ultra-regimented society.

East Germany has the highest family allowances in the world to boost its low birthrate, which is barely at replacement level. Both husband and wife work. The workday starts between 6:30 and 7:00 a.m. and ends at 4:00 p.m., adding up to about 48 hours a week. Children are awak-

ened early, deposited in daycare centers, and then picked
up at 4:00 p.m. by tired parents who still have the work at
home before them. This work-dominated living is hard on
family life.

After a baby is born, the mother can take one year off
with pay; after that the State places the child in a pre-
school daycare center every workday morning until three
years of age, when he advances into a three-year school
program. The Catholic Church is allowed a number of
kindergartens. These and one seminary are the sum total
of formal Catholic education allowed.

A badly composed chemical Pill is used widely for birth
control, with very harmful effects; East Germany cannot
afford the expensive female hormones usually used for such
Pills. Because of the low birthrate, contraception is not
urged by the government. As of now, there is little sterilization.

There is an estimated one abortion for every live birth,
and by law every woman is allowed one abortion per year
and no more than three in her lifetime. But if you become
pregnant after you have had your abortion for the year,
there are always "social indications" or "risky pregnancies"
that excuse the killing of the child.

The word *euthanasia* is like a red flag before a bull,
conjuring up memories of the hated Hitler. However, there
is a professor in Leipzig who talks about making dying
more comfortable. Life on the whole is severely regi-
mented. Few can afford TVs and even fewer the videocassette players so common in West Germany. Currently
the one seminary in Erfurt has 100 students, whereas in
1966 there were 250.

Because of the regimentation, depression and loneliness
are common and great problems—hence the alcoholism—
and this in the country with the highest standard of living
behind the Iron Curtain! Spies galore, sometimes even
dressed as priests, sneak into West Germany to undermine
her, to gather intelligence, and to stir up and support the
peaceniks—who increasingly intone, "Ami go home."

WEST GERMANY: THE CHURCH AND ABORTION

This keystone of NATO has the lowest birthrate in the
world. The law allows virtual abortion on demand any
time in all nine months. The estimated number of doc-
tor-committed abortions yearly is 400,000, with 450,000
babies born, for 60 million people. This year there are 5.7

percent fewer children in school than last year! The Pill-happy Germans are fast turning to sterilization. More than one-third of the almost five million foreigners are Moslems, who now have the majority of children in the schools of large German cities.

German bishops are paying dearly for their dissent from *Humanae Vitae*—a dissent fomented by university theologians such as Jesuit Karl Rahner. Fr. Rahner's private letters, recently published in the Swiss Catholic journal *Orientierung*, seem to indicate that he did not believe, as seems to be the case with his colleagues and students such as Metz, Böckle, Bocklet, Schiller, Auer, Gründel and others, who have polluted the theological streams of Germany and the world. I was astonished to learn that "liberation theology" had its origins in the Frankfurt school of atheists and Freemasons such as Marcuse and Block. Never trust in intellect without virtue, warned Cardinal Newman. (Goebbels, Hitler's mouthpiece, was a PhD.)

Privately, most German bishops will admit that their dissent was a tragedy, but none has had the courage to admit it publicly. A pastoral by the bishops some months ago rejected the test-tube-baby process, fetal experimentation, surrogate parenthood and artificial insemination. Some say these evils are the direct fruit of the bishops' doing what we are taught may never be done: divorcing the procreative and unitive meanings of the marital act; and so the bishops are now implicitly rejecting their own dissent to *Humanae Vitae*. But no bishop will say that out loud.

(Over the border, the Austrian hierarchy has sanctioned the morality of test-tube-baby production.)

Meanwhile, several bishops are awakening to reality, namely the bishops of Münster and Fulda, thanks to the incredible exposés of Elisabeth Backhaus and the priest-theologian Johannes Bökmann, whose excellent journal *Theologisches* is widely read.

The shortage of priests in West Germany's 22 dioceses is great. Three thousand parishes have no pastors. More and more lay deacons and theologically trained laymen conduct a Word Service (*Wortgottesdienst*) here and there. In the archdiocese of Cologne last year, 58 priests died and only 11 were ordained, whereas in the past as many as 80-90 were ordained. Between 1962 and 1975 the number of priests dwindled by one-third. In 1983, 231 priests were

ordained, fewer than one-half the number in 1963.
Religious orders have suffered a similar fate. As in the
USA, Germans never discuss a leading cause, sinful birth
control.

Germany has three major political parties, the Christian Democrats, the Social Democrats and the Liberal
Party, plus a small, annoying group of environmentalists,
abortionists and extreme liberals known as the Green
Party. The right-to-life movement is so weak that abortion
is never an election issue. If the Left dominates politically
in the future, it may mean the end of NATO, no more
atomic weapons on German soil, and an invitation for the
Soviets to move in. There is good evidence that the Communists bankroll the Green Party and the anti-nuke demonstrators.

Nowhere is Planned Parenthood as free as in West
Germany. Here PP openly speaks of abortion as an inherent part of birth control, the legitimacy of homosexuality, alternatives to the family, and no restrictions whatsoever on sex. PP is directly involved with the Green
Party leftists. Thanks to PP, Germany has undoubtedly
the worst sex education in the world. Most parents either
do not care or do not know what is happening in their
schools.

Known as Pro Familia (!), PP organized in 1952 when
the Germans were still recovering from the war. Heavily
financed by the government ever since, these relentless
antilifers are now trying to set up centers in every state
for pregnancy testing, contraceptive counseling, sterilization
and abortion, all under one roof.

Pornography and prostitution are legal. Doctors can
hand out the Pill and commit abortions on minors at will,
without parents' knowing it. Eighty percent of abortions
are done for "social indications." Before she can legally
abort her baby, a woman must visit an approved counselor.
Ninety percent go to PP's centers.

One of the most horrendous scandals of the Church in
Germany is its acceptance of money from the government
to run these dreadful counseling centers, thus involving the
Church directly in abortion! Prolife centers such as Birthright are almost unknown. Amniocentesis is virtually
mandatory for women 35 and older; if the doctor does not
suggest it, he will be sued if a defective child is born.

West Germany, like six other countries including Mexico, Denmark and Sweden, does not penalize suicide. Be-

cause of the devilish way the German abortion law is written, it could easily apply to euthanasia also, to which Germany is wide open. They have an active euthanasia society, thanks to famed "Catholic" jurist Albin Eser. By the year 2000 there may be three retired Germans for each one working. The pressure for euthanasia will be immense.

Many of Germany's problems can be laid at the feet of the agnostic theologians whose moral teaching amounts to a mix of humanism-evolutionism-situationism (Gute Erwagung).

HOLLAND: HATRED GREETS THE POPE

In this nation of 15 million people and an alleged 10,000 Bible groups, there are an estimated 120,000 abortions each year. One hospital reported 600 "menstrual extractions" weekly. The birthrate is 1.8 children per completed family, making necessary the importation of more than 300,000 foreign workers, more than a third of whom are Moslems.

Approximately 50 percent of the Dutch use the Pill, 30 percent are sterilized, and 15 percent use the IUD. Few know that the Pill and IUD are abortifacients, although some say "one cannot tell or know." University students and other young people "live together" freely, following the teaching and example of some priests. Estimates of the number of Catholics who still accept full Catholic doctrine run as low as five percent. One bishop gave $40,000 to the Moslems to build a mosque, many of which are in evidence. Some Catholic churches allow Moslem prayer services.

Critical informants thought it was good that Pope John Paul II came to Holland, where the crowds were small and derogatory signs were evident; the visit smoked the termites out into the open.

The Pope joked that the proffered $4,000 reward for his assassination was not much for killing a pope. Patiently he faced rebels who want the Church's blessing for homosexuality, fornication, adultery, divorce, "living together," abortion, women priests, married priests and liberation theology. On (anti-Catholic) TV the pope was portrayed dancing with scantily clad women. One sign said, "Pope go Rome." Old Dominican priests, in habit, held up pictures of Franciscan Leonardo Boff, Brazil's silenced "liberation theologian."

An estimated 50 percent of the 14-year-old girls in
Holland are on the Pill, given them by doctors who do not
have to notify their parents. Annulments are granted
freely in every diocese. The one orthodox seminary has
produced more priests than all the schools of theology
combined (thank God). In the latter the young often lose
their faith. PP is strong, and raw, physical "sex education"
bordering on pornography is the norm. Good parents are
at wits' end to know how to teach their children the faith.

The situation in Holland is far worse than good Catholic writers in American Catholic papers, such as the *National Catholic Register*, report! By careful appointments,
though, the Pope now has five of seven bishops on his side.
The recent appointment of Bishop Jan ter Schures to Holland's largest diocese, Den Bosch, was actively opposed by
30 of the 31 deacons and virtually all of the priests.
Breakaway Archbishop Marcel Lefebvre has four well-attended parishes and wants to establish a seminary. The
once-powerful Catholic Pontifical University at Nijmegen
has removed all crucifixes; recently students held a sit-in
to demand that the university not even be called "Catholic"
but "a Christian university."

Most of the incredible theological situation in Holland
is due to the Dominican theologian Fr. Edward Schillebeeckx, a homosexual with a police record of exposing
himself in his home town in Belgium. Before the Pope
arrived, a huge tent was erected with large letters proclaiming "Free Sex." This group was addressed by Fr.
Schillebeeckx, who is the hero of so many American rebel
theologians. Like Hans Küng—according to his pastor—
Schillebeeckx offers Mass only when he can put on a show.
A confrere of Schillebeeckx who is a theologian in his own
right insists that Fr. Schillebeeckx no longer believes. I
asked why he stays in the Catholic Church. "Because the
Church gives him a platform to undermine and destroy,
like the predicted evil prophets in the Bible." Confession
in Holland has come virtually to a halt, except in one or
two dioceses.

THE POPE DEFENDS LIFE IN BELGIUM

This land of 12 million, with 500,000 foreigners (including many Moslems), has thousands of abortions, but they
are clandestine; the law still forbids them.

At a three-hour Mass, the Pope displayed his genius in
shifting from French to Flemish with ease. Reflecting

events in Holland, one sign read, "Do Not Touch My Pope."
As in Holland, the Pope stood his ground, condemning
contraception and sexual license.

He reminded young and old alike that it is never easy
to be a Catholic. Between the lines he told them they had
to decide whether they wanted to be Catholic or not. He
warned the Belgian bishops to make sure that "professional
theologians" do not "create a parallel Magisterium."

Young people, the Vicar of Christ insisted, must shun
". . . the promise of easy, immediate pleasure, unbridled
sex, drugs of all kinds, artificial gadgets, expensive fashions, thought-destroying noise, illusion-mongers and dream
merchants—every modern idol which fosters our egoism in
all its aspects." He observed, "We must find a cure for the
spiritual weakness of Christians. The Christian fabric of
society must be remade."

On national TV, the Pope reminded the justice minister
that human life begins with conception and should be
legally protected thereafter. The official arrogantly told
the Pope there were other views that needed to be respected. In Belgium, though, the crowds were large and ap-
preciative, and the Pope joshed with the youth as he always does. Shamefully, the students at the so-called Catholic University of Louvain pointedly told the Pope that
they wanted their sex and he should get off their backs.

One Belgian bishop made an interesting comment to a
colleague who teaches NFP. He said that of course it was
a tragedy that the Belgian bishops dissented from *Humanae Vitae,* and the demographic results prove it. But, he
argued, if the bishops condemned contraception now, after
making it a matter of "conscience," they would lose all
credibility. (Would they?)

The bishop argued further that people have to learn
NFP ever so gradually and thus be weaned away from the
seamy garment of contraception-sterilization-abortion-euthanasia. But obviously there is no time for such weaning.
All of the developed nations except Ireland are now dying.

UNITED KINGDOM: PROLIFERS AND PRELATES

Because of low birthrates, this country is a mixtum-ga-
therum racially. Among the millions of immigrants are
countless Moslems with their mosques. They give the
pagan English a lesson in religion and churchgoing.

The Catholics—fewer than four million—go to church
more than the 33 million baptized Anglicans. There is a

steady conversion of Anglican priests to Catholicism, a point of no little concern to Anglican officialdom. But the latter should not be surprised: every English bishop in the House of Lords voted for the Abortion Act in 1967. They have since come out for women priests, homosexuality and permissive divorce. Most likely these cowardly ecclesiastical wolves in sheep's clothing will vote for the proposed animal-rights bill. (One could cynically say they would be more useful as chaplains to the many animal-pet hospitals one finds along the German autobahns.)

The Anglican hierarchy, remember, was the first Christian body in 20 centuries to come out for contraception (in 1930). Ever since, it has been downhill for the Anglican Church. A few months ago they gave their blessing to contraceptive fornication for engaged couples.

Catholic episcopal leadership is lacking in England. The Benedictine Cardinal and Primate has said imbecilic things about the IUD, the test-tube-baby problem and other sins. As elsewhere, many English young people join fundamentalist sects and occult groups.

Victoria Gillick, a Catholic mother of nine children, waged a single-handed campaign in the courts to stop doctors from passing out the Pill to girls younger than 16 without parental consent. She won! There is now a gigantic effort to reverse this decision in a higher court. Large billboards in London streets show a pregnant child with the caption, "Must little girls grow bigger like this?" Lies and more lies and the crudest propaganda are used to make it legal for girls to obtain the Pill at age 10 and be aborted at 11 without parental knowledge. This child-sex lobby claims falsely that pregnant 11-year-olds have committed suicide because they were denied contraception and could not get abortions without their parents' knowledge or consent.

The British have more videocassette machines per capita than any other nation, the Germans being second. Many British Catholics foresee that they cannot depend on Catholic schools to educate their children in true Catholic doctrine. So they are forming an organization to put on videocassette the essential teachings of the Church, the Sacrament of the Mass, salvation history, Catholicism's rich cultural history, and (not least) the best apologetics to convert the new pagan in the street.

SWITZERLAND EMBRACES DEATH

On June 9 we lost an important national referendum on abortion by a margin of two to one, 19 cantons (states) against seven. Swiss TV refused to show *The Silent Scream* because "it would arouse the emotions." (To arouse the emotions by pornography on TV is okay, but God forbid you should show the truth.) We tried to get the film on Bavarian TV, which the Swiss view. We also gave the film to Germany's second TV channel in Mainz, for the same reason. Switzerland is another abortion-mad country. And it has more than one million foreign workers. Goodbye Switzerland and Europe!

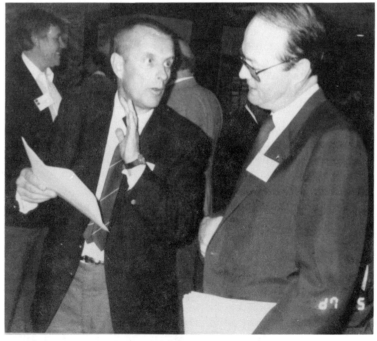

Dr. Philippe Schepens (Belgium), the head of the World Federation of Doctors Who Respect Life, discusses plans with HLI's Mike Engler.

SOUTH AFRICA: THE TRUTH

(No. 15—September 1985)

Fifteen hours on the plane out of New York and you are in Johannesburg, capital of the Republic of South Africa (RSA).

This immense, rich, fascinating, but troubled country has 30 million people: 20 million blacks, four and a half million whites, two and a half million "Coloreds" (i.e., mixed parentage), and 900,000 Asiatics.

The Afrikaaners, who are white Dutch Reformed Calvinists, are the largest religious group and hold most of the power. The Zion Christian Church is the largest black church, with four million members. Only four percent of the people are Catholics, mostly blacks. Recently 8,000 Moslems, many of whom are ex-Catholics, built a five-million-dollar mosque.

South Africa's contracepting whites are no longer replacing themselves, having barely two children per completed family; the blacks average five, the "Coloreds" 3.29, and the Asiatics 2.7. For the whites, the handwriting is on the wall!

In 1975 the government passed a very tight abortion law and legalized sterilization. These, of course, were aimed at the blacks, who mostly shunned them, while the whites use them. The regime has proposed that 200,000 people be sterilized annually.

When the government reported 600 legal abortions last year, Planned Parenthood lied (as usual) by claiming there were 200,000 "backstreet abortions" per year. Despite international and PP pressures, the government recently opposed abortion on request—perhaps because of HLI's prolife efforts there, says a prolife leader. However, the government is ominously studying a "population development program."

Preoccupied with apartheid, the bishops have done little to build resistance to the coming slaughter of their nation's babies. Five years after *Humanae Vitae*, they issued an incredible dissenting statement. The current president of the South African Catholic hierarchy, Durban's

Archbishop Denis Hurley, has publicly contradicted the Pope on contraception.

HLI Reports recently published his ludicrous remarks excusing the pro-abortion record of Senator Ted Kennedy, who visited South Africa in search of black American votes. More recently, Hurley sponsored a talk on human rights by a politician who had called for abortion on demand in parliament!

The bishops operate a Committee to End Conscription, because they say the army only props up a thoroughly evil government. Angry Catholics complain that the bishops have appointed virtually no chaplains in the armed services to care for Catholics. The same bishops have yet to promulgate Rome's decree permitting the Latin Tridentine Mass. Liturgical abuses seem to be fewer than in the USA, though, and group confession is rare.

Thinking Catholic people keep asking the bishops why the RSA cannot defend itself better against the frequent incursions of the Communists.

The RSA, despite its sins, must be the most lied-about country on earth. The international liberal media report only the bad, never the good things the government does. No one can justify the evil of apartheid, but only naive leftists, and too many bishops, think you can get rid of it overnight without the bloody chaos that now reigns in Angola, Zimbabwe and Mozambique. Those dominoes near South Africa are now in Communist hands, while Marxist terrorists ravage neighboring Botswana and Southwest Africa (Namibia).

In Angola 30,000 raping Cuban troops have dismantled virtually all factories and shipped them to Cuba, at the same time destroying Catholic churches and schools. Angola, once a food exporter, is now starving. In Zimbabwe, Robert Mugabe's North Korean-backed stormtroopers are massacring the nation into a one-party state. And strategic Mozambique is ruled by East European Communist "advisors," giving the Soviets ominous control over the supertankers that bring the West's oil from the Persian Gulf around the Cape of Good Hope.

The countries of southern Africa have a land area the size of continental USA, with one-third of the population. The region is a treasure house of minerals essential to Western defense and industry.

The once-flourishing Catholic Church is persecuted severely, especially in Mozambique and Angola. You do

not hear facts such as these from American media,
though— not even from the Catholic press.

The West has only the Republic of South Africa to
prevent a Communist takeover of this immensely rich and
strategically located bottom third of Africa. It is said that
the South African military is so professional and so well
armed (probably with atomic weapons) that they could be
in Cairo within 10 days.

Meanwhile, the government is educating the blacks as
fast as possible with special educational programs on TV.
It has brought the "Coloreds" and Asiatics into a three-tier
parliament, has desegregated trains, is starting special
literacy programs, is improving already fairly good health
services, etc.—but it feels it can move only so fast with 20
percent of the people illiterate.

Some Catholic lay leaders say the present government
is doing more for the blacks than the "one issue" bishops
who rave against racism constantly while saying nothing
about what is destroying the nation inwardly—lust, contraception-sterilization-abortion, no-fault divorce, and now
pornography. The prelates teach little about chastity, NFP
and respect for all life.

In light of the unique situation in South Africa, Reagan's policy of "creative engagement" seems sensible. The
Communist strategy in the developing countries is the
same everywhere: destabilize and destroy colonial (and
post-colonial) governments before native populations are
ready for self-government. The white populations of South
Africa's Marxist neighbors could escape across the nearest
borders, including the RSA's. But the South Africans have
nowhere to go, They will stay and fight, hoping that
Washington, London and the UN will not make another
Zimbabwe or Nicaragua out of their country.

I stayed five days with the tireless and intelligent Dr.
Claude and Glenys Newbury, who between them gave 153
prolife talks last year! I know no doctor and wife in the
whole world who fight the antilifers more effectively, more
wisely. They are not afraid to stand up to the abortionists
and talk to them about God and morality.

Along with the American Life Lobby, HLI sponsored
the sixth Protect Life in All Nations (PLAN) conference in
Nairobi, July 5-8. More than 100 leaders from 13 countries took part. The goal was to unite Africa against the
antilife monster invading that continent from the dying,
pagan West.

It was a delight to see so many missionary nuns and doctors and priests with whom we had communicated for years. I passed out 17 films, plus a ton of the best literature.

A black African bishop spoke eloquently against contraception-sterilization-abortion, adding that God commanded us to increase and multiply and to subdue the earth, but that we had not subdued it, since obviously there is plenty for everybody. When he finished, an Austrian got up and invited him to teach the European bishops! In the developing world, the bishops are loyal to the Holy See, and it makes a huge difference.

The site for this conference could not have been better chosen, because the notorious 10-day women's conference sponsored by the UN followed. We briefed the Kenyans on what to do at this meeting and how to do it. Kenyans have the highest birthrate in the world: seven children! Can you see why the UN has its antilife meetings here?

Both minor and major seminaries in Kenya are filled to overflowing. The hardest working, most apostolic, most loyal priests and nuns and bishops in the world are those from the mission countries of the developing world. With the West dying out, the future of the Catholic Church can only be here—as I keep telling anyone who will listen.

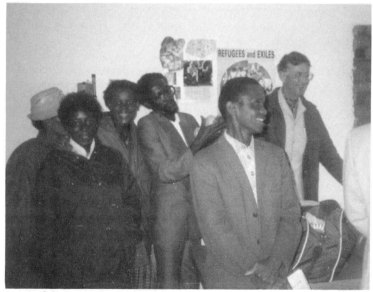

A prolife meeting in Soweto.

CHURCH FLOURISHES IN AFRICA

(No. 16—October 1985)

This continent is the world's second largest, but it is rather empty, having fewer than 500 million people in 52 nations. But Africa has the highest birthrate in the world, an unparalleled three percent-plus—growing five times as fast as Europe and North America, twice as fast as the world overall, and doubling every 20 years.

Despite surging Islamic fundamentalism, the Church is truly flourishing; every seminary and novitiate is filled to overflowing. The black continent boasts more than two million baptisms and more than a million converts each year.

In 1901 Africa was one percent Catholic; in 1951, 7.5 percent; today, 13 percent—more than 65 million. By the year 2000, Africa will have 100 million Catholics. There will be more Catholics in Africa and Latin America than in Europe and North America. From every indication, Africa in the 21st century will be the most vigorous segment of the Catholic Church. Catholics in Europe and North America dwindle by 7,200 every day, whereas African Catholics increase by 16,400.

The African religious climate is most favorable for Catholicism. Unlike Latin America, there is no "liberation theology" and much less competition from other churches.

KENYA: BISHOPS vs. POPULATION CONTROLLERS

This one-party "democracy" has 20 million people in 245,000 square miles. The average family size is more than seven children, amounting to a 4.1 percent annual population increase, the world's highest.

Kenya has five million Catholics, 2.5 million Anglicans, at least that many Moslems, and a sprinkling of Protestant communities, with Seventh-Day Adventists and Presbyterians predominating. She also has many native religions.

Proof of Catholicism's vigor are the five major seminaries with almost 1,000 seminarians, the numerous minor seminaries, the burgeoning novitiates, and the Catholic schools, hospitals and dispensaries.

Every developed nation and international company with an interest in Africa has an office or laboratory in Nairobi. Here, too, are the African headquarters of the sex-pushing International Planned Parenthood Federation (IPPF). And here is every major population control group, including the Kenyan Family Planning Association (KFPA), the Pathfinder Fund (PF), the New York-based Family Planning International Assistance (FPIA), the World Bank, the American Association for Voluntary Sterilization (AVS), and others.

Most of them are fueled by millions of dollars from the United Nations Fund for Population Activities (UNFPA), the U.S. Agency for International Development (USAID), the Population Council, the Ford Foundation, and other American foundations. The family-destroyers have targeted Kenya as the model, the guinea pig, for African population control.

It would take too long to describe the satanic infiltration, the countless seminars and devious "population development" campaigns, financed mostly by U.S. taxes through USAID. This is the worst form of colonialism; it is infecting Kenya with a contraception-sterilization-abortion culture that is destroying the healthy sexual taboos and restraints which until recently held the line against VD, divorce, prostitution and all the other evils that stem from uncontrolled sex.

Abortion is still illegal, but it is widely committed, in secret and without punishment. Sterilization is rampant and is often inflicted without informed consent. Service clubs such as the Lions Club sponsor sterilization camps that reportedly do 900 operations a week.

In Nairobi (as well as in Baltimore) Johns Hopkins Medical School has trained Kenyan doctors in the latest methods of sterilization since the early 1970s. They have also taught midwives and nurses to fit abortifacient IUDs. Bad effects are overlooked; anything to bring down the population! Because "sterilization" has a bad ring, they call it "surgical contraception."

Once I visited, as if I were a sympathizer, IPPF's immense African headquarters. Twice I went *incognito* to a base clinic and learned that Pills are given freely to incoming teens and a packet of 30 condoms to every teenage boy. IUDs are fitted by specially trained nurses. Depo-Provera (or the German Depo-Clinovir), a potion too dangerous for American women, is injected freely into Kenyan women, as evidenced by the many Upjohn containers.

Thank God, the Kenyan Catholic bishops have fought magnificently against this antilife onslaught. Nairobi's Maurice Cardinal Otunga, a convert who comes from a large polygamous family himself, has been known to preach for two hours on *Humanae Vitae* at Holy Family Cathedral. The bishops have issued several good statements and have totally confronted the government.

In Nyayo National Stadium I was delighted to hear the Pope condemn contraception and abortion in the near presence of President Moi, KFPA's patron! (I thought of the American bishops, most of whom are afraid to do likewise in their cathedrals.) Proclaimed the Pope, "Antilife actions such as contraception and abortion are wrong and unworthy of good husbands and wives."

(Cardinal Bernardin was there, too. What did he think when he heard this, having sacked a good priest from the Chicago Archdiocesan Pro-Life Office because he sponsored a Mass and Holy Hour of reparation for the sin of contraception? Such liturgies, wrote the Cardinal, were "too negative and too narrowly focused.")

The Kenyan bishops are the first hierarchy in the world to have warned their people about the abortifacient nature of the Pill and IUD. (A decade ago I wrote to *all* the bishops in North America begging them to do so; I received five polite replies and two pertinent ones.)

With 300 trained teachers, the bishops are fast promoting NFP and marriage preparation courses. When KFPA got eight weeks of training in contraception-sterilization put into the curriculum for the public health nurses, the Catholics were able to substitute NFP for any objectors.

Although 55 percent of Kenya's land is semi-arid like California, 18 percent is arable, but only a fraction of that (17 percent) is actually farmed. An expert missionary priest-farmer told me that a five-mile strip along 210-mile Lake Victoria could be irrigated and farmed to feed the whole of East Africa. Instead, the money goes to murder babies, poison wombs, spread VD and destroy family life.

I spent nine days in Kisii, a unique area of 40 by 50 miles with the highest rural birthrate in the world. One of Africa's great missionaries works here, Fr. John Kaiser, a Mill Hill Father and former student of mine, who has built 22 churches and even more schools.

He has baptized more than 15,000 people in 21 years—including more than 500 adults since January! In his *parish* of 35,000 souls, there are 44 Catholic grade schools, 18 mission stations (one of them serving 8,000-9,000 people), 10 Catholic high schools, including two boarding schools, one dispensary and maternity hospital, and a polytechnic school! All of this is run by one priest, a deacon, a religious brother, five native nuns, and a small flock of lay catechists, who are the backbone of African Catholicism.

In Kisii they raise an average of eight children on two acres with an average income of $400 a year! I have never seen more babies and teenagers in my life. I have never seen them better behaved, either. In fact, you rarely hear a baby cry in Africa. I saw five homemade toys in seven weeks. The real toy is often a little brother or sister on the back.

In the diocese of Kisii there are 30 parishes (with many mission stations and schools), 500,000 Catholics, 50 priests, some 200 native nuns, 52 seminarians and a large number of catechists. The bishop is desperately looking for money while building the only Catholic teacher-training college in the nation. "Only in this way can we save our young," he said. "Government-trained teachers lead the youth astray with contraception and sex education." In his city a huge sterilization center was being built. Foreign money has paid for 10 sterilization "theaters," easily converted into abortion centers.

Meanwhile, living in thatched or tinned huts, these gracious and humble people love their children. They live mainly on a mush of maize and beans boiled with hot water, with a little meat now and then, and some milk. Visiting, speaking, eating and praying with them was an experience I shall never forget; it was the best retreat I ever made. Two NFP teachers—one a nun and former student of mine, Sister Mary Pauline—roam the diocese to teach NFP. Throughout Africa, women, who do 60-70 percent of the out-of-hut work, suffer horribly from rape, polygamy, prostitution and drunken husbands.

I had a great talk over dinner with the bishop of Kisii, the Most Rev. Tiberius Mugendi, who put it all in a nutshell: "Because we are poor and so helpless to fight back, the population czars lord it over us, ruining our families and youth."

NIGERIA: CATHOLICS FIGHT ANTILIFERS

This oil-rich nation is about 10 percent Catholic and 30 percent Moslem. No Catholics in Africa are better educated than Nigeria's Ibos, whose native priests took over when 300 mostly-Irish Holy Ghost Fathers were kicked out by the government in the 1970s. These Catholic Ibos wield an enormous influence in public life.

One of Nigeria's seminaries is the largest in the world, with more than 1,000 seminarians! The Nigerian bishops recently founded the National Missionary Seminary of St. Paul to produce missionaries for the whole world. Like the Kenyan bishops, the Nigerian hierarchy is very orthodox and loyal to the Holy See. They have done much to promote NFP, with our friend Sister Leonie McSweeney, a medical missionary/authoress, leading the way. Unlike the bishops of the West, Nigeria's prelates have condemned contraception and sterilization strongly.

I found that the African bishops understand very well how contraception is the gateway to abortion and many other abuses, and how it is destroying the family and Church in the West. The population controllers (mostly through PP) are deeply entrenched in Nigeria, though; they virtually run the health and education departments with much foreign money. PP has been accused of giving a Mercedes-Benz to a powerful Catholic government official to win him over to its way of thinking, the deathstyle of the sex-obsessed West.

The 100 million Nigerians are the sleeping giant of Africa: one of four Africans belongs to the powerful nation. I promised many films and much literature.

AT THE U.N. WOMEN'S CONFERENCE IN NAIROBI

Almost 13,000 women delegates swarmed into Nairobi and buzzed for two weeks. Pseudo-feminism, every kind of immoral birth control, manic and artificial equality with men, and every other aberration and perversion were hawked. It was really an international anti-American, anti-Israel and antilife/anti-family propaganda meeting— with a typical PP agenda. Woe to the world if these home- and children-hating women have their way!

Attending were every noted population-controller and every type of secular feminist, from Betty Friedan speaking from under a tree (someone said at least she got down from it) to Simone Weil, who as health minister masterminded abortion liberalization in France. President Reagan's pro-abortion daughter Maureen led the U.S. delegation, which contained not one prolifer. The Canadian government, excluding all prolifers as being anti-women, paid some $350,000 to send a delegation of 40 antilifers who stayed at the most expensive Hilton Hotel.

As the eminent English Catholic convert Valerie Riches observed, "Today we do not live in democracies; we are ever so subtly manipulated." She infiltrated the meeting, as did other prolifers such as the articulate Gabrielle Avery of Oregon, Babette Francis of Australia, ALL's Jim Deger, Sara Brown (the head of HLI's branch in Scotland), India's Dr. Mascarenhas, Eileen Moran of New Zealand, Ireland's Bill Sherwin, and yours truly. We annoyed the antilifers with prolife/family literature (although we had too little), and especially with well-written news releases, which were published surprisingly often.

To make a good impression, the Kenyan government took all the prostitutes, beggars, vendors and poor off the streets and into the jails during the UN meeting and the following Eucharistic Congress. As usual, of course, the pacifists and Communists had a field day propagandizing, especially against the USA and Israel, the bogeymen at these international meetings, which always swarm with Reds.

I destroyed PP literature and placed prolife literature in key locations at the UN meeting. I was overwhelmed by the lies, distortions, deception and wickedness—all tools of the Father of Lies. The best thing Maureen Reagan did was tell her father there should be no more such meetings. The Soviets promoted the idea of having another in five years.

AT THE EUCHARISTIC CONGRESS

This 43rd International Eucharistic Congress was the first held in Africa below the Sahara, in Nairobi, a city of well over one million. Whereas the UN women's conference drew some 13,000 from foreign countries, the Pope once more showed the world that he is the greatest drawing card of all, with more than 200,000 attending a public Mass he offered.

In connection with the Congress, I addressed the priests of the archdiocese of Nairobi for two hours, speaking about the worldwide antilife movement and how to counter it.

At the exhibit hall of the Congress, Bill Sherwin showed our films in two halls, always crowded. People kept coming to the very end. We also gave out huge amounts of prolife/pro-family literature that we shipped over in advance. As a secular newspaper complained, "Prolifers had a field day at the Congress."

In his sermon on peace, Cardinal Bernardin of seamless-garment/crazy-quilt fame never mentioned the greatest war of all time, the war on the unborn! But what would you expect from a Cardinal who does nothing about pornographer Fr. Andrew Greeley, who allows dancing platforms to be built in several Chicago churches, and who permits a Sunday Mass for active homosexuals promoted by Dignity and the *Chicago Catholic*? Maybe there will be a Mass for fornicators next.

TANZANIA: TARGET OF THE BABY-HATERS

Freed from Britain in 1961, this immense country of 365,900 square miles is resource-rich but severely undeveloped. It has a fast-growing population of 21 million people, the most literate in black Africa.

Tanzania has 27 dioceses with six million Catholics, three major seminaries, more than 250 seminarians, many minor seminaries, 30,000 mostly native nuns, 800 native priests and 600 missionary priests. Among the 2.3 million Protestants, the Anglicans and Lutherans predominate. There are two huge Swiss-German Benedictine mission abbeys in Ndanla and Peramiho. Each has a large printing plant and many schools on campus, including trade schools. They do magnificent work.

During my two-week stay the bishops met. They saw my four abortion films and were shocked. Mainland Tanzania has no TV ("Thank God," said a nun-superior). So cut off is Tanzania that not one bishop had heard of *The Silent Scream*. They asked me to send them as much literature and as many films as I possibly could to educate their people.

There is no talk about legalizing abortion yet, but it is committed in secret by doctors (Cuban, Soviet, Chinese, etc.), midwives and quacks. Then there are the many amateur abortions one finds in all the developing nations, induced by herbs, medicines and gadgetry. Premarital sex, sterilization and abortion seem to be exploding throughout Africa, thanks to the antilife invasion from the West.

The UNFPA has targeted Tanzania as a priority country for population control. The many governmental "Mother and Child Clinics" are strategically in place. Each has two PP counselors handing out contraceptives and abortifacients, including the deadly Depo-Provera. I visited one of these with a prolife Indian doctor; we examined abortifacient Pills and IUDs from many developed countries. As two nurses described the sordid operation for us, he seemed as appalled as I. To see the great number of mothers and babies treated so inhumanly reminded me of the poet's lament, "There are sorrows too deep for tears."

The average Tanzanian family has 6.5 children. The country has gone backward under Socialism. It once exported food, but today the people are poor and malnourished.

In Tanzania the Catholic Church is flourishing and vocations are many. For example, one native religious order that began in 1968 already boasts 39 professed sisters, 19 novices and many postulants! Parishes, some with 40,000 souls, have an average of 15 mission centers where Mass is offered as often as possible.

Two abbots told me that the old social system and moral restraints are breaking down. Asked what the solution might be to excessive population growth and related problems, I responded, "Socio-economic development, the end of polygamy which Christianity alone can achieve morally, later marriage, resistance to PP's fornication 'education,' and serious preparation for marriage-with-NFP."

The great task is to save the family. "But how?" an abbot asked me despairingly. Fornication begins early; VD is rife. One doctor told me he knew of 43 deaths from AIDS. Abortion is increasing. Two Swiss missionary nuns in charge of a large dispensary told me that in some hospitals 30 percent of the beds are occupied by illegally aborted women. A high percentage of their 250 outpatients per day were VD victims.

I spoke at length with a German farm couple who had tried over four years to teach the natives to farm. They told me, "Tanzania could be a paradise if it were developed and if people were educated." I spoke to a farmer-scholar-scientist monk who developed sun hemp, a burgeoning new plant with a great potential as a cash crop. It also has good possibilities for stopping the cornborer. When I asked him how many people Tanzania could support if properly developed, he pointed to several valleys that could feed the whole country.

When it comes to prolife literature and audiovisual aids, the Tanzanians have NOTHING. I promised the bishops and other leaders much, leaving four films and fetal development models at the great Benedictine mission abbey of Peramiho.

I have learned profound new respect for the missions. How thrilling to see so many Catholic hospitals, dispensaries, mission schools (usually the best), selfless native religious, and weather-beaten missionaries! The Catholic Church is truly the greatest promoter of physical and mental health in the world, and the Number One defender of women, children and the family. Today the chief causes of women's deaths are all of the hideous varieties of birth control, to say nothing of the many forms of VD that result from the irresponsible sex explosion. The Church alone has the solution.

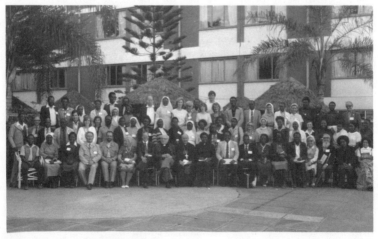

Prolifers meet in Nairobi.

THE KILLER PILLS

(No. 17—November 1985)

In September I invaded Europe again for two weeks to (1) nail down scientific proof that *all* current "birth control" Pills abort at some time, (2) prove that aborted babies are being used to make cosmetics and for other purposes, (3) attend the Eleventh World Congress of OB-GYN in Berlin and, above all, the subsequent two-day secret meeting of the doctor-population-controllers, and (4) lay plans for a requested new HLI branch headquarters, now being set up in Utrecht, Holland, for continental Europe.

HOW THE PILLS KILL

Ann Landers, who has 60 million readers, recently denied flatly that the Pill aborts and that aborted babies are used commercially. She is dead wrong on both counts.

All current Pills abort *at some time*. Current medical literature, documents of Pill companies and scientists, written responses from Pill executives to specific questions, and even the testimony of the Pill's inventors leave no doubt about it. In the 1950s, Planned Parenthood's medical people admitted that even the old high-dose Pills sometimes aborted.

Of course, we are talking about the so-called first generation of Pills that created the first revolution in "birth control." Now comes the second generation or revolution: the first "foolproof" abortion Pill, the French RU486 Pill—already approved by the UN's World Health Organization to kill babies in the Third World and reportedly used widely in Red China.

This satanic potion is in a late stage of development. In San Diego, American women are being paid $1,200 to act as guinea pigs. This and similar Pills (researched by the Population Council and soon to come from Upjohn) are taken for only four days, when a woman usually menstruates. If she is pregnant, she aborts; if not, she merely sheds. The new Pill is most effective in the first seven weeks of gestation, but it can also be used to kill older babies. This is home or bathroom abortion, soon to descend on us!

Stockholm's infamous Karolinska Institute has produced abortive vaginal suppositories to kill babies after pregnancy is confirmed; they are already in use in Germany.

Very recently Schering of Berlin, the first company to produce "birth control" Pills in Europe, and which today sells one-fourth of all Pills worldwide, announced a new "Morning-after Pill." The Morning-after Pill, which PP has been touting and which is used widely by college students, amounts to taking several traditional Pills within 48 hours to kill a possible new life.

Mothers also use the IUD in these circumstances; PP calls this "post-coital contraception." The IUD has been known to be abortifacient for decades. It also causes a great deal of infection, sterility and life-threatening tubal pregnancy. (Remember the Dalkon Shield and the thousands of lawsuits against its producer, A.H. Robins?) The whole struggle in the British Parliament over legalizing fetal experimentation in the first 15 days of pregnancy turns on finding an early chemical means of abortion.

Did you know that in 1965 the American College of Obstetricians and Gynecologists arbitrarily declared that pregnancy begins with the completion of implantation, about 14 days (!) after conception? They redefined conception to justify current and future Pills as well as the IUD, which PP also calls "intrauterine contraception." Medical societies in other countries followed suit.

What a fool Pope Paul VI would be today had he approved of the Pill in *Humanae Vitae*! And what excuse have the bishops, priests, ministers and rabbis who give their blessings to these *billions* of mini-murders?

THE ABUSE OF ABORTED BABIES

I have no doubt that aborted babies are being used for cosmetics and other industrial and medical purposes, as well as for Mengele-style experiments. A member of the parliament of Hesse in Germany, Roland Rösler, has investigated these horrors relentlessly, with some success.

Recently the Viennese papers published a flurry of articles on fetal abuses, to the embarrassment of the abortuaries, the companies and the middlemen involved—and not least the government, which admitted loopholes in the law and shamefacedly promised their closure. A large specialty store in Meckenheim advertises fetal parts in its catalog. In *Les Trafiquants de Bébés à Naître*, now translated into German, a French jurist and a well-known journalist tell a grisly tale of fetal use for cosmetics, particularly in France and Germany.

As early as the middle 1970s, four medical centers in England experimented with aborted babies, some still alive. In 1974 the great English gynecologist Dr. Ian Donald, who "invented" ultrasound, told me of witnessing modern experiments at Sweden's Karolinska Institute on large, living aborted babies, cringing with pain. (Why not use them, if abortion removes only "the products of conception" or "a meaningless clump of cells"?)

The whole subject is bedeviled by the legitimate use of the human placenta or afterbirth, the secrecy and word-games of godless researchers (often funded by your tax money), and theologians such as Jesuit Richard McCormick and Catholic (?) University's Fr. Charles E. Curran, who justified fetal experimentation at a government hearing.

Another confusing point is that collagen, a substance used in cosmetics, can also come from animals. The cosmetic industry's headquarters here in Washington insists that no human collagen is used in this country. The Food and Drug Administration assures us it knows of no abuse in the USA and asked us to report our findings to it.

THE NIGHTMARISH OB-GYN WORLD CONGRESS

More than 5,000 specialists from 92 countries attended this conference, which was like six days in hell. The bastardization of gynecological medicine by antilifers is fearsome! Legalize abortion, and the killers soon take over the professorships in medical schools, plus high positions in the media, medical societies and publishing houses, while pushing prolifers out. At this meeting abortion was openly embraced for "the health care of the mother." No questions were allowed. No prolife statements were made. Not a peep was heard about NFP.

"Ethics do not stand still—they have to move with technology," intoned test-tube-baby pioneer Dr. Robert Edwards. "I have no question in my mind that we must have a freezing program for embryos," he stated, "because we take all the egg cells available, attempt to fertilize them all and only replace three; it is unethical to replace everything." "Some clinics," he revealed, "have put back all that were collected—as many as 16—and that to me is unethical. The policy, therefore, should be to replace the minimum needed, freeze the others, and use the abnormal ones for research. [N.B., Fr. Charles E. Curran] The current risk of multiple pregnancy from IVF [*in vitro* fertilization] is 30 percent, and that is very high." Edwards concluded, "I cannot accept the 'absolutist' view of the beginning of life. I am a 'gradualist'—the rights of the embryo mature as it grows." He emphasized the need for scientists to "educate" the public on the issue.

The assembled gynecologists moaned that teens have 30 percent of all births in the USA and 55 percent in Malawi. They deplored the epidemic of herpes, new forms and strains of VD in both sexes, the potentially explosive AIDS, and increasing tumors and cancers in women (especially cervical cancer in teens, caused by early intercourse with multiple partners). But they had only more "sex education" plus abortifacient Pills, IUDs, injectables, implants and "post-coital and menses-inducing drugs" (read: early abortion-murder) to offer!

The president of the gynecologists, an Egyptian, reported his investigation of "birth control" in Red China: "The most common form of contraception there is also the most drastic—sterilization (50 percent) followed by the IUD (40 percent)." He said nothing about the estimated 30,000 babies aborted in China every working day.

In 62 sessions devoted to the reproductive system and "birth control," the future methods were described, including: long-acting vaginal rings, new injectables and implants feeding steroids into the female system, new IUDs, anti-pregnancy vaccines, female immunization against sperm, "safe, simple, early non-surgical abortion," but above all, simpler forms of "surgical contraception."

Twenty-five million Chinese women use IUDs. The Chinese sterilize women by putting chemicals or pellets into their fallopian tubes, it was revealed. Soon there will be 100 million sterilized women in the world (there are 15 million in the USA already). Sterilization was proclaimed as the wave of the future. For this, one professor recommended "medical mobile flying squads" for the developing countries.

The exhibits told the story even more eloquently: an overwhelming number dealt with new low-dose, "acne-removing," "skin-friendly" birth control Pills. A forest of new and old IUDs hung all about. But what struck me most was the number of medications to stop female infections and to cure infertility problems which the medical profession itself had directly caused. First doctors ruin women's fertility and then they seek to restore it by giving women more pills. Today one of eight marriages in the West is infertile, owing to natural or intentional causes.

I asked several people behind display counters how their Pills work. (I nearly always find them uninformed; they are only there to sell.) The naive ones discuss neatly the threefold action of the Pill, thus unwittingly admitting its inherent abortifacient character. Some, more clever, suspect what I am driving at and become devious.

Of course, these money-grabbing sex engineers, these all-knowing doctors and medical professors, have the solution to the "overpopulation" problem, which they are happy to solve while lining their dirty pockets. In the conference's major reports the contradictory and inconsistent figures given did not bother anyone. The real solutions were never addressed. When medicine loses its ethic, doctors become morals-free biological mechanics.

But the two-day "Christopher Tietze International Symposium on the Prevention and Treatment of Contraceptive Failure" which followed took the cake. It was sponsored by groups such as PP's Alan Guttmacher Institute, the International Women's Health Coalition, the International Planned Parenthood Federation, the Rockefeller Population Council (with which Tietze was affiliated), and the UN's dubious World Health Organization, virtually all fueled at least in part by U.S. taxes.

I had paid my conference registration fee early. Months later, not wanting me, the organizers returned my money (with interest!). So I went there as a fully credentialed journalist instead. I was stopped at the door; it was a private meeting, they explained. "But on a public subject, with tax money?" I asked. "A tax-paying citizen and the public have a right to know how their money is spent." Pause—consultation—consternation! I tried to get through the door, but did not make it. They threatened to call the police. That seems to happen everywhere I go.

Trying to persuade me to go away peacefully was one of the Gamble boys of Pathfinder Fund fame. They have spent millions of Procter and Gamble's profits and tax-exempt foundation funds, and received $11 million this year from USAID to spread contraceptives, abortifacients and injectables to kill babies and ruin family life in the Third World.

Lecturing at this meeting were the absolute worst of the medical population controllers: Drs. Lippes, Stubblefield, Rosenfeld, Sai and others, financed by PP and your tax money. The topics: contraceptives for all; remedies for failed contraception ("menstrual extraction," Morning-after Pills, injectables such as Depo-Provera for the poor, and induced abortion); the latest in abortion technology; cost of and access to abortion; training "motivators" to find "acceptors"; freeing women from the yoke of childbearing; and so on. Holding forth on the glories of abortion was the president of the world congress, who is from Moslem Egypt, where abortion is forbidden.

Always remember, the only way the population-controller-imperialists can destroy the birthrates and families of the poor is by *force*—and they are using it in all manner of subtle ways in the Third World, as I observed again during seven weeks in Africa last summer.

Ironically, the memorialized Christopher Tietze (whose favored dress at international meetings was a black turtleneck sweater with the sex symbols on a neck chain) was never enthusiastic about the abortifacient Pills and IUDs. Until something better came along, he said frequently, the best means of birth control was the condom with backup abortion. Against people such as these, most bishops, priests and intellectuals have little to say—if they even know what's going on.

PROLIFE NEWS FROM WEST GERMANY

This talented nation of 60 million is in serious trouble. Germany has the lowest birthrate in the world today, an unbelievable one child per family (1.2 counting the children of the foreigners). Needed for national survival: 2.2.

It has been proven that only one of every 10 German abortions is reported; there may be 500,000 surgical abortions annually. Last year the Germans had 113,000 more coffins than cradles. Because of "die anti-Baby-Pille" and "das Anti-Baby-Kondom," the nation will be 117,000 soldiers short of its quota for NATO in 1986! The lavish family allowances and tax deductions for children which will start next January will not solve the problem. Meanwhile, so many "guest workers" have come to Germany that West Berlin is now the world's largest Moslem city after Istanbul!

In 1974 the godless Socialists legalized abortion for any reason in the first three months of pregnancy. In 1975 the German Supreme Court declared the law unconstitutional but decreed, in a devilishly deceptive document, that abortions could be committed for certain "indications," and even suggested some. (This document has become the model for other countries.)

In 1976 the Socialist government, using all the talent Germans have for deceptive obfuscation and convoluted language, passed an "indications" law leaving the way virtually wide open for abortion on demand from implantation to birth pangs. The Socialists deliberately accepted the gynecologists' false and arbitrary decree that life begins at implantation so they could allow the abortifacient Pills, IUDs, Morning-after Pill, PP's "post-coital contraception," and the future abortion Pill for home abortions.

Moral theologians and episcopal advisors such as Frs. F. Böckle and J. Gründel and Catholic law professors such as Albin Eser never informed the bishops about the law's implications. Before a doctor may kill her baby, the pregnant woman must be officially counseled by a social worker and a doctor, but *nondirectively*; the decision is *always* left to her. Once counseled, and with proof of counseling in hand, she may go to an abortionist and have her child killed at the taxpayers' expense, whether there is an "indication" or not!

Much of this outrageous so-called counseling, which amounts to direct collaboration with abortion, takes place at counseling centers run by the badly advised bishops. Thus they unwittingly collaborate with the abortionists, while receiving millions of deutschemarks for their counseling centers. Ninety percent of the "counseling" is done by money-making PP, known in Germany as "Pro Familia"; their abortion mills are very busy.

Before anyone blames the bishops, let me say that the German Supreme Court commentary on the Socialists' law was so devilishly subtle that two prolife American law professors, Robert E. Jones and John D. Gorby, wrote a rather favorable (although very erroneous) critique of the German decision in the *John Marshall Journal of Practice and Procedure*. It was distributed widely by Americans United for Life!

Meanwhile, the German equivalent of our Bishops' Committee for Pro-Life Activities, *Wahle das Leben* (founded in 1982), has embraced the seamy (er, seamless) garment concept with a vengeance. Rather than work to remove the whole abortion-on-demand law, they, like their American counterparts, maintain that we should strive only to lessen its effects and to be positive in offering help.

They recommend a "consistent life ethic" of reducing deaths on the highway, environmental protection, justice issues, war and peace concerns, "und etwa Abtreibung" ("and perhaps abortion").

By using utilitarian consequentialism (Guterabwagung)—a cross between situation ethics and pragmatism—prominent German moral theologians and some bureaucrats in the national bishops' conference have at one time or another justified masturbation, contraception, sterilization, homosexuality, test-tube-baby production as long as it involves husband and wife, abortion under certain circumstances, and euthanasia.

However, the German bishops *have* awakened to reality and now know they have been deceived. Josef Cardinal Höffner, President of the German Catholic Conference, immediately condemned Schering's new Morning-after Pill. He stated on TV that the German *Königstein Erklarung* (dissent from *Humanae Vitae*) is not the last word, and that the whole abortion law must go—as well as the Church's scandalous participation in abortion-facilitating counseling centers. He also condemned eloquently the theology of liberation (hatched in Germany, largely by Karl Rahner), the idea of women priests, and euthanasia. Other bishops, too, have spoken out strongly against the antilife evils.

What will the German bishops say when they finally learn that all Pills abort at some time? A few years ago the humble Höffner also commented that, when it came to NFP, Germany is an "underdeveloped country." This year the German government has made available three million DM for research and the promotion of NFP. The great Austrian authority on NFP, Dr. Josef Rötzer, is totally occupied teaching NFP with other good people in the dying German-speaking countries.

Strangely, the German bishops have left open the whole question of the morality of the test-tube-baby process when it involves husband and wife, even though the Church condemns it as "immoral and absolutely illicit." Like the 12 other hierarchies that dissented from *Humanae Vitae*, they are in a difficult position. If one may morally separate the unitive from the procreative aspects of the marital act as *Humanae Vitae* said one may not, then one objection to test-tube-baby production for husband and wife falls away. No doubt this is why—contrary to the directives of the Holy See—the Austrian bishops have pronounced *in vitro* fertilization and embryo transfer morally right for the married.

Friedrich Cardinal Wetter of Munich, speaking for the German bishops, seems to have no idea that every successful test-tube-baby operation involves masturbation, some 90 abortions (N.B., Fr. Richard McCormick), and other inherent evils.

Meanwhile, the potential plague of AIDS has hit Germany with 272 confirmed cases. The half-dozen school children with the disease are segregated. Government health and other agencies are recommending the condom frantically as protection against AIDS. In August, condom sales increased by one-third; they are expected to double by the end of the year. In a Germany and Europe where syphilis reigns, chastity is little practiced and rarely preached.

The theology of liberation is invading the seminaries, while strange theologians indoctrinate ever more nuns in ever more seminars. The first volume of the much-revised new *German Catechism for Adults* contains its share of subtle ambiguities for intellectuals to exploit, especially in the area of theological anthropology. Still, the catechism must have considerable merit, because the once-Catholic theologian Fr. Hans Küng attacked it immediately. The second volume, dealing with morality, is awaited with trepidation by orthodox Catholics.

HOLLAND: PLUSSES AND MINUSES

In this country of many abortions and staggering loss of faith, I was privileged to have an interview with the young Primate of Holland, Adrianus Cardinal Simonis of Utrecht. The subject was our plan to establish a new European branch of HLI there.

To the consternation of the leftists, Pope Paul VI handpicked the openly prolife Fr. Simonis to be the archbishop of Rotterdam when the latter was a 39-year-old parish assistant. Speaking in German, the pleasant Cardinal immediately agreed with my idea of a new European branch, but he said he knew of only one Dutch doctor willing to fight abortion—alas, our board advisor, Presbyterian Dr. Karl Gunning. What a contrast with the Holland of only 45 years ago, when not a single Dutch doctor would cooperate with the Nazi euthanasia program!

Holland once produced even more missionaries than Ireland and had four Catholic daily newspapers. But

Holland today has fallen deeply into "arrogant paganism and needs fundamental evangelization," the Cardinal warned. He bemoaned his lack of a seminary. (There is only one in Holland.) When told the Pill is an abortifacient, the Cardinal volunteered that the Dutch are concerned only with the health aspects of the Pill.

The 15 million Dutch commit more than 100,000 abortions annually, and there is much "abortion tourism." They also commit active euthanasia, i.e., direct killing of patients, permitted by an appalling Supreme Court decision. The subject is discussed widely; the Socialists are for it and so are the unchristian and undemocratic Christian Democrats. In a poll, 89 percent of adults saw nothing wrong with it. A pro-euthanasia law is imminent. The old and very ill fear going to a hospital. The Dutch bishops have warned of a "descent into barbarity."

Premarital sex is common in Holland; an estimated 50 percent live in common-law marriages. Informed, orthodox Catholics estimate that perhaps five percent really believe all the essential teachings of the Church. Now that five of seven bishops are loyal to the Holy See, the tide is turning ever so slowly.

MORE PROBLEMS IN IRELAND

Many people ask me about Ireland. The Irish wrote protection of the unborn (from fertilization onward) into their constitution two years ago, by a two-to-one vote in a national referendum. But their birthrate is dropping fast because of increasing contraception and sterilization. It is now down to three children per completed family. Still, it is the only good, reproductive birthrate among the world's developed nations.

Several months ago the government passed a very bad bill on contraception, which can only lead to increasing promiscuity. With government encouragement, sex "education" is attacking the school children. Pornography is increasing. About 4,200 girls a year are referred to England for abortions by PP-types. The media and government are exceedingly antilife, anti-family and anti-Catholic.

Amazingly, but perhaps typically for our age, Fr. Enda McDonagh, a Curran-like dissenting theologian who once taught at Notre Dame, recently organized a seminar on in vitro fertilization at the national seminary of Maynooth. Virtually all lecturers were notorious pro-abortionists, including an American. Abortion doctors have machinated to "produce" three successful test-tube babies. There is a loud clamor for a national referendum to legalize divorce, now forbidden by the constitution. Even so, the Irish have the world's highest weekly church attendance—more than 90 percent.

PRAY FOR BELGIUM

Two prominent prolife leaders came to the Brussels airport to discuss prolife strategy with me. Eighty percent Catholic, this country of nine million and Ireland are the only European countries that have not legalized abortion. All attempts have failed so far, despite several doctors' openly proclaiming they commit abortions, and despite the noisy propaganda of feminists who boast of killing their own babies. Fortunately, NFP has a good foothold in some dioceses.

Belgium has a low, non-replacement birthrate. There are now 400,000 foreigners. Many of them are Moslems, who now have one-fourth of the country's grade school children. In some classes there is not a single child of Belgian-born parents. Two prolife organizations have a combined 30,000 members, among whom are 1,000 rather inactive priests.

One prolife group scheduled a day's seminar in October for Belgium's 5,000 priests, to be addressed by the French Fr. René Bel, the German Fr. Otto Maier and yours truly. As of early October only a handful had signed up, including the prolife bishop of Ghent.

"Don't the priests see what's at stake?" I asked. "Can't they see what's happened in neighboring countries, how Belgium is choking with affluence but dying for lack of children?" The answer: "The government pays the priests a good salary; the eating and living is good. So all must be well. They don't know the problem. There are exceptions, of course."

I told them to write to each bishop and describe what is really at stake, what is happening in neighboring countries, what needs to be done—and beg them to tell every one of their priests to attend. They said they would.

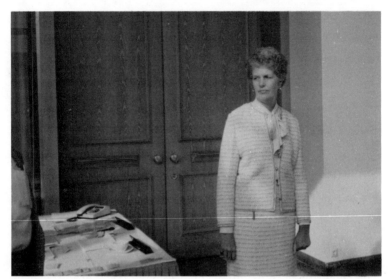

The door to the Tietze conference in East Berlin was guarded.

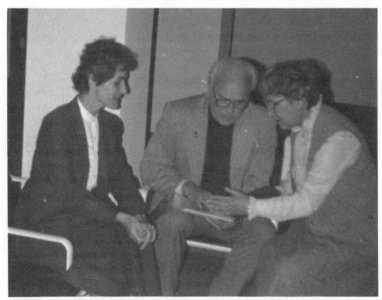

Germany's great activists, Heidi Lebert and Frau Elisabeth Backhaus.

PROLIFE WORK IN BELGIUM

(No. 18—December 1985)

After 10 days in California (where I preached at 10 Masses and addressed two prolife banquets), I flew to Europe to assist Frs. Otto Maier of Germany and René Bel of France with a day-long seminar on abortion in Mechelen, Belgium.

Pro-Vita of Belgium had invited all the bishops and 5,000 priests. Fifty-two priests came, plus some lay people. Much HLI literature was available, and it was appreciated. It always astonishes me how little priests know about NFP and about how contraception-sterilization-abortion is destroying their flocks and the Church. The Pill-happy Belgians (80 percent Catholic) now have fewer than two children per completed family.

Belgium and Ireland are the only European countries that have not relaxed their abortion laws. No one knows the number of illegal abortions in Belgium, but they are considerable; and plenty of Belgian "tourists" travel to neighboring countries to have their preborns murdered.

Because of language difficulties, once fully Catholic Louvain University has broken into two; doctors commit abortions at the medical schools of both campuses. Priests assured me that "Catholic" doctors also kill unborn babies in various clinics. One doctor has admitted killing 1,800 babies; he is in and out of court, keeping the issue alive, to the abortionists' glee.

The median age of priests in Belgium is 60 years. The bishops are weak and seem befuddled; only one publicly condemns contraception and fosters NFP. Belgium's best hope lies in the Flemish and Walloon prolife movements and in the brave few who fight sex education and teach NFP.

A Belgian prolife leader has proposed that HLI collaborate with and guide Europe's prolife groups in boycotting Upjohn. Upjohn's huge factory outside of Brussels produces the injectable abortifacient Depo-Provera, which is too dangerous for American women but is sent to the poor countries of the world (mostly with your tax money), where women suffer terribly from it.

NEW H.L.I. H.Q. IN HOLLAND

This country has lost more of its Catholic heritage than any other in Europe. Planned Parenthood crows that the Dutch are the world's most successful contracepting nation. The Hollanders are the closest to passing a law allowing active euthanasia. The government has also proposed legalizing sex between adults and children as young as 12!

I finalized arrangements for our 13th international branch—HLI Europe—headed by long-time prolife activist Fr. Joannis Koopman, SSS. The headquarters are in Nijmegen. Its aims are: (1) to enhance and coordinate prolife work in continental Europe, with programs resisting contraception-sterilization-abortion-euthanasia; (2) to promote NFP positively; (3) to improve marriage preparation programs; and (4) to educate the young in a truly Christian sexuality.

Our very first project is to organize a coordinated boycott against Upjohn. After initial financial help from us, this branch will finance itself. Some 40–50 Europeans will attend our Second International Symposium on Human Sexuality in Montreal next April.

GERMANY'S DUELING BISHOPS

At the end of the annual German Catholic Bishops' Conference, the elderly president, Josef Cardinal Höffner of Cologne, condemned not only Schering's new Morning-after abortion Pill, but also all "Pills-before," including all contraceptives. He said they are directly contrary to the Church's explicit teaching in *Humanae Vitae*, in the solemn pronouncements of all recent popes, and in 1,900 years of unbroken Catholic tradition. The only moral method of birth control for Catholics, said the Cardinal, is NFP.

But then, at a session of the diocesan synod of Rottenburg-Stuttgart, Bishop Moser contradicted his brother bishop, as happens so often these days. The German bishops, he said, took their stand in their 1968 dissent from *Humanae Vitae*.

Moser claimed he told this recently to Pope John Paul II in the presence of four other German bishops and that the Pope made no comments! (I was advised not to believe the latter.) There was thunderous applause from Pill-happy laity and priests. He then made the incredible assertion that "conscience is the law of all laws." Someone should remind him of Pope Pius XII's remark, "Conscience is a pupil, not a teacher."

Everyone is waiting to see what will be said or decided at the German synod next February—especially in the aftermath of the Extraordinary Synod in Rome. Said a papal nuncio, "The great problem of the Church in the West is the division of bishops within and between countries." At the Roman synod there will surely be a struggle between the liberals, whom some call Modernists, and the orthodox, for whom much-suffering Cardinal Ratzinger has spoken so eloquently.

(I spent three days in Rome consulting with various authorities. One high Vatican official observed that individual bishops of the USA, Canada, England (Benedictine Cardinal Hume) and France want to lessen or even break the authority of the pope; they do it by attacking not the pope but his curia. While in Rome I addressed the generalate, staff, seminarians and sisters of the Holy Cross order, who aim to revive knowledge of and devotion to the angels.)

Good German Christians, including priests and bishops, reacted angrily to Catholic Chancellor Kohl's recent appointment of a pro-abortion and feminist professor to head the health ministry. She has proclaimed that the German abortion law is here to stay, and has proposed that girls and women be given the Pill at government expense to reduce the number of abortions! (O Lord, deliver us from naive intellectuals.)

Many Germans think this latest appointment, plus the success of the Socialists and the pro-abortion, environmentalist Green Party in state elections, spells Kohl's doom. (For the first time the Greens, in the state of Hesse, have been voted a share of power.) A takeover by these anti-American, godless leftists, who gave Germany virtual abortion on request, would pull Germany out of NATO and drive atomic weapons from her soil. The specter of the treacherous leftist Willy Brandt is ever-present, too.

One of Germany's best newspapers, *Die Welt*, published an awesome map of Soviet "binary" poison-gas depots in the Communist countries surrounding West Germany. When released, the gas is more or less harmless; but then when bombs are detonated, the gas creates a mile-wide death zone where nothing can survive. There was speculation about whether the Americans had such weapons or

the means to counter them. Who will keep the Soviets
out?

While I was in Germany, parliamentarian Roland
Rösler gave me a small mountain of documents, some
secret, on the use of aborted babies for experiments, cell
therapy and cosmetic manufacture. There is no doubt
(sorry, Ann Landers) about such horrors, committed in
deep secrecy in collaboration with abortion mills—and in
collaboration with the lying German media, surely some of
the most wicked in the world.

PLUSSES AND MINUSES IN JAPAN

Since 1948 the Japanese have killed more than 65
million preborn babies. Today there are more than two
million abortions yearly among 121 million people. For
medical reasons and for fear of promiscuity, the government never approved the Pill and IUD. In 1974, the num-
ber-two official in the health ministry told me, "All authentic foreign medical reports on the Pill show the Pill to be
bad medication."

The chief means of birth control is still the condom
with backup abortion. Some 20 percent of the Japanese
still use the old Ogino rhythm method, which is the Model
T of NFP. For years HLI has worked with the great prolife missionary, Fr. Anthony Zimmerman, to upgrade NFP
practice in Japan. Because there is little so-called sex
education in Japan, and because family life is close-knit,
there is comparatively little fornication and therefore comparatively few teen abortions—fewer than 30,000 last year.
Most abortions are committed by married people, in contrast to the USA.

Massive abortion has given the Japanese a completed
family size of 1.7 children, far below the replacement rate.
Unlike Western nations, Japan cannot import labor, because she is an island nation with a difficult language.
The *only* way the pragmatic Japanese can have any future
as a nation is to curtail abortion. A prolife group with
three million active members and a large number of parliamentarians are interested in repealing the abortion law's
economic-grounds clause, which accounts for 90 percent of
the abortions.

Contraception and abortion are the two chief reasons
the Catholic Church in Japan is stagnant and slowly dying, maintains Fr. Zimmerman. For years he has tried to
goad the bishops into action. For two decades they refused

Fr. Zimmerman's suggestion to come out with a national
pastoral against abortion.   Meanwhile, the suffering Japanese women, who are ashamed of their many abortions,
bring little statues of Buddha to shrines to atone for their
sins and to give rest to the souls of their aborted children.

H.L.I. AND FEMINISTS IN DYING CANADA
   Abortion came to Canada in 1969, thanks to "Catholic"
Prime Minister Pierre Trudeau.   It is virtually "on demand," although the killing must be done in a hospital and
must be approved by a committee of three doctors.   In
1983 the adoption of the Canadian Constitution and the
Charter of Rights offered a chance to restore protection of
the unborn.   But Toronto's Emmett Cardinal Carter naively believed Trudeau's assurance that the Constitution
would not increase the slaughter.   Carter gave way, thus
wiping out the noble efforts of the prolifers.   Canadians
long for a prelate cut from the same cloth as Cardinal
O'Connor of New York.
   With a staff of eight, our branch in Montreal is truly
flourishing under the genius of Sister Lucille Durocher,
C.S.J.   She predicts that our international symposium next
April will draw 800 participants from 25 countries.   Montreal is in stagnant "Catholic" Quebec Province, which has
one of the lowest birthrates in the world and more than 10
free-standing abortion mills.   This beautiful, cool, sunshiny
city needs a strong prolife injection.
   A committee of Canadian Catholic women and bishops
have produced an incredible secular feminist study guide
entitled "Women in the Church."   It was approved after
revisions last summer by the Canadian hierarchy.   The kit
contains 12 two-hour workshops on a range of feminist
subjects, complete with highly selective readings from
Scripture, astonishing quotations from Canadian episcopal
statements, methods a la "values clarification," and 12
feminist recommendations.
   On November 2, 300 people (mostly women, with more
than a sprinkling of nuns) attended a one-day feminist
workshop in Ottawa where the kit was discussed at length.
Dr. Mary Malone, a married ex-nun and professor of theology at the Toronto School of Theology and a Catholic
seminary, addressed and guided the meeting.   The only
theologians she quoted were pro-abortion feminists such as
Rosemary Reuther, Mary Daly and Arlene Swidler.   "I've
learned to be disruptive in the Church," Malone boasted.

Indeed, she was.   She likened women's position in the
Church to that of blacks under apartheid.   Even lesbians
had their input.

"When only the ruling group [read: pope, bishops,
priests] gives input on what constitutes equality," Malone
intoned, "it is an exploitive situation."   Repeated themes:
"the exploitation of women," their "limited authority," the
"blatant inequality of women in the Church," the "unjust
patriarchal structures," the "hierarchical structure of the
Church where priests and bishops make all the important
decisions," etc., etc.

The accusation that the kit seemed pro-contraception
and pro-women-priests had been denied earlier.   But any
rational observer could only conclude from it and the workshop that these are indeed what underlies all the anger.
In fact, Malone commanded, "Insist on ordination."

In discussing the functions and roles of women in the
Church, *not a word* was said about a woman's role as wife,
mother, child-bearer (in a country that is dying!), primary
educator, etc.   The concept of male-female complementarity
was rejected totally because it is based on "false sex differences."   Pope Pius XII's saying that a mother is the
heart of the family was ridiculed explicitly.   Other villains
were Sts. Jerome, Augustine, Bernard and Thomas
Aquinas.

When contraception came up, Malone said that each
woman can hold and state her own views and "experiences," a buzzword voiced repeatedly.   When abortion
surfaced, the response was that larger questions were
under discussion.

Malone maintained, almost blasphemously, that Pope
Paul VI "offered [women] the role of being either Mary or
Eve—on a pedestal or in the gutter."   St. Teresa of Avila
found a way, so Malone said, to get around "the structure"
of the Church: "She had a vision" and secured "permission
to disobey superiors."   St. Catherine of Siena wanted power
as a laywoman; so she, too, had a vision: go straight to the
pope.   "She used the structure to straighten out the
Church."

All too few were the women brave enough to respond
to such malignant distortions of history and Malone's theological garbage.   Mother Teresa, who works within the
hated structure of the Church and is more powerful than
any prelate in the Church short of the pope himself, was
totally ignored.   One can only gasp at the total blackout on

Humanae Vitae and *Familiaris Consortio* in a day-long
meeting of Catholic women discussing their role in the
Church—in a dying nation!   But even more insidious and
dishonest was the selective quoting from official Church
documents.

A female pastoral assistant in a parish moaned that
there is "no room for advancement."   She is allowed to
prepare the liturgy and to do some counseling and administration but may not preside over the ceremony—where
only male priests may consecrate the bread and wine.   She
foresaw the day when all baptized Christians (non-Catholics, too?) would take part in Church policy-making and
lead the congregation in worship.   "The patriarchal structures are going to have to topple," she warned.

Speaking later on "Mary, Sign of Hope" at Windsor
University, Malone suddenly became rather orthodox.   She
knows what to say, when to say it, and to whom.   Theologian speak with forked tongue.

Perhaps the Canadian bishops will help the Malones of
Canada.   According to Toronto's *Globe and Mail*, the Holy
See asked the Canadian hierarchy not to publish their bold
joint statement based on a questionnaire sent out by the
Holy See with reference to the Extraordinary Synod.   It
was leaked; the *Globe and Mail* published it.   The statement calls for a dilution of papal authority via a *permanent* synod which would share authority with the pope and
the curia.

Ukrainian Archbishop Maxim Hermaniuk of Winnipeg
actually suggested such a permanent legislative synod.   He
said every form of government has a legislative and executive branch.   "The Roman Curia would have the executive
power," he conceded, but "the proposed permanent Synod of
Bishops could be composed of members elected by the
existing Synod of Bishops (perhaps 20) with six-year terms,
and another five appointed by the Holy Father."   Such a
reorganization would have a real impact on the Universal
Church, he was sure.   It sure would—but how much
Church would be left?!

What if such a permanent synod—dominated by dissenting European bishops—had existed in 1968 when birth
control was the issue?   It took an inspired, farsighted,
lonely *pope* to save the entire Church from the scourge of
contraception-sterilization-abortion-euthanasia.

Even today, most bishops of the dying West seem not
to see the significance of Pope Paul VI's *Humanae Vitae*,

judging from their statements and pastorals. Surely Europe's 12 dissenting national hierarchies must take some responsibility for the state of that dying continent. The Canadian bishops are partly to blame for Canada's dismal birthrate, too. And yet these prelates covet the Vicar of Christ's authority!

But our good neighbors to the north have even more problems. Toronto's *Catholic New Times* (Canada's *National Catholic Reporter*), whose editorial board includes various women religious, a Jesuit and a Redemptorist, attacks the Pope for condemning polygamy in Africa and for not understanding the true nature of sex and marriage.

Worst of all, though, is a two-hour "documentary" film, *Behind the Veil: Nuns*, put out by the feminist wing of the anti-Catholic Canadian Film Board. The film was made with the collaboration of Benedictine nuns who now claim to have been deceived. A feminist nun shows this film at every opportunity. The central theme: the suppression of women and the tyranny of men. This thing has to be seen to be believed.

For years I tried to interest the official Canadian Catholic Women's League in NFP, but to no avail. With the appearance of *Humanae Vitae* in 1968, Serena, the pioneer NFP group, offered their help to the Canadian hierarchy. The bishops ignored them.

Go where you may in this world, the underlying disagreement, like a festering sore, is artificial birth control. The crisis of authority in the Church began with *Humanae Vitae*. The resulting collapse of the Catholic Church in the West, the genocidally low birthrates, the empty seminaries and novitiates, the rampant VD, the abortions, the escalating divorce and overcopulation—these seem to make no impression on most Western bishops, priests, intellectuals and theologians. As St. Paul warned, spiritual blindness is one of God's severest punishments.

HERE COMES "ONE MORE CHILD"!

A few years ago a Croatian pastor in Yugoslavia saw his baptisms declining rapidly and parishes going through their death throes. So he started a movement called "One More Child." In a few years his baptisms increased 40 percent. The movement went national and the Pope blessed it.

HLI wants to make One More Child international, starting in the USA and Canada. In Europe and North

America the faithful decrease by 7,000 every day. (In Africa, Catholics *increase* by 16,000 daily.) The USA's birthrate is below replacement level, with only 1.8 children per completed family. Canadians have only 1.7 children (2.2 are needed for national survival).

SUICIDE OF THE DUTCH CHURCH

(#19—March 1986)

In the last few months, I have visited Canada, Holland, France, Mexico and Germany, working with the world's greatest people, prolifers.

In Europe I did more research for our upcoming document proving that *all* so-called contraceptive Pills abort at some time. I also saw unassailable proof that aborted babies are used for various Nazi-type purposes. Here is a peek under the rock, courtesy of Dominique Lapierre's recent best-selling novel (based on fact), *City of Joy*:

> The opulent dowager of Nizamudhin Lane was carrying on the very latest of Calcutta's clandestine professions: the sale of human embryos and fetuses. The mainsprings of the industry were a network of foreign buyers who scoured the third world on behalf of international laboratories and institutes for genetic research. The majority of these buyers were Swiss or American. They used the embryos and fetuses either for scientific work or in the manufacture of rejuvenating products for a clientele of privileged people in specialized establishments in Europe and America. The demand had provoked a fruitful trade for which Calcutta was one of the central sources. One of the recognized providers of this unusual merchandise was an ex-pharmacist named Sushil Vohra. He obtained his supplies from several clinics that specialized in abortions, and he looked after the packaging of the consignments which left for Europe or the USA, via Moscow on the Soviet airline, Aeroflot's, regular flight.

Our booklet *The Deadly Neo-Colonialism*, which exposed foreign "aid" antilife crimes, has really set the World Bank and USAID on their ears. The Bank held a special meeting over it, the first such ever, trying to defend itself. Many congressmen had been asking tough questions. Our editor, John Cavanaugh-O'Keefe, has told you all about this meeting in our international newsletter *HLI Reports.* John helped lead the brave prolifers who stopped virtually all abortions in the Washington area on the January 22 anniversary of *Roe v. Wade.* His sit-ins and picketing paralyzed five of the nine murder mills and caused the other four to close out of fright!

BATTLING FEMINIST-ABORTIONISTS IN CANADA

In November I exposed the global death movement at a city-wide meeting in Windsor, Ontario, sponsored by the Knights of Columbus. I also spoke to two high schools, preached at Windsor University, was the main speaker at the annual prolife ecumenical service in an Anglican Church, picketed an abortion "hospital," exposed a Planned Barrenhood teen-sex-advice center, and scurried across the river to preach at all the Masses in a prolife Detroit parish that has *two* great priests.

Women's groups in Canada are fighting a battle royal. The official Catholic Women's League has been infiltrated to its highest offices by a sinister coterie of secular-thinking feminists. Led by the tireless G. Landolt, a women's group named REAL (Realistic, Equal, Active, for Life) opposes those antilife/anti-family feminists without appealing to religion.

Another group, Women for Life, Faith and the Family, opposes the highly questionable "Women's Kit" approved by the bishops. They are also battling the movement for women priests, whose guiding spirit is the conniving ex-nun and historian Dr. Mary Malone, professor at the University of Toronto School of Theology and at St. Augustine's Seminary there.

With only 25 million people, the immense land of Canada is very underpopulated. But the mania for contraception, the abortifacient Pill and IUD, sterilization and surgical abortion goes on. These abuses are catching up with the Canadians, who now have an aging population and must import about 125,000 immigrants annually. The low birthrate, plus too few foreign markets for Canada's vast farm product, equals a declining dollar.

As in the USA, sterilization has become a scourge. Between 1974 and 1984, the health department reported 1,368,299 men and women sterilized. The peak year was 1978–79, with 105,509 tubal ligations and 40,069 vasectomies. The latest figures show that doctors are running out of victims for this veterinarian way of birth control. Meanwhile, to make things worse, the government has just reduced family allowances. (Of course, it supports militant feminist groups, but not prolife women.)

In Quebec, Canada's most Catholic and populous province, public school nurses must by law train all 14-year-olds in all forms of contraception, refer girls for the abortifacient Pill, and even take them to the abortion chambers without their parents' knowledge. This happens in "Catholic" schools as well.

Will the Quebecers have a future without Sisters? In the early 1960s, no region in the world had a higher percentage of women religious. Quebec's population was then six million. According to the *Ratzinger Report* (p. 101): "Between 1961 and 1981, the women religious, as the result of departures, deaths and decline in recruitment, have been reduced from 46,933 to 26,294. Hence, a drop of 44 percent, with no end in sight. New vocations, in fact, declined 98.5 percent in the same period."

Furthermore, most of the remaining 1.5 percent are "late vocations," not young ladies. Only Holland has a worse record.

At lunch, the Papal Nuncio in Ottawa was most supportive of HLI; he wished us well in the International Symposium on Human Sexuality to be held April 23–27 in Montreal, at which we expect 750–1,000 people.

THE SUICIDE OF THE DUTCH CATHOLIC CHURCH

The incredible, unique and almost total demolition of Catholicism since 1960 in this country of 14 million has been recorded in a 124-page *Documentation on Dutch Catholicism on the Eve of the Papal Visit*. This blockbuster, written by a loyal Dutch Jesuit, was given to all journalists before the Pope's visit to Holland. It is shocking to read; you are constantly reminded of how the rest of Europe and North America seem well on the way to a similar tragedy. One section shows how Dominican Fr. Edward Schillebeeckx has been undermining the Church since 1964.

In no European country in recent times did the Church flourish more than in the land of windmills and tulips. At one time Holland produced more missionaries than Poland or Ireland. In 1939, when Dutch Catholics were only two percent of the world's Catholics, they contributed 11 percent of all priest/missionaries. In 1954, 7,000 Dutch priests, bishops and sisters were at work in overseas missions.

At home, the Church flourished. It had its own national Catholic radio/TV network, schools, hospitals, etc. Holland had become the showcase of Catholicism. It had also become one of the 10 richest nations—which may have led to the crash.

Since 1960, the number of priests and religious has dropped to less than half. The number of newly ordained priests dwindled from 318 in 1960 to 16 in 1977. From 1965 to 1975, 1,700 priests and 4,300 religious deserted. By 1981, more than 2,100 priests out of 8,000 had left. Comparatively, this is twice as many as in the USA and three times the world average!

In the frenetic yen for "renewal," the Dutch combined 44 major seminaries into five special schools of theology— where students lost not only their priestly and religious vocations, but often their faith. Fifty-five minor seminaries simply disappeared. Today half the students are female, most of them ardent secular feminists. Many of the theological graduates, both male and female, have become married pastoral workers. Today one of every four pastors is a non-ordained lay pastoral worker, often a woman. Fr. Schillebeeckx taught that a special priesthood does not exist.

Hundreds of married priests and ex-nuns teach theology at all levels or have high pastoral positions, contrary to papal directives. Twenty-seven ex-priests, all married and some divorced, teach in the five theological centers.

Most religious communities are in such an advanced state of decomposition that they would not know what to do with new candidates if they had them. Novitiates have been cancelled almost everywhere, except in the Jesuit and some contemplative orders. A Dutch lad who wants to be a priest has to go abroad or become a monk.

In no other country of the world has what is called "the third way" (cheating on one's vow of chastity by having an intimate man-woman relationship) received such full, although unofficial, legitimation. Even some of the highest authorities in the Dutch provinces approve, especially the Franciscans and Capuchins. Unbelievable books promote "functional love" and "affective relations" between celibate men and women religious, leading to "autonomy" and "pluriformity."

Some of these authors were later elected religious superiors, even provincials! Do weak and sick religious communities elect weak and sick superiors? It seems to be characteristic of our times. Almost any informed Catholic could cite examples in the USA.

Holland's so-called Catholic schools and institutions have become utterly corrupted. Nuns live in separate apartments and sport the latest hairdos and fashions. Priests live scandalous lives, being married or divorced—or just openly living with women in that "alternative lifestyle" we used to call "shacking up."

PP and the huge Dutch drug company Organon provide the schools' sex/contraception books. The idea, obviously, is that the more fornication you stir up, the more Pills you sell. Meanwhile, 15,000 Dutch nuns who are 65 or older suffer silently as they watch the work for which they gave their lives being systematically destroyed.

The Dutch crime rate has escalated, while the Sacrament of Reconciliation has virtually evaporated. Catholics now have the highest crime rates, reflecting the turmoil in the Church. The liturgical abuses can only be imagined. Coached by Fr. Schillebeeckx, some 13,000 ex-priests, exnuns, and male and female pastoral workers have taken over the administration of the Church, the Catholic media, the schools of theology, the mission training centers and the parishes. They have used the resources of the Church to destroy authentic Catholicism and obedience to the pope. Once "free" from Rome, the Church withered fast, so that the pope needed courage to visit a land of protesters and mockers.

When the push came for legal abortion, not one prominent rebel Catholic lifted a finger—and that includes Fr. Schillebeeckx, who assured his followers that abortion was merely a matter of "conscience," that cover-all for so much evil today. Recently the Dutch bishops admitted that at least half of the 56 "Catholic" hospitals had applied to the government for licenses to commit abortions on demand.

Holland's Catholic TV, radio and press are brutally critical of Rome, the pope and true Catholicism. Thus, an orthodox bishop often finds it impossible to include authentic teaching in his own diocesan paper. The "little" Catholics who still believe—farmers, small businessmen and workers—are at wits' end as to how to educate their children in genuine Catholicism. Some have founded their own schools. As Adrianus Cardinal Simonis told me personally, the Netherlands needs a "fundamental evangelization." So does most of the West, I am afraid.

The harm done by the famous *New Catechism*, which was not without merit, was incalculable. Later editions never included the corrections officially demanded by Rome, concerning the sacrificial character of the Mass, the Resurrection, the Virgin Birth and sexual ethics. Many Catholic theologians and religion teachers in other countries thought they were using the latest and best! (To their credit, the American bishops never gave the book an *imprimatur*.)

The classic example of what happens when power is taken away from the Church hierarchy was "the Simonis affair," which proved that power then goes not to the people but to self-serving cliques. When Pope Paul VI selected an orthodox parish assistant to be the Archbishop of Rotterdam (now Cardinal Primate of Utrecht), the opposition was unbelievable. But even worse was the rebellion against the appointment of Joannis Gijsen as bishop of Roermond in 1972. The Pope himself had to install Gijsen because Primate Cardinal Alfrink refused!

Gijsen immediately built the only seminary in Holland. In eight years he ordained more priests than all the wild theological schools combined. In fact, in eight years Jan Cardinal Willebrands ordained only four, among whom were several Vietnamese.

Simonis and Gijsen fought fiercely against the legalization of abortion. Willebrands, while condemning this sin morally, told the politicians that politically there were various possibilities! Today the Dutch have 800,000 foreigners in their land because of their low birthrate. They are also close to passing an active euthanasia law; they may do so this year.

To rebuild the hierarchy, Pope John Paul II has removed Willebrands and installed orthodox bishops at every opportunity. When the Pope appointed Gijsen's auxiliary bishop to head Holland's biggest diocese, Den Bosch, some months ago, the outcry again was total. Today the score is switched, as Holland's true Catholics say: five for the Pope, two against.

Is the Dutch tragedy repeating itself in the USA, Canada and the rest of the West? Disturbing signs abound: RENEW programs, weak bishops, the domination of leftist theologians in high places, a Catholic school system that is mostly not Catholic, witchcraft and homosexuality among many religious and their superiors, the pro-abortion ad by priests and religious in the *New York Times*, empty seminaries and novitiates, a liberal Catholic press that censors orthodox views, millions of contracepting or sterilized married couples, and more.

I accuse the NC News Service, the *National Catholic Reporter* and virtually all of the diocesan press of a conspiracy of silence in not publishing the full truth about the Dutch Church. Honest reporting might have helped prevent much damage.

FROM FRANCE, BAD NEWS AND GOOD

More than any other people in Europe, the French worry about their birthrate. It is consistently low despite the highest family allowances in the West. They worry even more about the almost seven million foreigners, especially about the nearly four million African Moslems, whose birthrate is three times that of their hosts.

The unsociable Moslems burden the public services, especially the hospitals, and some 25 percent of all prisoners are African Moslems. The French are not joking when they say Muammar Khaddafi could have a bridgehead in the southern city of Marseilles, loaded with Moslems and Communists. Fearing that their national identity will vanish, some French want the Moslems curbed or exported.

Dr. Emmanuel Tremblay, a French scientist, has calculated that if current trends hold, France will be largely a Moslem country by 2035 (thank you, contraception-sterilization-abortion).

Fewer than 20 percent of the Catholics in this "Eldest Daughter of the Church" attend Mass regularly; in Paris, even fewer than that. Still, the French demonstrated in the streets by the millions against Socialist Freemason Mitterrand's attempt to take over the Catholic schools. French parents complain bitterly about their children's not learning the essentials of the Faith. Meanwhile, PP and its accomplices have installed contraceptive sex "education" in the schools.

The theological situation in France is exceedingly confused; perhaps no bishops in the world resent Cardinal Ratzinger more than the French. Religious vocations are very few, but there is little clamor for women priests, this being mostly an American and Canadian aberration. The Masonic-humanist influence is long-standing and pervasive, although politically France has become very conservative.

I was invited to Lille to meet with some prolife leaders in an attempt to revive the sagging French right-to-life movement, which is riddled with dissension. Laissez-les-Vivre, the national group, has only 30,000 members, of whom only 10,000 are active.

Even though one out of three babies is aborted, and the birthrate is below the survival level, the bishops act as if the holocaust of the infants did not exist. So-called therapeutic abortions are committed freely in "Catholic" hospitals, with prostaglandin injections used for the later killings.

Nowhere has Archbishop Marcel Lefebvre's movement had more of a following than in France. I meet his priests all over the world and find them well-informed and very prolife, far more so than the average non-Lefebvre priest. Lefebvre's many followers were furious when the bishop of Lille refused to sell them a disused church—and then sold it to the Moslems for a mosque!

I met the Benedictine Dom Gerard Lafond at his abbey outside of Lille. He founded the Knights of Our Lady (encouraged by Rome), whose patron is St. Benedict and whose purpose is to restore Christianity in Europe. HLI and the Knights will sponsor a prolife seminar next August 14–15 at Chartres, where thousands of pilgrims come at that time.

REPORT ON THE SYNOD

History turns no sharp corners, a wise man said. "Habit is the flywheel of society," remarked James Watson. We should not expect any quick turnaround in the Catholic Church. Only time will tell. The forthcoming universal catechism based on Vatican II documents could be a much-needed guide for authors of future national catechisms. But who can guarantee obedience to it in a world of heretical theologians who claim quasi-magisterial status—and weak bishops who fail to correct them?

After pointing out some shortcomings in the American Church, Bishop James Malone, head of the American hierarchy and an admitted optimist, declared, "The Church in the United States is fundamentally on the right track in implementing the teachings and decisions of Vatican II." Yes, there have been some gains and benefits. But I could write a long tract for him on the unbelievable abuses that have happened—liturgical, theological and otherwise.

A few examples must suffice. First, and arguably worst, there is the collapse of religious life, the Church's frontline force, its educators. Seminaries and novitiates are nearly empty; many have closed. Witchcraft and magic are not uncommon in the religious worship of convents (see the December 1985 *Fidelity* for a horrifying 11-page exposé). Ten thousand priests, 30,000 nuns and 7,000 brothers have left their commitments since 1960.

Doesn't Malone know the doctrinal confusion and aberrations that exist in so-called Catholic colleges and seminaries? Let him start with Notre Dame! There are always exceptions, but most Catholic youth go all through "Catholic" schools without learning the essential doctrines of their Faith. Even Catholic schools are overrun with sex "education" programs that border on outright contraceptive training.

Between three and five million Catholics are divorced and remarried; their children are far more likely to be crippled emotionally and confused religiously.

The American birthrate is below replacement level because of contraception, sterilizations and abortions, with Catholics guilty nearly as often as their neighbors.

More than half of all married couples in childbearing years are incapable of bearing children; 30 percent of all couples married 10 years or more have been sterilized. Where is the bishop who will protest this fastest growing, sinful means of birth control?

Perhaps even Malone would be shocked if he examined today's "Catholic" marriage preparation courses. In one California diocese, a required course taught oral and anal intercourse as good and normal. And what about the increasing pregnancies among Catholic teens, not to mention the resulting single-parent families with their emotionally crippled children?

One can count on one hand the number of US bishops who speak out strongly for *Humanae Vitae*. Without adherence to that key moral teaching, in my view, moral regeneration is impossible. That is because its rich content guards the very heart of life and love, marriage and family, which are the bases of society and Church. And if one can blatantly disobey *Humanae Vitae* and fail even to teach or preach its essentials, why cannot one ignore the Church's other clearly defined moral directives?

The theological confusion reaches right to the top. At the Synod on the Family in 1980, I was astonished to hear so many bishops plead for remarried divorced Catholics to be allowed to receive Holy Communion! The Pope had to step in and stop them. At the recent Extraordinary Synod, four archbishops pleaded for the same aberration.

CANADIAN CONVENTS IN CRISIS

(No. 20—April 1986)

The nuns have been my heroes all my life. They put up with me through six grades, despite having to box my ears occasionally. Later, I got even, trying to teach them liturgy for two summers, during which I was also their chaplain. For 15 years I taught family sociology (marriage prep) in a nun-run Catholic college for women. For 10 years I was confessor in a large convent. A great Sister of St. Joseph, Sister Lucille, directs HLI's Canadian branch. Two of my own sisters are women religious.

So I thought I knew what was happening in convents. But having had little contact with nuns for the last 15 years, I find I was dead wrong: nuns are not what they used to be! I always did wonder why, out of 121,000 nuns in the USA, only one really stands out from the crowd in the abortion fight: Sister Paula Vandegaer of Los Angeles.

Of course, there are still thousands of wonderful nuns. But I have had much contact lately with women religious in the USA and elsewhere. And I am shocked by their naivete, their lack of understanding of the kind of society and Church we live in today, their rebellion—and yes, their loss of faith.

Only the last, it seems, can explain the witchcraft, the anger, the arrogant disobedience (even among superiors of large communities), the frenetic and scandalous demand for priestly ordination, the preoccupation with material things (fashionable clothes, hair care, luxurious separate living quarters, etc.), to say nothing of the heresies many are teaching (where they still teach).

A wise old Canadian religious priest told me the nuns have lost their clout, their role and their platform, by giving up so many of their schools, hospitals and other institutions to tackle all manner of "social ministries" which the laity perhaps can do better.

Having surrendered their presence at the cutting edge of society, they seem to have turned in on themselves and now feel confused, alienated and uprooted—as if someone had done them wrong. Countless nuns have joined the radical, angry feminists. Apart from the contemplative orders (whose many novices assure their futures), rare is the motherhouse or convent that has not breathed in the deadly feminist virus.

All of this is best exemplified in the Canadian National Film Board's incredible film, *Behind the Veil: Nuns,* which was shown on Canadian TV. You have to see this show to believe it.

Sister Lucille and I visited Mother Abbess of Montreal's cloistered Benedictine abbey, which played such a prominent role in this atrocious film. The producers had promised the sisters that the film would show the glories of female religious life down through the ages. What came out instead was a vicious travesty engineered by angry feminist nuns. When the abbess protested and asked for changes, she was lied to again and then ignored! The film board did not even have the courtesy to give them a copy.

On my recent reinvasion of Canada, HLI held a weekend seminar on family and life issues for women religious superiors and their councillors. Our goal was to draw nuns into the prolife/pro-family cause, where they are scandalously absent because they do not know the situation. Twenty-nine sisters attended, and they were most receptive.

The faculty (Fr. Lawrence Abello, SJ, Sr. Lucille and yours truly) described the world's sex-mess, stressed the need to teach solid doctrine, and explained the importance of chastity both in and out of marriage, especially via the responsible use of NFP. The truth shocked the sisters; so did our prolife films, which hardly any had seen.

Somehow the French Canadians, so proud of their culture (and rightly so), have forgotten that "culture walks on two legs." Quebec's socialized health services are arranging to provide free vasectomies to "rescue" the citizens from gouging doctors (veterinarians?) who charge $200 per victim. While in Ontario I helped picket provincial Premier Peterson, who is "personally against abortion." (Pilate was "personally against" crucifying Jesus.) Peterson did not keep his campaign promise to keep abortionist Henry Morgentaler's mills out of Ontario—and I told him so in a brief conversation.

What if the bishops of Canada, which is about half Catholic, had stood up to so-called Catholic prime minister Pierre Trudeau on abortion the way the Filipino bishops stood up to Marcos? They could have explained that abortion is not a sectarian issue, that it is a matter of civil rights, and that as moral leaders in a nation almost half Catholic they would never go along with baby-killing. What if the Canadian bishops had demanded of Trudeau that the 1981 Charter of Rights include the protection of all human lives from fertilization on?

These thoughts came to me when a good Canadian priest, thoroughly familiar with the abortion battle and Trudeau's tricks, told me that of all the world's hierarchies, Canada's had had the best chance of preventing legalized abortion.

ON THE MOVE IN GERMANY

Cardinal Ratzinger's famous report on the fallout from Vatican II had more influence in his native Germany, perhaps, than in any other country. At least, more and more German bishops are speaking the unpopular truths of the day, even if they are ignored totally by Curran-like theologians such as Böckle and Gründel. Cardinal Höffner said recently that 93 percent of German Catholics never go to Confession. Archbishop Dyba of Fulda says three-fourths of Germany's believers rarely or never go to church.

In a news conference, Höffner also condemned (1) Schering's new Morning-after Pill, (2) "the Pill-before" (as the Germans call it) and (3) *all* contraception. The German hierarchy's dissent to *Humanae Vitae* was invalid, he declared. (Some bishops contradicted him; the rest kept silent.)

Bishop Stimfle of Augsburg recently condemned the Pill in a pastoral letter. Whether he meant the Schering morning-after Pill, all Pills, or all contraception, was not clear; in Germany, "die Pille" often means all contraception.

Aktion Leben, the largest prolife group in Germany, has the bishops on the ropes: they insist that the bishops obey the pope, follow Höffner, and take back their dissent to *Humanae Vitae*, especially since it is becoming more and more well-known that all Pills abort, at least sometimes.

Someone has said that if there is anything we can learn from history, it is that we learn nothing from history. The Bundestag (German parliament) will demonstrate that this year by passing, almost certainly, a bill for passive euthanasia. This will, of course, soon become active (direct killing).

Dr. Julius Hacketal of Munich has been promoting euthanasia with satanic cleverness. Pro Familia (Germany's Planned Parenthood) has come out for it officially, even more than PP enthusiasts Ann Landers and Dear Abby have. There are now more than 50 national euthanasia societies in the world; next summer they will hold their third international meeting in Bombay; last year's meeting in Nice, France, drew more than 750 participants from 70 countries, including HLI's "observer."

The new national health minister, a secular feminist who is also vice-president of the German Catholic women's organization, has proclaimed that the abortion law is here to stay. Her remedy for abortion? The Pill, at taxpayers' expense. In the largest German state, Rheinland-Pfalz, the government offers the Pill free to all women who have two children, to reduce the numbers of abortions!

Only one-fifth of the Bundestag would sign a recent statement urging repeal of the abortion law. One parliamentarian, a Catholic Christian Democrat, told me personally that the 30 women in the legislature, virtually all radical feminists, are the problem.

A recent issue of the prestigious German counterpart of *Communio* gives evidence that much fetal experimentation goes on and that Europeans use aborted babies for cosmetic and industrial purposes. At Hadamar, where the Nazis began the killing of people who had defects, prolife Germans want to hold a gigantic, day-long demonstration on May 10 with Mother Teresa, Dr. Nathanson, exiled Czech Bishop Paul Hnilica, yours truly and others.

My open letter to Cardinal Bernardin in *HLI Reports* was published recently in Germany's most significant theological journal, *Theologisches*. *Theologisches*, I am told, is read by all German bishops and by the Pope. HLI rushed Prof. Don DeMarco's pamphlet *Fertility and In Vitro Fertilization* to Germany for translation and publication in *Theologisches* in the hope of stopping the bishops from approving *in vitro* fertilization involving husband and wife, as the Austrian bishops have. Valerie Riches' *Contraception's Legacy*, published by us, may soon flood the German-speaking countries from our branches in Holland and Germany. So, too, my booklet *And Now Euthanasia*.

ABORTIONISTS IMPOSE THEIR IMMORALITY

The Spaniards waited too long, thinking abortion "can't happen here." But no country has publicly protested the legalization of abortion as Spain has. Mother Teresa and the Pope drew millions of protesters into the streets.

In August 1985 Spain legalized abortion in cases of rape, defective baby, or pregnancy endangering a mother's health or life. Spain's National Conference of Catholic Bishops immediately declared that anyone "who cooperates physically or morally" in an abortion is "automatically excommunicated." (How can we get Kennedy, Cuomo, Ferraro, Fr. Drinan and certain nuns to Spain?)

The board of Spain's National Medical Association forced the Health Ministry to abandon a plan (tried unsuccessfully in Italy) that would have doctors with "conscientious objections" declare themselves. Further, the board advised doctors not to declare their personal views and to refuse each abortion case by case.

Threats of legal suits for homicide, plus pressure from medical superiors, have doctors afraid to commit abortions. Four doctors who committed them were sued. Nun-superiors of Catholic hospitals warned staff doctors that if they tried even one abortion, there were several doors leading out of the hospital. Many doctors in public and private hospitals are reluctant to abort even once, fearing they would then have to commit all the abortions, thus becoming known as abortionists and ruining their careers.

Enter 3,000 angry feminists, in a national pro-abortion conference in Barcelona, boasting that they had killed their babies. They insisted that doctors be forced to abort (no freedom of choice for *them*!), that women be given unrestricted abortions as a right, and that women have the right "to control their own bodies." (Most abortions come from bodies out of control.)

Technicians allegedly aborted two women's babies in adjoining rooms. They left equipment and two bottles containing "fetuses" on the table for all to see. A videotape of one of the abortions was shown. And so it goes in Catholic Spain, where the Socialist government is intent on quickly undoing anything smacking of Franco.

Fifteen years ago, I tried by correspondence to stir up the Spaniards to educate their nation, to build a resistance to what was sure to come. There were no takers. Could the Spaniards have thought, like the Belgians today, that the abortion monster would stay in England, France and Germany? As Pope Pius XII lamented, "Why are we always too late with too little?"

H.L.I.-MEXICO BATTLES THE ABORTION-PUSHERS

Recently I spent a week working in Mexico City, where I saw the appalling ruins of last year's double earthquake. The Mexicans told me perhaps 50,000 died—compared with the 8,000 reported by the government. The politicians had cut corners erecting huge buildings and pocketed the difference. These buildings collapsed easily. In one case, 15 floors of a government hospital dropped to the ground. On TV you saw the newborn babies rescued after a week in the rubble. God makes them tough! There were many little miracles like this.

HLI's branch in Mexico is truly flourishing under the genius of Angelina Muñiz. With her contacts and our resources, she has made HLI virtually *the* right-to-life movement in Mexico.

Angelina attended one of many extension courses at the autonomous University of Mexico. Only degreed persons were accepted. The highly trained teachers immediately made it clear that there are no moral guidelines whatsoever, that nothing is wrong in the area of sex—not even bestiality, incest and abortion.

They urged changes in sex roles to achieve total "equality" in true secular feminist fashion. They called for sex "education" in the government schools, with universal contraceptives/abortifacients and back-up abortions. They ridiculed "rhythm" as old-fashioned, unprogressive, unworkable and contrary to human freedom. Old, "suffocating" values must be destroyed.

Angelina, unafraid and fluent in four languages, insisted on giving her talk on NFP. The class immediately proclaimed NFP "too restrictive," although many found it fascinating. She then conned them into seeing *The Silent Scream*, which proved a total shock.

After recovering, the teachers furiously denied its authenticity, saying that early suction abortions do not involve crushing the baby's head, etc. They called the film "manipulative and unscientific." But although they hated the film and Angelina, they all wanted to copy it. In the end, she won over most of the class; her phone has been ringing ever since with many requests for courses in NFP. In Latin America you can still count on basic Christian instincts.

Mexico's no-holds-barred population control program began with the 1974 World Population Conference at Bucharest. Out of this came CONAPO (Consejo Nacional de

Población), which in 1981 hatched into the PNES (Programa Nacional de Educación Sexual).   This outfit produced four incredible volumes entitled *La Educación de la Sexualidad Humana* (Education in Human Sexuality). Totally devoid of any reference to morality or religion, full of "sensitivity training" and "values clarification" to break down "prejudices" and "tired values," there could hardly be a more sinister program.

Tragically, there is little available in Mexico to counter this satanic onslaught.   So Angelina is hard at work producing a Spanish-language course in Christian sexuality which emphasizes chastity, NFP and serious preparation for Christian marriage.   Earlier we had financed a complete course in NFP, including all teacher training materials; Angelina has sold 91 of these sets.   The bishops are very pleased with her work and that of her collaborators.

The sinister extension course described above is taught throughout Mexico, which suffers under one of the world's worst governments, riddled with Communists, Freemasons and godless Socialists.   Although abortion is still illegal, the government almost need not legalize it, several observers told me, because many abortions are already being committed—even at the government hospitals.

Hampered by governmental hostility toward religion, the bishops can do only so much, the Cardinal explained to me.   We have supplied Mexico's prolifers with some $30,000 worth of projectors, Spanish-language films, videocassettes, slides and literature so far.

In the last few months, at least 20 million Latin Americans have seen *The Silent Scream* (thanks to the generosity of HLI's donors).   That includes at least seven million Argentines, thanks largely to our great collaborators Pedro M. Garcia, a busy economist who finds time to run the League for Decency from the city of Rosario, and Victor T. Taussig, a businessman who heads HLI's branch in Buenos Aires.

The incomparable Magaly Llaguno, a highly educated Cuban lady who works for HLI in Miami, got *The Silent Scream* shown on national TV in Chile, Ecuador and Peru. She edits *Escoge La Vida*, HLI's excellent newsletter which we publish for the world's Spanish-speaking people.

Magaly keeps telling me we must concentrate our time and resources in the developing countries of the world, especially in Africa and Latin America, where we can still win.

POPE QUOTES GANDHI ON CONTRACEPTION

How shrewd of the Pope to cite India's hero Gandhi in condemning artificial, inhuman methods of birth control in that sensitive country! "The act of generation should be controlled for the ordered growth of the world," he quoted. Then he asked, "How is the suspension of procreation to be brought about? Not by immoral and artificial checks." Rather, the Pope observed, "Gandhi declared that the answer lay 'in a life of discipline and self-control.'" When was the last time you heard a bishop talk like that?

P.P.'S LEGAL EFFORTS TO STOP H.L.I.

In May 1985, I joined picketers at a PP abortuary in Concord, California, whose landlord is a waffling Catholic businessman, Maurice Moyal. While I was joshing with the police (who I find always have trouble with a Roman collar in front of a killing chamber), an aborted teenager stumbled palefaced out of the abortion mill and collapsed. I rushed to her aid, kneeling at her side. A blustering officer, obviously on PP's side, shouted at me, "Get away from there or I'll put you in jail!"

I did leave the scene (slowly), but only because I had to preach eight times in a parish that weekend, which is hard to do from behind bars.

The officer's order was unjust and immoral, but also illegal. He deprived the young woman of counsel, and violated my First Amendment rights to conduct my ministry and render aid in an emergency. He and the city could be liable. Prolife lawyer Frank X. Driscoll is suing the City of Concord for me. I have promised the Lord that if we win I will spend the money on saving babies, educating youth and training seminarians in Africa.

Earlier in 1985, in Ottawa, radio talk-show host Lowell Green had me on his popular three-hour program on station CFRA. I was out to expose the evils of PP and said, "Having seen their operation worldwide, I maintain that PP is the most wicked organization on earth, destroying the youth, the family and society, etc., etc."

Green, a PP enthusiast, asked whether I really wanted to say that. "Yes," I said, and repeated it, offering to send proof to any doubters. Two weeks later, in DC, a courier handed me two documents from an Ottawa law firm, threatening to sue both HLI and me for libeling poor PP. According to Canadian law, such warnings must be fol-

lowed up by a certain date. On the last day, PP's lawyer
wrote me that they were withdrawing the suit but would
sue in the future if I did not stop defaming noble PP.
They do not seem to realize I do not scare easily—and
have only poverty to sue!

I understand PP also sued the radio network for $1
million. Apparently they settled out of court, with PP
given "equal time" to tell the world how wonderful they
are. That is how PP blackmails and neutralizes the media, when necessary.

On my way to Mexico, I stopped in Miami to debate
PP on Miami's biggest radio talk show, the three-hour
Steve Cain show on WNWS. PP did not show up. I wonder why! The controversial Cain is semi-prolife but will
not admit it in public; he invited me back to discuss euthanasia.

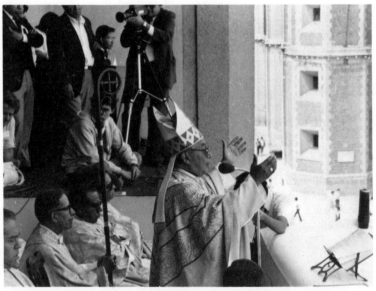

*Cardinal Corripio-Ahumada (HLI advisor) celebrated Mass at
the Shrine of Our Lady of Guadalupe, encouraging prolifers to
stand firm against Planned Parenthood propaganda.*

CURRANISM AND THE AMERICAN CHURCH

(No. 21—May 1986)

In his sensational *Ratzinger Report*, the Cardinal Prefect for the Sacred Congregation for the Doctrine of the Faith remarked, "It is incontestable that the last ten years have been decidedly unfavorable for the Catholic Church." He described the period since Vatican II as "a progressive process of decadence." Several years ago a high Church official told me that "the real problem of the Catholic Church in the West is the problem of bishops and theologians."

Nothing demonstrates this better than the Curran scandal. For more than 20 years, this theologian has (1) actively and publicly led the attack on *Humanae Vitae*; (2) boldly spread far and wide, through writings, speeches and interviews, his scandalous views on abortion, contraception/abortifacients, premarital sex, homosexual acts, masturbation, sterilization and divorce; (3) poisoned thousands of future priests and parents with these twisted ideas; and (4) embarrassed the Holy Father, at whose pontifical university (Catholic University of America) Curran does his thing.

Yet this Pied Piper of Error has received open, active resistance and correction from only one American bishop, the late Joseph V. Sullivan of Baton Rouge, who forbade him to speak to the Catholic students of Louisiana State University. Archbishop Jean Jadot, the "progressive" apostolic delegate at the time, opposed Sullivan. So did the provincial archbishop, initially. Sullivan became the pariah of the American hierarchy.

That was bad enough. But when Sullivan took his case to Rome, his immediate superior there, Sebastian Cardinal Baggio, refused him an audience with Pope John Paul II! Thanks to Franjo Cardinal Seper, Ratzinger's predecessor, Sullivan was able to give his account and dossier on Curran to the Pope. The Holy Father supported the bishop and accorded him the special honor of giving a conjoint blessing to the thousands in the audience hall. Sullivan again demonstrated that "the brave walk in single file, while cowards hide in crowds."

On October 12, 1985, the Pope told the Filipino hierarchy that bishops are "entrusted with the task of proclaiming and defending the whole of the Church's teaching
in all its authenticity," and they must "be vigilant that
others who preach and teach in the name of the Church
should not be allowed to distort that teaching." Therefore,
he concluded, bishops must sometimes correct their "collaborators" because "a false compassion" will only end in
"undermining the truth and destroying the very harmony
that it claims to preserve."

Cardinal Ratzinger has faced Curran with "the whole
of the Church's teaching" and has told him to recant his
errors or be declared a theologian not fit to teach Catholic
doctrine, like Germany's Fr. Hans Küng. Even more astonishing than Curran's offenses is the brazen attempt of
Cardinal Bernardin to protect him.

Bernardin, whose "consistent life ethic" does not require
one to oppose contraception/abortifacients or sterilization,
went to Rome recently to work out a compromise, as did
Archbishop James Hickey of Washington before him. Six
hundred other theologians, including Jesuits Richard Mc-
Cormick and Walter Burghardt, say Rome is picking on
Curran and that countless American theologians hold the
same views. (They should *all* be disciplined.)

Meanwhile, Curran claims that all he did was to raise
legitimate questions about noninfallible teaching (all of
which binds in conscience, according to canon law and the
documents of Vatican II). If that were all he had done, it
would be bad enough. But he want far beyond that.

For Curran, no human acts are intrinsically evil, given
his theory of the "fundamental option," his strange "principle of compromise," the doctrine of "proportional reason"
and his version of "situation ethics."

Besides, since when do peers decide orthodoxy in theological matters, as if the Church were a mere human
project? If we in the West cannot even count on most of
our bishops—whose vocation is to guarantee purity of
doctrine—what can we expect of our theologians? No
theologian has the right, nor is it his role, to organize a
national (let alone international) dissent to long-standing,
official teachings of the Church—particularly on grave
moral issues. I could go on and on—but who cares, notices
or worries, let alone *acts*? Meanwhile, Bishop James Malone, president of the American hierarchy, proclaims, "The

Church in the United States is fundamentally on the right track."

Nor are we now beset with mere dissent, a "nice guy" dissenter or "dissenting theologians"; rather, we are faced with open rebellion by radical, disobedient, all-but-schismatic theologians acting in concert.

Take, for example, Curran's defiant conduct with David W. Tracy and abortion-waffling theologian Leonard Swidler. With 19 hours of phone calls, they mobilized 75 American theologians to sign a statement of support for Fr. Hans Küng within 24 hours of learning that Rome had declared him unacceptable as a Catholic theologian.

Contradicting the Holy See and the German hierarchy, the statement read, in part, "We publicly affirm our recognition that Hans Küng is indeed a Catholic theologian." So what if Küng has clearly denied official Catholic teachings on papal infallibility, the need for baptism, the Real Presence and even eternal life! (To see Curran and his rebel colleagues in action, read the Image paperback *Küng in Conflict*.)

BISHOPS EMBRACE MILITANT FEMINISM

The Church in Canada, particularly in the Province of Quebec, is fast becoming like the self-destroyed Church in Holland. Quebec has the lowest birthrate in Canada and the nation's only free-standing abortion centers. It also has the highest suicide rate in the industrial world.

Twenty-nine of Quebec's 35 Catholic bishops met in March with 86 laywomen and 13 laymen for a weekend study session to enhance the role and power of women in the Church. They concluded that the Church should extend an unconditional welcome to the remarried divorced, unmarried couples, single-parent families and others living in unconventional family situations—even, said Bishop Adolphe Proulx, to homosexual couples. There are so many exceptions to Church laws, Proulx asserted, that "there is really nothing to prevent anyone of good faith from receiving the sacraments," including Holy Communion. Has he been reading Curran-like theologians?

The conferees adopted the following resolutions, among others, by overwhelming majorities: (1) that paid women's-affairs coordinators be appointed in every diocese by May 1987; (2) that the Assembly of Quebec Bishops remain vigilant and open to the question of ordination of women and that it take the question all the way to Rome; (3) that

other steps be taken to increase women's power, including
their involvement in the training of priests, equal participation of the two sexes in liturgical celebration (altar girls
are common in Canada, contrary to explicit Church rules),
and the placement of more women in decision-making
positions; (4) that women be consulted before the Church
speaks out on sexual issues, including contraception and
abortion (the women delegates made it clear that contraception and abortion must be treated as separate issues, in
no way related); (5) that steps be taken to remove "sexually discriminating" terms from language used by the
Church. Amazingly, Quebec City's Louis-Albert Cardinal
Vachon commented, "My heart is profoundly comforted" by
these proposals!

As long ago as 1983 the Pope asked the world's bishops
to end the talk about women priests. "The bishop," he
insisted, "must give proof of his pastoral ability and leadership by withdrawing all support from individuals or groups
who in the name of progress, justice or compassion, or for
any other alleged reason, promote the ordination of women
to the priesthood."

In true radical feminist fashion, a biased female history
professor poured it on the bishops. Needed: "a parallel,
subversive power, another power" to that of men. Con-
tested: "the whole idea of authority and hierarchial structure." Predicted: Feminism will leave nothing as it was
before; not the family, not work, not social organization,
not the spiritual, not relations between the sexes. Admitted: Women have finally realized that the so-called sexual
revolution was at their expense, replacing the notion that a
woman belongs to one man with the notion that she belongs to all of them. Hallucinated: "It's difficult to imagine
that one can oppose contraception and abortion at the
same time."

To placate the feminists, there was no concelebration.
The Holy See's rules state clearly that extraordinary ministers should be used only in extraordinary circumstances,
yet the women helped distribute Communion. This was
judged an extraordinary situation, so the bishops received
Communion from women, according to reports.

In 1976 Archbishop Philip Pocock pulled all Catholic
agencies out of Toronto's United Fund (UF) when the latter
accepted Planned Parenthood. To their eternal honor, the
archbishops of Edmonton and Vancouver later did similar-
ly, with good results.

Despite the good example of these proper stances on collaboration with an "unspeakable crime" (as Vatican II called it), Ottawa's Archbishop Joseph Plourde recently declined to do the same. Officials of UF asked Plourde what he would do if they accepted PP. In no way, countered Plourde, would Catholics or others opposed to abortion pay for it. UF warned that PP might sue. Then they suggested "negative designation" at the time of donation— something that has never worked in any city. Plourde tumbled to the idea.

Obviously, the UF officials wanted his assurance that they would continue to handle the Catholic charities' huge fundraising business, even if they admitted PP to their combined campaign. By accepting their ploy, Plourde gave them that assurance.

Whether PP would actually have filed a lawsuit to force its way into the UF campaign, or would have won it, is totally irrelevant, because no court could force the Archdiocese to stay in UF with PP. PP gloated over its cheap victory, bought with a mere threat. When Plourde gave the green light, these unborn-baby-killers and youth-corrupters gained public respectability on a par with the Catholic Church itself. Plourde indirectly gave them official community acceptance, made them an official part of UF, and handed a generous cut of the unknowing citizenry's generosity to the most wicked organization on earth.

Stung by the storm of charges that he had approved PP, Plourde ran an ad in the Ottawa *Citizen* trying to defend himself. He claimed he had never approved of giving money to PP and therefore did not support them; but he overlooked the fact that he had indirectly given UF the green light to accept PP and to enable citizens to fund this evil juggernaut, which is destroying youth, family, Church and society.

PP does more than promote abortion. It gives abortifacient Pills and contraceptives to children without parental knowledge or consent. Thus, it causes more fornication and becomes an accomplice in the statutory rape of minor girls and the criminality of their fornicating boyfriends. It fosters sterilization. Its publications condone homosexuality, masturbation, oral and anal sex, pornography and even bestiality.

Surely Plourde does not approve of these horrors. Just as surely, he missed a great chance to educate the community about the evils of PP and to damage their working funds seriously—to say nothing of their horrendous "sex education" programs. PP is due to receive "only" $44,000 this year; this, however, will surely and continually increase if precedents elsewhere are any indication.

In any case, CARAL (Canadian Abortion Rights Action League), UF and PP were delighted over PP's admission into UF, according to an article appearing in the *Citizen* a few days later. PP's executive director boasted, "We know we have a lot of supporters out there." And so satanic PP won again, this time in the capital city of Canada, where they had little foothold.

ON MOTHER ANGELICA'S SHOW

On March 18 I was interviewed on TV by Mother Angelica, the extraordinary cloistered Poor Clare nun who succeeded, with faith and trust in God, in doing what the American bishops could not do with money—erecting the nation's first Catholic cable TV network. An almost $4-million-a-year operation, this miracle in the woods near Birmingham, Alabama, is still growing. Mother Angelica is now broadcasting six hours daily by satellite in 39 states. She covers 10 million homes with a daily audience of three to four million over her Eternal Word Television Network (EWTN).

Our discussion of abortion and HLI's work ran a little more than an hour. Hardly had we begun, though, when the devil knocked us off the air for seven minutes by hexing a part of the equipment which rarely malfunctions. Mother Angelica observed calmly that this was the first time the Father of Lies had succeeded in putting her off the air in five years of bringing the authentic Christian message to millions.

Like all holy ones in the hands of God, Mother Angelica is a very unusual person, simple and unsophisticated. Superior of her community of 15, she spends five hours daily before the Blessed Sacrament, which is always exposed. She wears a back brace without which she could not stand, and a foot brace without which she could not walk. Although she seems to be in constant pain, no one has ever heard her complain; she always has a smile for everyone. In all my contacts with sisters and convents, I have never met a group of nuns who so loved their superior.

Mother Angelica and her nuns emerge from the cloister only when necessary for God's work. They also run a large

Catholic publishing operation.   She employs 22 persons besides her own community.

Like St. Benedict, Mother Angelica thinks one must pray *and* work—but always pray *first*, so one's unselfish work can be the genuine reflection of prayer, that is, communion with God. There is room for only one more member in the community; serious applicants are carefully referred to other convents.

Like me, Mother Angelica believes God has lots of money and will fund a worthwhile religious project if there is enough prayer, penance and sacrifice behind it. That is why she bristles when anyone talks of budgets, which might constrain God's infinite generosity.

It was my privilege to share in praying the Office at 6:00 a.m. and to offer the Holy Mass at 7:00 a.m., with curtains opened to welcome 25 lay worshippers on the other side of the altar from the nuns. The singing was angelic, and was accompanied by an excellent violinist, two soft guitars, a quiet set of drums, and a strange-looking little organ played by Mother Angelica.

THE FEDS, FETAL COLLAGEN AND COSMETICS

A third letter of inquiry from HLI to the Food and Drug Administration concerning human collagen led to a long telephone conversation with a fine Catholic gentleman working in the division of cosmetics and technology.

He said they have had some 8,000 letters from consumers asking whether collagen from aborted babies is used in making American cosmetics. The FDA has made some 450 investigations in the USA, and they are moving to require American cosmetic firms to specify on their packages whether the collagen is human or animal. He seemed to know little about European cosmetics.

KISS GERMANY AND THE WEST GOODBYE

Evil as Curran's teachings are, and scandalous as our bishops' toleration of them may be, German theologians such as Gründel, Böckle and Auer have gone much farther, unchecked and unhindered by their prelates.

The frightening results can be seen in a prestigious recent poll of German Catholic thinking: only 23 percent of practicing Catholics feel obligated to obey the pope in serious moral and doctrinal matters; only five percent of adult Catholics actually accept the full authentic teaching of the Catholic Church. Most of the young are ignorant of the Faith and therefore are more or less lost to the Church.

Thanks to the subtlety of the abortion law, the German Catholic Church is paid for its direct involvement in abortion through the "counseling" system (leftist theologians justify this easily).

For consistently exposing this and other horrors, a fine Pallottine priest who works with HLI was dismissed from his chaplaincy. They are allowing him to continue his prolife work on his own, but only because he is too well-known for them to treat any more shabbily. He is the tenth active prolife priest in the world whom I know personally who has suffered persecution like this. In the Western Church, disloyal theologians such as Curran, McCormick and McBrien are allowed to propagate their errors in the name of "academic freedom," while loyal priests are silenced, fired, exiled, ridiculed, defamed, and robbed of livelihood. But then, did our Lord not predict as much?

In his *Die Verhütete Zukunft* (The Contracepted Future), the well-known French historian Pierre Chaunu has exposed the sinister "population explosion" propaganda that led to the current war on people. He draws a frightening picture of the long-range consequences of low birthrates, which he predicts the corrupt West will succeed in bringing about worldwide.

According to Chaunu's calculations, for example, by the year 2080 Germany's present 60 million inhabitants will have shrunk to 10–12 million. At that rate the industrialized nations, which have 25 percent of the world's people today, will have only 8.8 percent a century from now. The handwriting is on the wall.

Look at the present demographic disaster in the West, created by the contraception-sterilization-abortion that accompanies the copulation explosion. Never in the history of Christianity has there been better evidence that what the Church has always taught about sexual morality and marriage, summarized in *Humanae Vitae*, is correct, true and indispensable. Depart from it and you get sexual chaos, mass murder of babies, and dying nations. But with Curran-type theologians infesting the Church, and with bishops approving or tolerating them, how can this self-destruction be stopped?

CATHOLICS AMONG THE WOLVES

The Wanderer (27 March 1986) ran HLI's exposé of the incredible Rome-bashing weekend seminar on modern "Catholic" marriage, sponsored by "Catholic" Dayton University and baptized by Bishop Raymond A. Lucker. Five of the participants at the seminar were signers of the recent *New York Times* full-page pro-abortion ad. Rebel Catholics hawked a petition of support for Fr. Curran. We infiltrated that meeting and several others recently. Here are capsule reports on two of the worst:

—Fifteen hundred PP types came to Washington for the annual convention of the Children's Defense Fund (CDF). One of the most urgent topics was, in effect, how to contracept-sterilize-abort the racial minorities out of existence in the United States.

The various PP-type speakers were beside themselves over the high level of premarital intercourse, pregnancy, illegitimacy and abortion among blacks. They were almost in a panic because Catholic Hispanics, already 7.2 percent of the population, are growing five times faster than the general population and will be the largest minority in the year 2000. The "solution" proposed? More immoral "sex education" and "comprehensive health [read: abortifacients/-birth control] centers" in the high schools.

You would be shocked at the hatred of Catholics, the Church and the Pope poured out at these meetings. And you will be saddened to learn that pro-abortion former Congressman Fr. Robert Drinan, SJ, offered the invocation at CDF's breakfast! He sat at the head table and applauded the "Planned Parenthood Players'" dirty skits on stage.

Fortunately, Sr. Barbara Spears, OSP, field rep for urban parishes in Washington's archdiocesan Office of Religious Education, did not appear as scheduled; she was supposed to invoke a blessing on the "congregation" at the noon luncheon the same day. How Satan uses so-called Catholics these days!

—Even worse was the speech of "Catholic" Ms. Frances Kissling, executive director of the pro-abortion, *Playboy*-funded Catholics for a Free Choice, at the National Family Planning and Reproductive Health Association Convention. The lying and distortions were incredible. Receiving honorable mention from this Church-hater were Fr. Richard McCormick, SJ, of Georgetown University's Kennedy

Center, Fr. Charles Curran, the U.S. Catholic Conference's Fr. Bryan Hehir, South African Archbishop Denis Hurley, and the 12 national hierarchies (out of about 130) who dissented to *Humanae Vitae*.

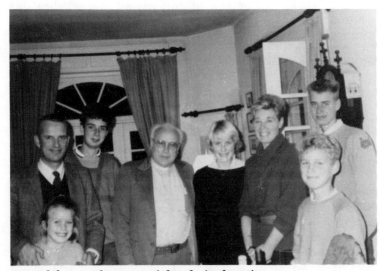

Dr. Philippe Schepens and family (Belgium).

700 CONTRIBUTE TO SYMPOSIUM

(No. 22—July 1986)

From 22 countries, 35 states and all 10 Canadian provinces, almost 700 leaders and activists came to our Second Annual International Symposium on Human Sexuality in Montreal, 23–27 April. The networking, information-gathering and cross-fertilization was intense.

Many conferees told me that there was not one talk that was not good. Some insisted that, after a lifetime of attending meetings of all kinds, this was by far the most impressive conference they had ever shared. They were astonished at the quality and variety of speakers and participants, all leaders and activists totally committed to life, family, Church and pope.

John Cavanaugh-O'Keefe of HLI, Joe Scheidler and a hundred others picketed an illegal but government-tolerated abortion mill that kills 5,000 babies annually. For once the media, both French and English, were rather fair to us. The symposium and demonstration received national TV and front-page newspaper coverage, as an estimated six million Canadians heard the prolife/pro-family message.

The symposium was a deeply spiritual experience. We began it with a Mass, had two Masses daily and ended with a Mass. At the closing Mass, Chief Andrew Delisle of the Iroquois-Mohawk nation shared with us the beautiful prayer he had offered before the Pope earlier. Many prayed the Rosary daily.

The Mexican Catholic hierarchy has officially invited us to hold the third symposium in Mexico City from 29 April to 3 May 1987. Mexico's bishops are wisely and totally prolife and pro-family. Unlike some bishops elsewhere, they know their people's high birthrate gives them a place in the future.

In Montreal we presented HLI's second International Human Life Award for doing the most in the past year to save the unborn, to Christine de Vollmer of Caracas, Venezuela. Her great work and that of her organization has made Venezuela the most prolife country in Latin America.

With the help of Mrs. de Vollmer, other prolife leaders in Latin America, and our branches in Mexico City and

Buenos Aires, HLI will use the Mexico City symposium to
organize the whole continent and subcontinent against the
population controllers. Like me, Christine and other leaders in Latin America believe we can still save that continent from the abortion imperialists of the wealthy West,
where the Church is fast dying.

Our goal is a major escalation of our war to save the
family in that Catholic continent which, with Africa, will
have some 70 percent of the world's Catholics in the year
2000. To do this we will need lots of financing, because
Latin America is poor; but God has lots of money.

EPISCOPAL PARALYSIS IN CANADA

You should know that our record crowd in Montreal
came despite the boycott of Auxiliary Bishop Leonard J.
Crowley, who is in charge of 43 English-speaking parishes
in French Montreal. Bishop Crowley seems to be more at
home with radical feminists and homosexuals than with
prolifers.

For example, Crowley was the TV spokesman for 29
Quebec bishops who met with some 100 radical feminists
and, with the approval of those radicals, passed the dangerous resolutions listed in *Special Report No. 21.* That
meeting, said a famous Canadian Catholic, was "a complete
affront to the Pope."

The bishop had this to say to all his pastors about HLI
in the April issue of his *Newsnotes:*

CONCERNING HUMAN LIFE INTERNATIONAL

I wish to inform you that I had been invited to
give the opening prayer at the Symposium in Montreal on April 23. I wrote to Sister Lucille Durocher, Director of Human Life International Canada, and stated "that I am unable at this time to
associate myself with Human Life International, as
I cannot support the objectives and the manner in
which this organization operates. There has been
an evident lack of respect towards persons and
their right to their reputation; also I cannot agree
with the limited perspective taken by the organization on the whole area of human life. The written
statements against my fellow bishops who are
judged without a hearing are repugnant to me.
Furthermore, Respect for Life (Respect de la Vie,

Mouvement d'Education) has the approval of and is financed by the dioceses.

What is one to make of a bishop of a dying church in a dying country who tells his priests and people not to attend a totally orthodox international meeting boasting the largest gathering of pro-family/prolife experts ever assembled anywhere? The many thousands across the world who know what HLI does will see through his statement; like us, they will feel sorry for him and will pray for him especially.

In a year of prolife/pro-family work in Montreal and in the province of Quebec, we have detected comparatively little prolife activity in this, the most Catholic province of Canada. Even worse, Quebec has the nation's lowest birthrate and tolerates Canada's only free-standing abortion clinics, which are contrary to federal law. Recently the Quebec government agreed to pay for vasectomies as a health service. Quebec prolifers have told us they receive only $3,000 annually from the bishops and little episcopal encouragement. (HLI donated $74,000 to its Canadian branch in one year.) The Canadian national hierarchy has issued seven statements on respect for life since 1967. But episcopal statements, even if many people read them, are no substitute for actions. Besides, the last statement was a "seamless garment" document.

The recent statement of the Pope seems a kind of rebuke: "An extreme sensitivity akin to a holy reaction is felt when attempts on life are made in the form of famine, war, and terrorism; yet, one cannot find this feeling of sensitivity when faced with abortion, which takes the lives of innumerable innocent beings" (12 February 1986).

In all sincerity and charity: pray for Bishop Crowley, who boycotted HLI but recently made himself a part of a national weekend conference of Dignity, an organization of Catholic homosexuals (mostly active). He offered Mass for them. (Our investigative reporter was excluded from the conference. What are they hiding?) In his homily Crowley said, "If He made you different, He has given you gifts that no one else has. We are what we are."

"Which gifts?" some Canadians asked. Others asked when Crowley will offer a Mass for unrepentant fornicators or adulterers. What prompts these questions is the overwhelming evidence (and the Biblical truth) that homosexuals are not born as homosexuals, that homosexuality is a

learned aberration/perversion/sin which a bishop should not
encourage in any way, although he should be prudently
pastoral in helping the afflicted sinner to reform.

The president of Dignity/Canada commented on Crowley's action: "It makes a powerful statement of ministry
[that] bishops should be providing to homosexual people.
It breaks new territory. It makes it easier for the next
bishop."

In all fairness to Crowley, in the first of two long
articles the Dignity conference engendered, he did say
beforehand that "obviously, the Church disagrees with
homosexual practices." But a world authority on healing
for homosexuals who has a program called "Courage" tried
to contact Crowley and got the runaround.

In 1984 a pornographic play, *Les enfants n'ont pas de
sex?* (Children Have No Sex?) was making the rounds in
elementary Catholic schools in Montreal, pegged as "sex
education." Parents, teachers and some nuns objected, and
turned to Bishop Crowley for advice. He said it was up to
the parents to oppose it, and if they did not approve, to
keep their children home on the days it was shown.

Later he told an objecting nun that there was nothing
he could do because the government claims "bishops and
priests know nothing about sex; it is up to the parents to
fight it." Does Bishop Crowley really believe these battles
can be fought without leadership from the hierarchy?
These days, bishops had better be well informed about
human sexuality and above all about sexual morality. The
Pope seems to know a great deal about the subject!

Bishop Crowley accused HLI of "an evident lack of
respect toward persons and their right to their reputation,"
and complains that "written statements against my fellow
bishops who are judged without a hearing are repugnant to
me."

On the advice of our board, we will offer Bishop Crowley two pages in our next semi-private *Special Report* and
1,000 words in our very public international newsletter
HLI Reports, so he can point out to us where we have
been untruthful, unfair or whatever. We did not attack
Crowley personally; we merely commented on what he has
done and said publicly. We never judge. We always try
hard to publish only what is accurate and just. We will
retract and make amends if we miss the mark.

But these days one is reminded of St. Thomas Aquinas'
13th-century dictum, "If the Faith is in imminent peril,

prelates ought to be accused by their subjects, even in public." Or, as St. Pius X remarked about 75 years ago with reference to the Modernism of his time, "The greatest obstacle in the apostolate of the Church is the timidity, or rather, the cowardice, of the faithful."

We appreciate Montreal Archbishop Paul Gregoire's "best wishes."

While in Canada I debated a female abortion-doctor for 30 minutes on TV. The show will be screened in September in Quebec, Ontario and the Maritime Provinces. I was also called in as a consultant to the Law Reform Commission in Ottawa, which has been given an impossible mandate to come up with some kind of abortion reform which will please everybody.

I also had a good two-hour session with the Catholic School Commission of Greater Montreal, who came out with a good *Humanae Vitae*-type statement on sexual morality, which their French counterparts are ridiculing in the name of "pluralism." Thanks to Gordon Taylor, a Protestant Member of Parliament, I was able to speak to a small group of prolife MP's on abortion and euthanasia.

HOLLAND—SCHISM, EUTHANASIA, ISLAM

On 8 May 1986, 10,000 members of the liberal, schismatic National "Catholic" Association met for the second time in Den Bosch. Although invited, all the bishops refused to attend this amalgam of ex-priests, nuns, leftists, intellectuals and others who claim they are the People of God and do not need Rome. Confirming them in their views was the Dominican Fr. Edward Schillebeeckx, who "preached" to them, beginning with "My dear People . . ." I saw his sermon on TV. If it contained any authentic Christianity I failed to detect it, but his followers gave him a rousing ovation.

A young Filipina urged the audience to change the Church from the bottom because *they* were the real People of God and must be a catalyst, as were Filipino Catholics recently. Besides repeated complaints that the bishops' absence showed stupidity, there was dancing, hugging and other signs of solidarity with homosexuals, nuns in and out of habit, and much else. This was more or less the same group—then 12,000—who met to reject the Pope beforehand more than a year ago before he came to Holland. (Fr. Schillebeeckx coached that gathering, too.)

Then came the Eucharist, celebrated with a priest and vested women at the altar. With the whole mob, they read the words of a strange canon, including the words of consecration, over piles of noncanonical bread. (After all, Fr. Schillebeeckx had assured them long ago that they were all priests.) They sang songs written by a priest who had married a nun, fathered two children by her, and then (no doubt with love) divorced her. A nun-feminist out of habit preached a message of glorified humanism.

Meanwhile, on "Catholic" TV, which is controlled by these schismatics, a pro-abortion lady-chairperson who is all for free sex called the affair "a grandiose celebration," while hoping a dialogue with the bishops could begin. But because of costs, she expressed doubt that another demonstration would take place.

"Women in the Catholic Church," a small organization that meets bi-monthly, works with the bishops to convert Holland back to authentic Catholicism. Because Confession is almost unheard of, Adrianus Cardinal Simonis recently wondered out loud in his packed cathedral how many of those communicating were actually prepared spiritually.

The great bishop of Roermond, Joannis Gijsen, is establishing a full Family Life Center emphasizing NFP, marriage preparation, educational courses for Catholic parenthood, and other family programs. He has half of Holland's 175 seminarians in his orthodox seminary, which he established to teach the authentic Catholic faith. Although 35 percent of the schools are Catholic in name, their teachers are mostly non-believing or non-practicing, with many ex-priests and ex-nuns teaching "theology."

On the good side, the Christian Democrats won convincingly in a recent national election. Even better, the newly elected government is not likely to pass an active euthanasia law in the near future, even though the Dutch Supreme Court paved the way for it. During the previous administration, a private member's bill called for such direct killing in some cases.

But according to London's *Financial Times* (18 February 1986), up to 10,000 deaths recorded annually under "natural causes" in Holland are in fact a direct result of euthanasia. Dutch prolifers confirm this. I recall my shock in 1975 when Dutch prolife doctors told me that euthanasia was by no means unknown. Perhaps you had the same feelings recently when the *60 Minutes* TV show featured these Dutch medical murders.

Incidentally, the 500,000 Moslems in Holland have built the world's first mosque for women in Amsterdam, financed by various Islamic countries. It will be the spiritual center of Moslem women's groups in Western Europe. According to the leader of this "prayerhouse," the mosque will give Moslem women an opportunity to witness to their faith and to study the Koran and their tradition. Islamic culture centers and mosques function in many cities and communities in Holland and throughout Europe.

H.L.I. HELPS HEROIC BELGIANS

This country of 10 million Catholics is the only continental European country which has not yet legalized abortion. But an election is coming, and the new government will almost certainly try to do so. Belgium is totally Catholic on paper, but only 25 percent (at most) attend Mass weekly.

There are two national prolife groups, but the bishops consider them "extremists" and, except for one bishop, do not work with them. When confronted, the bishops say abortion is a "political" issue and everyone knows the Church is against abortion. They give abundant evidence that they do not realize the horrors that befell neighboring countries that embraced abortion, or do not seem to care. Meanwhile, the 800,000 Moslems increase and multiply, making up to 25 percent of the population of Brussels.

Prolife leaders with whom I have often conversed at length assure me that not one Belgian priest is actively involved in prolife work. Paid by the State, priests live comfortably, naively thinking that the abortifacient Pill is the great remedy for abortion. They know little or nothing about NFP, except in one small diocese where the bishop knows what needs to be done. Thanks largely to Cardinal Suenens, a Charismatic, the Belgian hierarchy dissented from *Humanae Vitae*. Prolife leaders believe the present cardinal rejects that prophetic encyclical of Pope Paul VI.

The same leaders gave me at least two weeks of work sending them documents and data with which to arm prolife parliamentarians to stave off the worst. Unlike most bishops and priests, these courageous, informed lay people know what will come to Belgium if abortion is legalized; they see how Belgium could be a great example to the world in refusing to take part in abortion, the greatest war of all time. But already many from this "Catholic"

land of few children go to surrounding countries to have
their babies killed.

BIG SINS IN LITTLE LUXEMBOURG

The German-speaking countries of Austria, West Germany, Switzerland, Luxembourg and Lichtenstein all have
more coffins than cradles, suffering virtually the lowest
birthrates in the world and having many foreigners, about
one-third Moslems, who have large families.

There are some fine bishops and priests, of course, but
in general it would come as a total shock to a serious,
practicing American Catholic to learn the incredible moral,
theological, religious and episcopal situation in these hedonistic countries. Counting all abortions, there are more
baby-murders than births in these lands, unbelievably
poisoned by uncontrolled theologians far worse than Catholic University of America's Curran, Georgetown University's McCormick and Notre Dame's McBrien.

Like individuals, nations learn little from their neighbors. So wealthy, Catholic Luxembourg now has an un-
usually low birthrate. One of three marriages ends in
divorce; many of the youth are guilty of the "alternative
lifestyle" we used to call "shacking up." Churches are
virtually empty, as are novitiates and even parish houses.
The median age of priests and religious is 62 years.

The Luxembourgers outdid the West Germans by passing an even more permissive abortion law. (Parents have
to repay the health service for killing their child, though.)
Out of a population of 350,000, one-fourth of whom are
foreigners, the Movement for Preborn Life has only about
3,000 members.

ABORTIONISTS PROFIT FROM RED FALLOUT

While I was in Europe the papers were filled with the
fallout from Chernobyl. Only after the Scandinavian skies
were loaded with radioactive particles did the Communist
authorities admit to the tragedy. The German newspapers
say the Soviets evacuated 255,000 adults, plus all of the
children.

Pregnant women in Germany flocked to the abortion
mills. Pro-abortion Health Minister Rita Süssmuth, who is
also Vice President of the German Catholic Women, gave a
clear directive, however, that abortion was not called for.
She said the level of radioactivity was too low, no matter
what local doctors advised. Despite her pro-abortionism,

she is still concerned about her country's tragically low birthrate.

LOYOLA HONORS KILLER OF 18 MILLION

If Planned Parenthood ever invites me to address its national convention, I will better understand why "Catholic" Loyola Marymount Law School in Los Angeles invited U.S. Supreme Court Justice William J. Brennan, Jr., to be its commencement speaker on June 1.

Brennan, as you know, was one of the two justices most responsible for the 1973 *Roe v. Wade* decision that has put to death more than 18 million innocent preborn babies. (The other was Blackmun.) Arguably the bloodiest and must unjust judge of all time, "Catholic" Brennan has voted pro-abortion repeatedly since then.

But LMU of Los Angeles has rolled out the red carpet for other leading advocates of child murder as well. On 12 March 1986, "Catholic" NOW President Eleanor Smeal spoke on campus, despite protests from faithful Catholics. She attacked *Humanae Vitae* and pushed abortion, abortifacients, contraception and sterilization. She insisted the unborn baby is "not a child" and is not living. She even said the federal government should force Catholic and other hospitals to commit abortion on demand. (Strangely, the Catholic press ignored her appearance at the school named for St. Ignatius and the Blessed Mother.)

According to a handout from Law School Dean Arthur Frakt, the Law School has had speeches by pro-abortion and anti-Catholic Sen. Fritz Hollings (D, SC) and by Rep. Patricia Schroeder (D, CO), one of Congress' worst abortion advocates.

Moreover, they gave the St. Thomas More Law Honor Society Medallion to Harvard Law Professor Laurence Tribe, one of the world's top abortion lawyers, "for his contributions to the legal profession." Tribe filed the abortion lobby's brief to block President Reagan's effort to overturn *Roe*. He is also leading the fight to overturn the last U.S. laws against sodomy. There is no room here to list the other abortion backers LMU has honored.

Catholics and Protestants protested Brennan's appearance with phone calls, letters, leafletting, a press conference and a prayer vigil/demonstration that attracted 75 people, including one priest. Hundreds of people attending the commencement made hostile remarks or gestures, often

obscene, at the prolifers. (One girl shouted, "F------
priest!")

Fundamentalist Baptists had an airplane overhead
trailing the words "PRAY FOR DEATH: BABY-KILLER
BRENNAN." Newspapers across the USA ran stories and
pictures.

Professor Michael Lightfoot introduced Brennan as "the
conscience of the nation." Brennan was applauded by
priests, religious and most of the laity present.

The great prolife activist Joe Scheidler flew in from
Chicago to interrupt and denounce a startled Brennan.
Security guards dragged Joe out violently, twisting his arm
painfully and breaking his bullhorn, presumably in the
name of dialogue, academic freedom and what Dean
Frakt's handout calls "intellectual intercourse." Also forced
out was Heather McCormack, a young mother who is one
of Australia's most dedicated prolife leaders.

The Los Angeles archdiocese refused to tell callers
Archbishop Mahony's position on Brennan's appearance,
although they did say he had written to Frakt.

May God have mercy on Catholic higher education.
And may no prolifer ever give another penny to a school
such as LMU.

GERMAN PROLIFERS vs.
PILL-PUSHING THEOLOGIANS

(No. 23—August 1986)

In this land of more coffins than cradles (and the world's lowest birthrate), prolifers sponsored a day of national remembrance on May 10, the 50th anniversary of the German doctors' first killing of mental patients, at Hadamar. With other speakers, I told some 1,000 demonstrators that Hitlerian thinking was indeed very much alive, not only in Germany but also across the world, where the war on the unborn kills many more in one year than died on both sides in World War II.

Four deadly weapons in this war on the preborn are the abortifacient birth control Pills, IUDs, injections and implants. For eight days a German lady researcher and I continued HLI's intensive investigations for a scientifically unassailable document proving that *all* Pills abort at least sometimes, as do IUDs, "contraceptive" injections (Depo-Provera) and implants (Norplant).

Much of our data has been supervised by German medical school scientists, checked and double-checked. Some of this proof goes back to 1962. Reliable Europeans told me long ago that a group of scientists visited Pope Paul VI to tell him that the Pill did not just work contraceptively. What a fool the Pope would have been to have approved the Pill and contraception!

Today we see that the real fools were (and still are) disloyal theologians such as Curran, McCormick, Häring, McBrien, and their many rebellious cohorts. A German woman has a letter from Fr. Häring, Curran's mentor, wherein the German theologian wrote that the condom was immoral but the Pill was acceptable because it "allowed normal intercourse." In those days Häring also wrote that the Pill merely puts the ovaries "in repose"!

Germany's foremost rebel moral theologian is Fr. Franz Böckle, who is much farther off the orthodox track than Curran. As early as 1976 he admitted, on the basis of the evidence, that 20 percent of the low-dose, combination birth control Pills fail to suppress ovulation—and therefore abort.   But he justified their use morally on the basis of proportionalism (Guterabwagung).

When Böckle celebrated his 65th birthday recently, the usually orthodox Cardinal Höffner congratulated him profusely, even though no moral theologian in Europe has done more harm.   So an orthodox theologian protested this strange contradictory behavior and sent Höffner a great talk given by the Pope to 123 orthodox theologians who met recently in Rome—a speech which clearly contradicted Böckle's teaching.

Amazingly, the Cardinal wrote back calmly to say that indeed the Pope was right, that unless there are absolute moral norms (which Böckle has denied for years), the whole of morality collapses!   No wonder the faithful are utterly confused and the Pope keeps saying that they have a right to be given clear moral norms.

Another nightmare: in the March 1986 issue of the prestigious German journal *Renovation*, the German Catholic Doctors' Organization published an incredible justification of the Pill and the IUD for the guidance of, and at the request of, the German hierarchy!   The document is already being completely refuted scientifically and morally by honest Germans.   The faces of the bishops and Böckle-type theologians will be red indeed, as it becomes clear that the doctors and theologians deceived the bishops—and are still deceiving them.   And the dissent of 12 national bishops' conferences (mostly European) from *Humanae Vitae* will be even more embarrassing and scandalous than it was in 1968.

GREECE LEGALIZES ABORTION, H.L.I. RESPONDS

This June the anti-American Socialist government of Premier Andreas Papandreou legalized abortion for the first three months of pregnancy.   The mothers do not have to give any reason, and the taxpayers pay for the murders. Both Orthodox and Catholic Churches protested in vain, steamrollered by the usual antilife tactics, arguments and lies.

Papandreou's American-born second wife is an ardent feminist.   This summer she addressed the viciously pro-abortion convention of NOW in Denver.

In 1968 I spent 15 days in beautiful Athens lecturing to US Air Force chaplains.   In hours of discussion with an American gynecologist who cared for American and some Greek wives, I learned that the most common gynecological problem in Greece was miscarriage—a result of women's having two or three abortions before marriage. According to international abortion literature, at least one Greek child is killed for every successful birth, and most likely more.

Greece, with its 2,000 islands, is the size of New York State. Of the 169 inhabited islands, Crete is the largest. It has 500,000 residents, including 50,000 Americans who mostly mind missiles aimed at the USSR. Greece has almost 10 million people; a below-replacement birthrate of 1.9 children per completed family (you need 2.2 for survival); an aging society; a 55 percent unemployment rate; and government-controlled communications media.

Greece's population is 98.5 percent Greek. An amazing 97 percent belong to the Greek Orthodox Church, but only about 50 percent attend Mass weekly, and most stay only a few minutes.

The punishment for abortion is three to five years' deprivation of Holy Communion. Since World War II, two million have emigrated; one million went to Europe, mostly to Germany. The Orthodox Church has always allowed divorce, which complicates ecumenical efforts severely. Not much seminary training or theological sophistication is required of Orthodox priests, which may explain their abundance. Also, many function only on Sunday. Most Orthodox priests are married.

Roman Catholics of the Latin Rite number almost 50,000, served by three bishops and approximately 110 priests, 50 nuns and 40 brothers. There are only about 1,000 Greek Catholic Uniates. They have their own bishop and are also united with Rome. The Islands of Syros (about 5,000 people) and Tinos (3,500) are almost entirely Roman Catholic; some 30,000 Roman Catholics live in Athens, a city of four million. Mixed marriage is a big problem.

The government pays the salaries of Orthodox priests. This made it difficult for the Orthodox Church to resist the Socialist government's reduction of religious instruction in public schools from five hours a week to one hour—and the same government's promotion of contraception on TV. Foreign Catholic priests are welcomed as tourists, but none may function in Greece for fear that they might make converts.

Tourism in Greece has all but dried up because of fear of terrorism. But in November I will spend 10 days there to set up HLI's fifteenth foreign branch, to start a prolife movement, and to flush out ubiquitous Planned Parenthood. The Greeks have NOTHING to ward off these family-destroyers and baby-killers.

HURRAH FOR THE IRISH!

They did it again! Three years ago the Gaels turned back the abortionists by a vote of two to one in a national referendum. In a new referendum on June 26, they voted three to two to keep their 45-year-old constitutional ban on divorce, thanks to the leadership of the Catholic bishops and the labors of alert lay people.

The laity made effective use of Stanford professor Lenore Weitzman's recent study, *The Divorce Revolution: The Unexpected Social and Economic Consequences for Women and Children in America.* This monumental work proved divorce has been a total disaster for women and children in the Western world. The anti-divorce people delivered a clever publication with excerpts from Weitzman to every home.

In both referenda, Prime Minister Garret FitzGerald's theologian advisor was Fr. Enda McDonagh, Ireland's Charles Curran. Like Curran, McDonagh teaches at a pontifical institution, Maynooth Seminary. The "progressive" FitzGerald may have committed political suicide by calling for the two referenda.

But not all is well in the Emerald Isle. Since 1980, when Ireland welcomed a record 74,388 babies, the decline in births has been disastrous. Today the birthrate is even lower than Northern Ireland's. Even so, at 2.7 children per completed family, Ireland is today the only developed nation with a good, reproductive birthrate.

Last year's PP-backed law permitting contraception for the unmarried has contributed to moral decline among the Irish. Working with FitzGerald's health ministry, PP is spreading its barnyard sex education. Sterilization is increasing, too. And PP and the radical feminists refer about 4,000 girls to England each year for abortions. Pornography is more and more visible. Ireland is no longer a Christian haven; even in the remotest glen, the farmers can tune in trash from four British and two national TV channels. Meanwhile, the Catholic bishops have denounced *in vitro* fertilization as immoral and dehumanizing.

MICHIGAN BISHOPS SAVE ABORTION FUNDING

When people no longer follow clear moral guidelines, grotesque things happen. I was lecturing in Michigan recently when Rep. Fred Dillingham added an amendment to the $1.4 billion state Medicaid bill, to delete the $6 million budgeted for killing some 19,000 preborn babies of the poor. Michigan's Catholic bishops wrote to every representative urging them not to vote for the amendment!

Catholic members of the House whom I consulted were stunned. Were the bishops sacrificing 19,000 babies to get the $94 million budgeted for their charities? Were they ready to commit or tolerate a great evil to do good? Some speculated that the bishops were trying to preserve pro-abortionist ex-nun Agnes Mansour's social services budget.

Dillingham, a Catholic, was so incensed that he telegraphed the Pope to ask what the Catholic Church really taught about abortion. The newspapers reported that Archbishop Edmund Szoka, chairman of the bishops' conference, was "infuriated" at this. He demanded an apology from Dillingham. To add salt to Szoka's wounds, Sr. Rose Michael, a prolife Loretto nun from Texas who claims to work for the Pope, personally lobbied the Catholic lawmakers. (Later, she was falsely accused of threatening them with excommunication if they voted to spend money to kill preborn babies).

Michiganders remarked on the spectacle of her hovering visibly in the balcony, in full habit, as legislators enacted the prolife amendment. In disgust, a pro-abortion representative said facetiously that the House might as well pass an amendment to spend $20 million more to pay for the care of the 19,000 "unwanted" children who would be born. A fellow legislator took this as a motion and seconded it, and it passed by a wide margin (with nun in balcony)!

Now the bishops had an ideal bill: $94 million for their charities, no money for abortions, and $20 million added for the children of the poor who would be saved. But did they write each House member urging them to pass it? No! Suppose the Medicaid bill had included six million dollars to kill 19,000 people over 80 years of age (or all of the Michigan bishops, as frustrated taxpayers suggested cynically)—would the bishops have acted the same way?

Eventually, pro-abortion Gov. James Blanchard vetoed the Medicaid bill. It was resubmitted without the prolife amendment, and passed. So Michigan will continue to be one of the 14 states which pay for the killing of preborn children. Obviously, when you abandon consistent moral principles, "seamless garment" morality can get even bishops into ludicrous and shameful situations.

ELEVEN STEPS TO SOLVE THE VOCATION CRISIS

At the American bishops' last national meeting, there was plenty of hand-wringing about the disastrous religious vocations situation. But only Boston's Bernard Cardinal Law seemed to get at the almost obvious roots: he listed contraception and abortion among seven causes.

The reasons for the vocations debacle do not seem difficult to discover. In the first place, countless young men and women who would normally consider religious commitment *simply are not there, because Catholic parents aborted or contracepted them.* They are unseen casualties of the sexual revolution.

When sex becomes fun and games, and chastity a strange virtue that is rarely taught, even more rarely preached and therefore comparatively little practiced, one should not expect our disappearing young people to desire the celibate state. Even many priests ignore chastity, judging from such scandals as the 50 homosexual priests in trouble with American courts because of pederasty.

Any abuse of God's awesome gifts of sexuality and fertility always strikes hard at the family. But it is from truly loving, unselfish families that most of the priests and religious of the past have come. Every worthy study of religious vocations I have ever seen, anywhere in the world, shows that priests and religious come mostly from fair-sized families with deeply believing parents. Persistently low Catholic birthrates foretell the future.

Visiting Canada recently, Cardinal Lubachivsky of the Ukrainian Catholic Church urged Ukrainian Catholics to help solve North America's vocations crisis by having more children.

Are there any bishops or religious superiors so naive as to think they will fill their seminaries or novitiates out of the wounded families of contracepting, aborting, sterilized or divorced Catholic parents, who today average fewer than two children? Well over 30 percent of American parents married 10 years or more, or with two children, have sterilized themselves! The figures for Catholics are virtually the same as for the rest of the population. According to census data, more than 50 percent of married American couples in their child-bearing years are now infertile.

What have our bishops said about (1) chastity, (2) contraception, (3) abortifacients, (4) serious and orthodox premarital education, (5) divorce, (6) sterilization and (7) natural family planning? Are they aware of the sorry state of the Catholic school system, at all levels? Do they understand how radical feminists are devastating Catholic belief? Have they noticed the cancer of secular feminism eating up the convents of active women religious, some of whom conduct Wiccan (witchcraft) rituals?

Sometimes I am tempted to think the vocation shortage is a punishment from God upon our hierarchy. They have actually helped destroy the family by failing to defend sexual morality, and by giving theologians such as Catholic University's Curran, Notre Dame's McBrien, and Georgetown's McCormick a free rein to speak, write, and teach against the clear directives of both pope and Magisterium.

Amid the hedonistic corruption of the fourth century, St. John Chrysostom put his finger on the problem: "When marriage is not esteemed, neither can consecrated virginity or celibacy exist. When human sexuality is not regarded as a great value given by the Creator, the renunciation of it for the sake of the Kingdom of Heaven loses its meaning."

If the bishops really want to solve the vocation crisis, they will have to (1) uphold bravely the Church's teachings on sexual morality and chastity; (2) prepare young people for marriage with orthodox pre-marriage courses that include NFP, as Poland's bishops do; (3) emphasize the blessedness of children as gifts from God; (4) rid the seminaries of all Curran-like theologians and also homosexuals; (5) discard psychological tests that screen out orthodox applicants for the priesthood; (6) make the Catholic school system and CCD truly Catholic again; (7) courageously implement the Holy See's directives in making Catholic universities and colleges live up to their name; (8) root out the secular feminism that is poisoning the hearts of so many women religious; (9) teach people to pray again; (10) invite the faithful to self-denial; and (11) lead everyone back to the confessional.

Pope John Paul II has said and written all of this eloquently, over and over. But you would never know it

from reading official diocesan literature or the censored
diocesan press. You have to read *L'Osservatore Romano*
weekly to see for yourself.

POPULATION CONTROLLERS FUME OVER H.L.I.

HLI's enemies are increasing their attacks on us all
over the world. But this only proves the effectiveness of
our work.

A recent blast came from population control fanatic
Werner Fornos, president of the multi-million-dollar Population Institute in Washington. Fornos ripped me and HLI
this March in a personal letter to my friend Frances Frech
of the Population Renewal Office in Kansas City:

> Father Paul Marx of Family [sic] Life Interna-
> tional has given us a preview of what anti-family
> planning fanatics think of Third World people. He
> opposes family planning because, if Third World
> couples can freely exercise their basic human rights
> regarding fertility, Catholic missionaries will be
> denied the opportunity to convert pagans! In Fa-
> ther Marx's eyes, Third World babies are mere
> pawns in some religious chess game.

The April issue of the Institute's *Popline* described HLI
as "an aggressive anti–family planning organization." On
the contrary, Mr. Sterilizer, Population-Controller-at-Any-
Price and Pro-Abortionist Fornos, we are FOR true family
planning: chastity before and in marriage, and NFP if
necessary. *You* should admit *you* are aggressively anti-
people.

The same *Popline* unfavorably reviewed and lied about
our stinging *The Deadly Neo-Colonialism*, which exposed
the coercive U.S. population program in Bangladesh. *Popline* also wailed about the growing prolife resistance in
Latin America and Kenya. We have poured more audiovisual aids and literature into that continent and that
country than any others. Much of this potent material
goes to our branch in Nairobi, but a great deal also goes to
seminary heads and veteran Irish missionary nuns who
spread it far and wide.

SIGNS OF HOPE
AMID JAPAN'S PROBLEMS

(No. 24—October 1986)

In 1948 Planned Parenthood and its cohorts sneaked the Eugenics Protection Law through the Diet (parliament) as part of an omnibus bill. Most members of the Diet thought they were voting only to abort babies who had defects. Since then Japan's 13,000 gynecologists—only they are allowed to commit abortions, because they are given special training—have killed more than 60 million babies.

As always happens when it is legalized, abortion in Japan has become a primary means of birth control, the others being the condom and the primitive calendar rhythm method practiced by some 20 percent. Likewise, as always happens, the killer doctors gained control of the medical schools and journals, thus increasingly corrupting the whole medical profession.

The average fertile Japanese wife now has three to five abortions in her married lifetime. With typical fatalism, the Japanese hide abortions away quietly. There is no euphemizing. The Japanese never talk about abortion; they are ashamed of it.

The wonderful Takato Honma, president of the Japanese Catholic women's group, has told HLI again and again how enormously (although silently) Japanese women suffer from having killed their children. The only solutions, she says, are chastity and NFP. But Japan's bishops drag their feet. They have never even issued a national pastoral letter against abortion.

The Japanese government, like the Soviet government, has never allowed the Pill or IUD, for medical reasons. Saline abortions are also banned.

Now Japan has the inevitable consequences of legal abortion: a nonreproductive birthrate of 1.7 children per family (you need 2.2 for good replacement), too few workers, growing layers of older people, and intermittent threats of euthanasia. Unlike Western Europe, the USA and Canada, Japan cannot introduce "guest workers" be-

cause her language is so difficult and because Japan is an
island nation.

Those 65 and over now make up 10.2 percent of Japan's 122 million people. Although that is still below Sweden's 16.8 percent and the USA's 11 percent, the Japanese
will quickly go to 20 percent within 30 years.

This will make Japan the world's oldest nation, thanks
to abortion. Unable to solve their demographic problem
with immigration, the Japanese will have to solve it in-
ternally with higher birthrates.

The Japanese have the world's longest life expectancy—
some 74 years for men and 80 for women—and the world's
fastest-growing over-65 population. To ease the financial
burden of the working-age segment, the government is
considering raising the retirement age from the current 55
to 65, and raising the age at which workers can receive
government pension payments.

HLI is in touch with a significant Japanese anti-abortion movement which has a great deal of support within
the government. We expect the pragmatic Japanese to
tighten their abortion law in the foreseeable future by
knocking out the clause allowing abortions for economic
reasons.

Although rich and industrially powerful, the polite
Japanese suffer from great spiritual poverty. Japan has
only 800,00 Christians, almost half of whom are Catholics.
But the Catholics now average fewer children than the rest
of the nation.

The hierarchy is lethargic and the Church worse than
stagnant. Father Anthony Zimmerman, SVD, Japan's
great and persecuted missionary (and priest and demographer), thinks the chief reasons are the massive contraception and abortion, which present serious temptations
to a struggling Catholic minority. Still, the Catholic
Church has an influence far beyond its numbers in Japan.

H.L.I. ARMS AUSTRIA'S PROLIFE RESISTANCE

This nation of seven million so-called Catholics has
more abortions than births, 20,000 registered prostitutes
(Austria's second-largest profession), a terribly dissident
hierarchy, 800 pastorless parishes and a theological situation that is as bad as Germany's or worse.

The Austrian bishops dissented from *Humanae Vitae*
twice. As a logical consequence, they recently approved *in
vitro* fertilization. Under the leadership of Ms. Grit Ebner,

the semi-official prolife movement almost promotes contraception—with the help of certain wild moral theologians
who are unchecked by the bishops. Many Austrian priests
and nuns march for peace and against nuclear weapons,
while ignoring the massive killing occurring daily in the
war on their unborn brothers and sisters.

It took the Holy See an entire year to find a replacement for Francis Cardinal König of Vienna. Finally they
chose Fr. Hermann Groer, a Benedictine monk. Those who
have known him personally for years report that he is
truly holy and genuinely pious but has no taste for conflict
and confrontation.

For example, as the national head of the Legion of
Mary, he forbade any members to march against abortion.
He has also said that contraception is a matter of conscience; what did he mean? Genuine prolifers feared the
worst when the newly elected archbishop remarked that he
would be guided by a far-left vicar general and the retired
König.

Genuine Austrian prolifers begged me to rush to Austria to instruct the newly elected Benedictine Archbishop,
as if I could work miracles!

The best-informed and most devout Catholics will tell
you again and again that König is a Mason or, at the very
least, has played into the Masons' hands. It is more than
rumor that he and the late Julius Cardinal Doepfner of
Munich flew to Rome in 1968 to try to talk Pope Paul VI
out of issuing *Humanae Vitae*. In his last years the German Cardinal realized his mistake, but it was too late,
because by then the Germans' sexual instincts had been
unleashed.

HLI sent the Austrians eight copies of *The Silent
Scream*. Martin Humer, Austria's greatest prolifer, has
used them with devastating effect. For years most priests
considered him "a fanatic." But through his large seminars, his very clever use of *The Silent Scream*, and one of
the best prolife newsletters in the world, the persecuted
Humer has finally won over many priests and leaders. He
is enormously resourceful as one of Austria's greatest pho-
tographers—and a workaholic.

The indefatigable Humer has also fought pornography
more successfully, perhaps, than anyone in the world. He
has been able to destroy literally millions of dollars' worth
of imported pornography. He has introduced the successful
picketing of abortion mills to Austria and put the Socialist

government on the spot by exposing the traffic in aborted babies.

FATHER MARX INVADES ABORTUARY

I do not have much time to picket abortion chambers, but picketing is a powerful weapon to save babies. It closes one abortion mill a month in the USA.

I have picketed about 10 times, including twice in Santa Barbara, California, recently. I appointed myself chaplain of the abortion mill, then walked in and announced myself as such. There was total consternation.

"As chaplain, I want to talk to the abortionist," I told the nervous receptionist. "He's out to lunch." "I'll wait for him." I asked how she could justify taking in this blood money. She was flustered: "I don't want to talk about it." From the back of the room came a woman who took one look at this strange priest-chaplain and as quickly disappeared.

A few minutes later, I left the abortion chamber to resume picketing and praying. Suddenly the abortionist stormed out, yelling about trespassing. I asked him calmly whether he would not discuss abortion with the chamber's chaplain; he slammed the door and locked it in my face.

The next week I carried a beautiful six-month-old baby named Monique into the same abortion mill. One young abortion candidate walked out after seeing this precious bundle. A somewhat older woman stared and stared at the child, perhaps regretting what she was about to do.

The abortionist, Daniel Joseph, is now threatening to sue the picketers, now that they are picketing his home, too. Abortionists hate that. Joseph kills second-trimester babies.

You would think the Catholic hierarchy would support a prolife activity as effective as picketing, and support Christians courageous enough to engage in it. That is why prolifers were so shocked and disillusioned by the incredible attack on activists by Benedictine Archbishop Rembert G. Weakland of Milwaukee, reported in the 3 August 1986 *National Catholic Register*.

Archbishop Weakland's accusations of "abusive" and "offensive" gestures by prolifers are untrue, shameful and irresponsible. (I know the prolife protest movement rather well, I think, supporting personally two of its great leaders, i.e., Joe Scheidler and our own John Cavanaugh-O'Keefe, who is the epitome of nonviolence.)

Astonishingly, Weakland condemns the picketing of abortionists' homes. Does he not know that such picketing has prompted several of these killers to stop, thus saving thousands of babies? It seems to be acceptable to Weakland to picket the owners of California vineyards, to picket for better working conditions or for more money—but not for life! There is nothing in Weakland's episcopal record to indicate he has taken the advice given in the American bishops' peace pastoral, which he played a large role in creating. This document called for a renewed study of the power and efficacy of nonviolence as a tactic for changing society.

Perhaps if Weakland had picketed even once he would never have written what he did. If he had read the confessions of Dr. Bernard Nathanson, once America's biggest abortionist but now prolife, he would know that even one protester outside an abortuary bothers the killer-doctor, the nurse who hands him the deadly tools and the receptionist who takes in the bloody cash. Weakland also criticized prolifers who hold peaceful sit-ins to save lives, or who dismantle the evil abortion machines.

This is the same Weakland who some years ago invited dissident theologian Fr. Charles Curran to instruct his religion teachers in Milwaukee. I wrote to Weakland at the time for an explanation, but did not receive the courtesy of a reply. And it is the same Weakland who justified the presence of ex-priest and pro-abortion Daniel Maguire on the theological faculty of "Catholic" Marquette University in his see city.

Weakland also allowed ballet dancing in his cathedral sanctuary, in his own presence. He told his priests to take "sexist" language out of the Mass without waiting for Rome to approve such changes. And Weakland's archdiocese has a highly questionable sex education program.

The most shocking part of the Weakland story is that he made his attack on prolifers at the request of a delegation of pro-abortion ministers.

We commend Bishops Leo A. Pursley and Andrew J. McDonald for their sensible pro-rescue statements, and we praise the several bishops who have picketed the death centers over the years.

PROLIFERS SHORE UP CANADA

According to a unique Canadian organization, the Birth Control Victims Association, the Canadian government has

not banned the IUD. Moreover, the government is trying
to legalize Upjohn's abortifacient Depo-Provera, which is
forbidden to American women but is used widely in some
80 countries of the world, mostly poor ones.

The abortifacient character of the IUD and its horrendous effects on women's health are well documented medically. Thirty-five thousand injured women have filed lawsuits and claims against the manufacturer of just one IUD,
the Dalkon Shield. Five years after the manufacturer
(A.H. Robins of Baltimore) was forced to withdraw this
devilish product from the American market, it was still
pushing it to the poor countries (with your tax money).

Although not a licensed pharmacy, Planned Parenthood
has been peddling abortifacient birth control Pills for profit
in Ottawa since 1970. PP admits the revenues provide
some 60 percent of its core budget. Of the $60,000 annual
gross, $40,000 is net profit. As in the USA, Canadian
taxes finance the dirty work of PP in ruining the youth,
family, Church and society. Sadly, Prime Minister Brian
Mulroney is trying to legalize homosexual activity in order
to win leftist support for his failing government.

We congratulate the Canadians in Toronto, and particularly Fr. Alphonse de Valk, for their pioneer organizing
of Teachers for Life. Three hundred attended their first
convention in Toronto.

Our flourishing Canadian branch will soon give birth to
a sub-branch in the Canadian capital, Ottawa.

We are still waiting for Montreal Auxiliary Bishop
Leonard Crowley's proof of the offenses he claims HLI has
committed, which we publicly promised to publish.

PRAY FOR FATHER HÄRING

Few theologians, in my view, have contributed more to
the problems of the Catholic Church than Germany's Redemptorist Fr. Bernard Häring.

In the 1970s Häring published an article in German
which maintained falsely that the practice of NFP led to
birth defects and more miscarriages. Fr. Walter Burghardt, the dissenting Jesuit editor of *Theological Studies*,
reprinted this article with some changes by Häring for the
American milieu. At the time I was organizing an International Symposium on Natural Family Planning at Minnesota's St. John's University.

I invited Häring to defend his excursion into gynecological medicine before the assembled NFP scientists of the

world. I even offered to pay his way. He refused to come, saying he was "too busy." We released a lengthy news release refuting Häring's unproven statements and distributed it in 32 countries.

Later I arranged for Dr. Thomas Hilgers to refute Häring in an article in *Theological Studies*, published only after a good deal of pressure. In addition, I offered a German translation of Hilgers' article to the German editor who had published Häring's original piece. It was never published; Häring was on the board of directors.

In the 3 August 1986 issue of *Christ in der Gegenwart*, Häring defends and glorifies his former student, Charles Curran. You have to read the article to believe it. Among other things, Häring says that Curran, apart from his dissent, really accepts the norms of *Humanae Vitae*! He emphasizes, irrelevantly, that Curran lives a life of virtue: "He lives the fundamental option for the poor and an almost radical version of Franciscan poverty."

Häring says nothing about Curran's opposition in this country, the harm he has done to the Church, or the effects of his teaching on students and teachers. He alleges that more than 700 American professors of theology and canon law stand solidly behind Curran and begs Rome at the very least to "compromise"! I have never seen that list of professors, and I am sure Häring has not seen it either. The rebel *National Catholic Reporter* was quick to publish the names of the dissenters of 1968, but for reasons of their own they have chosen not to identify the rebel theologians who agree with Curran.

H.L.I. INVADES BRAZIL AGAIN

This most Catholic country of 135 million people commits an estimated two million-plus illegal surgical abortions each year. The unwitting government suggests relaxing the law—which would increase the carnage. Country midwives, mostly untrained, commit many abortions, but so do doctors in special city "clinics"; the latter are not prosecuted unless they kill the mother as well as the baby.

To our knowledge there is only one NFP program in this vast, undeveloped country. It was organized by a magnificent nun through a hospital in Sao Paulo and has 18 branches teaching NFP. Recently, two Brazilian doctors visited HLI in Washington and told what they had seen: USAID, PP, the Pathfinder Fund and other anti-child forces pass out condoms and almost-free Pills. They steril-

ize people and insert IUDs—financed mostly by your taxes.
Too many Brazilian bishops seem unduly preoccupied with
liberation theology and poverty, overlooking the greatest
poverty of all, the deprivation of life through abortion.
At the invitation of several bishops, I am invading
Brazil for three weeks in September, along with New
York's Fr. Albert Salmon, one of our Latin American Coordinators. We are flying from city to city to organize a
prolife movement. We are sending Portuguese-language
copies of *The Silent Scream* ahead and will take along as
many as we can carry. Right now we are translating the
film *The First Days of Life* into Portuguese.

H.L.I.-ARGENTINA BATTLES DIVORCE

We are continuing to pour powerful literature and
audiovisual aids into Argentina. Right now our branch
there is doing all it can in a gigantic battle to prevent the
legalization of divorce in this Catholic country.

Fr. Angel Armelin, one of Argentina's great priests and
our co-worker, was in HLI's Washington office recently to
report. Argentine prolife forces believe strongly that if
they can stop divorce, the government will not dare try to
legalize abortion. So far we have lost in the House of
Deputies but hope to win in the Senate.

Most bishops have stood up to the government splen-
didly. Mostly under the leadership of our friend Bishop
Emilio Ognenovich, 80,000 people protested divorce in
downtown Buenos Aires—in bad weather, too. The government took note! Fr. Armelin showed me many large
ads published by the bishops and Catholic groups in the
metropolitan papers. These ads oppose the government
and point out the evils of divorce. We rushed the piece of
anti-divorce literature that was most effective in Ireland to
Buenos Aires.

The future of the Catholic Church and the world is in
Africa and South America, where more than 70 percent of
the Catholic Church will be in the year 2000. Today nine
out of 10 babies are born in the poor countries.

In 1950 the total population of the countries south of
the Rio Grande was 165 million, about the same as the
total population of the USA and Canada at that time. But
since then the population of Latin America has grown
much more rapidly than that of North America. In 1985
Latin America's population was estimated at 405 million,

compared with 265 million in North America. (Our Latin neighbors love their babies.)

According to the best estimates, by the year 2025 Latin America's population could be as high as 775 million, more than *twice* that of North America.

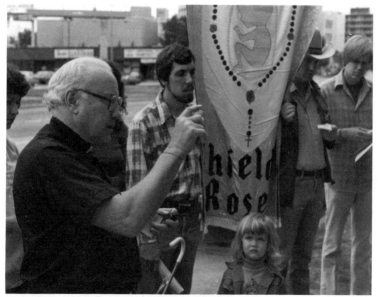

Exorcising an abortion mill in California.

OVERCOPULATION IN EUROPE

(No. 25—November 1986)

Every time I return from Europe I am tempted to depression. This once-Christian continent has become a Sodom and Gomorrah.

Europe has more coffins than cradles (except in Ireland), over*cop*ulation and under*pop*ulation, weak episcopal leadership, influential moral theologians who are far worse and more subtle than Fr. Charles Curran, rampant contraception, genocidal abortion, and the inevitable threat of euthanasia (the German parliament is discussing it).

Europe also has 21 million foreigners, of whom seven million are Moslems; these often have three times more children than the dying natives.

FRENCH BABIES, AN ENDANGERED SPECIES

Pope Pius XI's encyclical *Casti Connubii* (1931) was aimed largely at the French, who were making abundant use of the condom and withdrawal. Since then Masons, the godless Socialists, the secular feminists and Planned Parenthood have eroded France's moral fiber steadily. The French bishops' rejection of *Humanae Vitae* in 1968 seems to have assured France's national suicide.

Afraid to make a commitment, the young in France simply live together before marrying; it is almost the rule, even in "good" families. Divorce is common and increasing. There is little NFP.

In 1974, with all the usual lies, the French Socialists passed a strange, experimental, five-year abortion-on-demand law covering the first 10 weeks of life. They finalized this disastrous law on the last day of the Year of the Family in 1979. Today abortion may be committed at any time for "serious" health reasons or if the child has a defect.

Despite the highest family subsidies in the Western world, France has only 1.7 children per family, with millions of Moslems increasing and multiplying. Euthanasia has been mentioned in parliament; it will follow in time.

Only now are the French beginning to realize that the widely used Pill and IUD are abortifacients. As the Pill's harmful medical effects become more evident, doctors insert more and more IUDs. Although sterilization is still illegal, it is resorted to more and more. Prolife nurses told me they had personally seen doctors sterilize—without the woman's consent—mothers who had had multiple births. Mothers over 39 are routinely subjected to amniocentesis and are virtually forced to sign consent forms for abortion if their babies are found to have defects.

France's Catholic schools do not imbue the young with the Faith. Few people go to Mass regularly. The practice of Confession is all but dead. Seminaries and novitiates are more or less empty. Here and there the charismatic renewal is vigorous, though.

According to the law, a mother who wants her baby aborted must be counseled twice. Most of this government-paid counseling is done by PP and by the Catholic Centre de Liaison des Equipes de Recherche. I was told the latter saves only about five out of every 100 babies, abandoning the other 95 by signing the document, which has become a mere formality. The government parrots the abortionists' under-reported figure of 180,000 babies killed yearly, but the real figure is closer to 400,000.

Thus the "eldest daughter of the Catholic Church" has become a dying whore. The best-informed, active, prolife French priest told me he cannot understand the thinking of the fearful, do-nothing bishops. He agrees that only a moral rebirth through prayer and penance can save France and Europe.

While in France I brought films and two boxes of literature to the International Prolife Center in Lourdes. HLI has regularly contributed much material to this office for years.

ABORTION STANDOFF IN SPAIN

In 1985 Spain's ideology-mad Socialists, who are trying to destroy the Church, were able to pass only a restricted abortion law, against much resistance. Last year "only" 200 legal killings were reported. But thousands of Spanish women, coached by PP and homicidal feminists, go to England and France to have their babies murdered. Now the Socialist government wants to establish private abortion chambers to kill 30,000 babies a year at taxpayers' expense.

Every European country except Ireland and Belgium now permits the killing of preborn babies. The Green Isle may soon be alone.

ISRAEL'S ABORTION HOLOCAUST

Founded (or re-founded) in 1948, the Jewish state has 4.8 million people. Almost 40 percent are Arabs, counting those who live in the West Bank. Of these, 75,000 are Catholics, mostly Palestinians.

The average completed Israeli family has 2.8 children, but the Arab families (especially the Moslems), have more than twice as many children as the Jewish ones. Penalized in various subtle ways, many of Israel's Palestinians emigrate to Australia, Canada and the U.S. Because of lower (and declining) birthrates and increasing abortion, the Israeli government is much concerned about a future racial imbalance. The country is already surrounded by 100 million hostile, prolife, proliferating Moslems.

Even so, every health clinic displays a sign asking, "Is this child wanted?" Offensive sex education is required, and contraception is advertised on TV. According to foreign newspapers, Brazil and Israel are negotiating guidelines for adopting babies into Israeli families. *In vitro* fertilization (IVF) is increasing rapidly. Rabbis told me that "living together" and divorce are becoming frighteningly common.

When Israel began its modern existence, it inherited both the British and traditional Jewish prohibition of abortion. But illegal aborting began about 1952.

According to a study of the Institute of Applied Social Research, Israel's hospitals were committing 27 abortions for every 100 births, with at least that many committed privately. The Israelis have killed more than 1.2 million babies since 1948, the vast majority before it was legal. Thus they have one of the highest abortion rates in the world.

In 1978 the baby butchery was brought into the open. Then, with pressure from money-hungry gynecologists, the radical feminists and the Israeli Family Planning Association, the Knesset (parliament) passed a disastrous law: All requests for abortion must be referred to a committee of three: a gynecologist, another doctor and a social worker.

The committee was to judge each mother in terms of five clauses: (1) pregnancy over 40 or under 17; (2) pregnancy outside of marriage; (3) possible deformity of the

child; (4) mother's health, mental or physical; and (5) social
conditions. But as always happens, the killings escalated.
The committee soon degenerated into a mere formality.

In worrisome debates over how to raise the birthrate,
the Knesset has openly admitted what most know: abortions are committed for personal convenience and as a
means of birth control. When the far-right Orthodox rabbis pressured the government to eliminate the social clause
in 1979, women increasingly used the mental-health clause.

Israel is yet another country one can cite to prove that
widespread contraception always leads to massive abortion.
Far from reducing abortion, as a common myth would have
us believe, contraception increases it. In fact, the two sins
feed each other, because both abuse God's great gift of
human sexuality, taking it out of the proper and loving
role from which healthy family life should emerge.

Fewer Israelis use the abortifacient Pill all the time.
But they use the abortifacient IUD surprisingly often,
although I read and heard complaints of its bad health
effects. Sterilization is beginning, despite a strong Jewish
religious tradition against it.   The Israelis are too intelligent to use Upjohn's injectable abortifacient, Depo-
Provera. Mothers 35 and over are routinely subjected to
amniocentesis, by the way.

Free-standing abortion mills have appeared in the last
five years. One head of a large hospital freely admitted
that his institution would fail financially if it stopped
committing abortions. Killing preborn babies is big business in Israel, but the handwriting is on the wall for the
Jews—and they know it. The world's Jewish population is
declining rapidly. Of all religious groups in the U.S., the
six million Jews have the lowest birthrate, averaging barely one child per family.

In Israel as in the hedonistic West, sex has become
recreation; Israel has more and more fornication ("living
together") and divorce.

The young are out of control, with ever more alcohol
and drug abuse. As the head of Tel Aviv University's
Criminology Institute observed recently, increasing teen
alcohol abuse reflects the malaise of a society that has lost
its values.

"We are living in an era of hedonism," he continued.
"Our teenagers have no ideology. What values we had . . .
have all been lost. Small wonder that our youth turns to

alcohol and drugs." He might have added sex, the misuse of which is perhaps the most destructive of all.

Sensible Israelis founded the Society for the Advancement of Childbearing (known as "EFRAT") in 1962 to buck the deadly trends. Today it is under the leadership of Rabbi Mordechai Blanck, with whom HLI has been in contact for years.

EFRAT is an apolitical organization whose members represent all segments of Israeli society and all lifestyles and world-views. It is the only Jewish organization in the world working to encourage Jewish population growth, to prevent "unnecessary abortions, and to strengthen the Jewish family."

It does this through education, counseling, publishing and practical aid programs. It stresses preparing the young for marriage and parenthood, and both initiates and promotes laws that help and encourage large families. And what about euthanasia? I asked. "They just do it," snapped a prolife Israeli homemaker.

For years I have wondered why the Jews, so victimized by the Nazi Holocaust, should so eagerly engage in a greater one. The undeniable evidence that certain Jews have led the abortion movement in the U.S., France, and other countries has prompted me to ask my prolife Jewish friends for an explanation; never have I received a persuasive reply.

I put that question to Rabbi Blanck and his colleagues in Jerusalem after a long afternoon's discussion. They were intrigued and befuddled as I reeled off prominent Jewish abortionists and abortion promoters in the various countries, above all in the U.S. Again, their response was not satisfactory.

They speculated, though, that the very experience of the Nazi Holocaust may have hardened Jewish attitudes towards life. They noted that the chief advocate of liberalized abortion in the Knesset was a Jewish feminist, Chaike Crossman, who had suffered horribly at Auschwitz. (Another Jewish Auschwitz victim, Simone Weil, played the same role in the French parliament as health minister.) So the mystery remains as the worldwide decline of Jews continues, with unpredictable consequences for Israel once the prolife Moslem Arabs gain democratic ascendency in that country.

LAND OF THE PHARAOHS: PROLIFE

When you arrive the Cairo airport, the fetid air reminds you at once of the millions of gallons of raw sewage flowing from the port of Alexandria into the Mediterranean. This burgeoning city of almost four million people was once known as the "pearl of the Mediterranean." Egypt has almost 50 million people and grows by a million every eight months.

The country's land area is 387,000 square miles, 10 percent of which is arable. Cotton, rice, fruits and flowers are the chief exports. The many huge modern hotels on the Nile reflect the major revenue that tourism provides. Even so, Egypt imports $8 million of food daily. Plagued by high unemployment and a huge foreign debt, the land of the Pharaohs receives more than $1 billion in American civilian aid each year, and even more for military purposes, second only to Israel.

Egyptian women average five children. Outside the cities, nearly half marry before age 17; almost half the population is under 16. U.S. agencies have spent $16 million of your tax money in the last eight years providing abortifacient Pills and IUDs and all forms of contraception, but with comparatively little effect. After tragic medical experiences, the minister of health banned Upjohn's injectable abortifacient, Depo-Provera.

Egypt punishes abortion severely and discourages sterilization: both are "contrary to religious values." There is much poverty in the dirty streets, filled with cars and people. Contraceptives are virtually free, but the Moslems are little concerned with the flagging economy or the bursting population: "Allah will provide." Drug abuse, alcoholism, VD and homosexual activity are minimal.

This ancient, religious land, nourished by the Nile, has about 250,000 Catholics in six dioceses, with 13 bishops and five Rites. There are also 175,000 Protestants and seven to eight million Christian Copts who have many vocations, especially to their strict female orders. The rest of Egypt is Moslem. An estimated 14,000 Christians leave Christianity each year to embrace entrenched Islam.

Cairo, a city of 15 million, has 15 Catholic schools. The saintly Jesuit Fr. Leo Shea, an HLI colleague who is still active at 82, introduced NFP in 1981. Today it has a good foothold. A married couple works full time, lecturing up and down the Nile. Teachers are being trained and literature distributed. Several bishops have shown real

interest; one bishop divided his 160 priests into groups of
40 for a seminar on NFP.

But ignorance about NFP among people, priests and
teachers is immense in this Moslem land where the family
is all important, where children are begotten for Allah, and
where celibacy therefore seems odd. Among Roman Catholics, native vocations are few.

CAN A NATION REVERSE ANTI-CHILD POLICIES?

HLI-Singapore is the most flourishing of our 14 international branches, next to HLI-Canada. But Singapore is
another dying country, thanks to Planned Parenthood
policies which the government adopted and promoted.

Prolife Singaporeans love to tell us about their government's about-face on population. In 1974 I literally had to
sneak the first prolife films into Singapore. But now they
are most welcome, even to the government, which has
begun a Birthright-type counseling program to keep women
from aborting.

This little republic of 2.5 million people in 139 square
miles had one of the world's most stringent population
policies in the '60s and '70s. It was too successful, and so
the government has neutralized PP, whose facilities were
paid for by the International Planned Parenthood Federation, partly with American money. (In the July–August
1986 *Population Today*, PP claims dishonestly that it is
"winding down its activities, its objectives achieved.")

For more than two decades, loud had been the clamor
that no one should have more than two children; those
with a third were punished in various ways. PP and the
government eloquently promoted contraceptives, the abortifacient Pill, IUDs and sterilization.

The people took the advice only too well, while the
minority Malaysians increased and multiplied. In the Singapore *Sunday Times* for 6 July 1986, Professor Saw Swee
Hock questioned whether "there will be enough young
people to do national service and defend us" and whether
there will be enough working people to support the growing number of older citizens.

The minister of health pointed out that in 1967 Singapore had 50,560 births. Based on present fertility levels,
in the year 2000 there would be 37,000 births; there would
be only 29,300 births in the year 2030. He admitted frankly that Singapore could not defend itself in the future if
the situation continued.

I have news for him: it *will* continue, because once you ruin the birthrate with abortion and epidemic contraception, it is virtually impossible to restore it. That is the universal experience of Western nations. People will not have babies for the State. Hedonists will play with sex but will have few children. In the Singapore *Straits Times* for 4 August 1986, the deputy prime minister pleaded, "I would like to encourage young mothers who are here, those who can afford to have two or three children, to do so . . . even four, if you can afford it." In 1985 Singapore committed 23,512 abortions and had 42,500 births.

You can see the dimensions of the Singaporean demographic debacle from the numbers. In 1985 there were 8.7 persons 15–19 years of age supporting every person over 60. By the year 2000, the ratio will drop to 6.4. By 2020 there will be only 2.5 persons supporting each elderly person. The government is now reviewing its family planning policies. And Human Life International's branch is flourishing and most welcome.

Recently the health minister said, "I would welcome suggestions on how families can be encouraged to have two children and for those who can afford it, to encourage them to have more." Alas, the great, shrewd little Archbishop of Singapore, Gregory Yong, had good advice all along.

How well he fenced with the preceding Harvard-trained premier who inflicted the present developing disaster on Singapore! The Archbishop needed no convincing that contraception leads to abortion when I conversed with him in 1974 and again in 1982. I shall never forget his own eloquent reasons. Thanks to him, Singapore's Church and prolife/pro-family movement are truly flourishing, with many good programs and many converts.

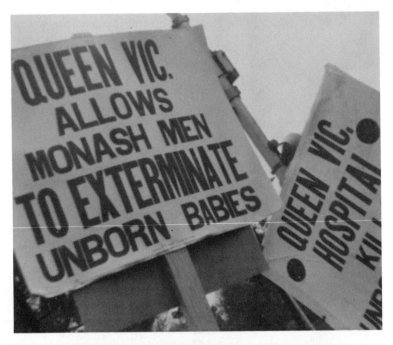

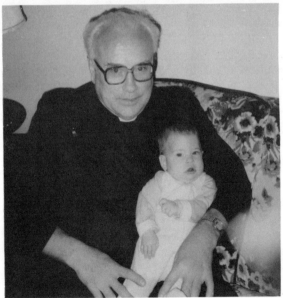

The fight for life is global.

15th BRANCH SAVING BABIES

(No. 26—December 1986)

This past September and October I spent three weeks in Brazil again and gave more than 40 lectures and film-shows in five of her largest cities. Fr. Albert Salmon, HLI's Latin American coordinator, accompanied me. Organizing the tour was Bishop Luciano Mendes, Secretary of the Brazilian National Bishops' Conference. This time things *did* happen; we now have a branch in Rio (number 15) and will soon have organized leaders all over the sleeping giant that is Brazil.

With 8.5 million square kilometers, Brazil is larger than the continental U.S. and covers two-thirds of South America. Her 133 million people make her the largest Catholic nation in the world, but she has no prolife movement—and the legalization of abortion is in the wings.

Brazil has a history of unstable though relatively non-violent governments, including a 21-year military regime which ended last year. But she has emerged as the eighth largest economy in the non-Communist world, currently boasting an eight percent annual growth rate, despite being saddled with the largest foreign debt of any nation: $107 billion.

Brazil is enormously rich in resources, but they are undeveloped. The poverty is appalling: one percent are very rich; four percent are rich; 15 percent are middle class; 40 percent are poor; and another 40 percent are extremely poor. Twenty million are illiterate.

The nation has 36 million very poor children, of whom seven million roam the streets homeless; 65 million children are deprived in part. More than 52 percent of all Brazilians are under 19.

With more than 12 million inhabitants, Sao Paulo is Brazil's largest city. A third of her people live in two kinds of slums: (1) *cortiços*, which are privately owned and rented houses, basements or covered between-walls areas in which 10–40 families may live, and (2) *favelas* or "misery villages" around cities, in each of which 500–1,000 families may exist.

One Capuchin parish I visited had more than 80 *cortiços*. In these, as in the *favelas*, a family may share one room in the midst of much "living together," promiscuity, VD, homosexuality and you-name-it. In the 69 countries I have visited, I have never seen so many obvious motel/hotel brothels as in Brazil. As one priest remarked facetiously, "The Sixth Commandment has never been taught in this country!"

Brazil is second only to the U.S. in AIDS cases, although the government is trying to hide the fact. (There are also many lepers.) And although it is against the law, hard-core pornography is now widespread in print form on the street, via cheaply rented videocassettes and on TV. Zealous missionaries agonized with me over how to apply moral rules in the unique, inhuman and thoroughly unjust conditions of this rich country whose people are mostly poor and deprived.

FOREIGN BABY-KILLERS SUBVERT BRAZIL

The average minimum monthly wage is $40. The average family has 3.9 children, although the birthrate is falling fast because of foreign-financed contraceptives, abortifacient Pills and IUDs (without prescription!), clandestine abortions and increasing sterilizations, often done without the victim's consent or knowledge. One foreign-sponsored organization, Pro-Pater, has $300,000 to sterilize men "for responsible family planning."

Most Brazilian husbands and wives work, when they can find work; 21 percent are unemployed despite the booming economy. Brazil is a religious and ethnic amalgam of Portuguese, blacks (descendants of slaves), Germans, Italians and Japanese (there are a million and a half of the last, with a large colony in Sao Paulo). Forty million are of German or Italian descent.

The law allows abortion in proven cases of rape and danger to mother's physical life, but it is not enforced. The estimated toll of babies aborted illegally is well more than two million per year. The UN's World Health Organization, which is pro-abortion and usually exaggerates, claims there are five million abortions in Brazil, one-tenth of the world's intentional ones. It is impossible to know whether more murders are committed by doctors in private clinics or by untrained midwives and even nurses.

In 1974 a deputy in the national congress proposed legalizing abortion; she got nowhere. In 1984 one state legalized abortion for rape and health. The bishops objected forcefully, and that state repealed the law the next year.

But the abortionists are more persevering than most Christians. Population controllers, fueled by foreign money, have been actively preparing the way for years. The government is making rumblings; recently radical feminists organized themselves and asked practicing Catholic President José Sarney for money to foster their aims. They got it.

One feminist national deputy is demanding abortion on demand, using the usual lies and tactics. The softening-up process is well under way. Almost every day the Rio de Janeiro newspapers carry sad stories about rape and other hard cases. The liberal newspapers, radio and TV distorted, in typical ways, the comments I made at press conferences. In Rio someone has started a pro-abortion, leftist daily newspaper, the funding of which is very suspicious.

The foreign-funded Family Welfare Society, known as BEMFAM (actually PP), and cohorts such as Family Health International and the Pathfinder Fund have been active very slyly since 1965. They have sponsored meetings and seminars for doctors, nurses, social workers and teachers on "population problems" and "totally voluntary" birth control programs. These foreign-financed groups and others have been largely responsible for the astonishingly widespread sterilization programs in Latin America, particularly in Central America, Brazil and Chile.

Last February the government started a national birth control program, complete with the usual trap of putting NFP on a par with contraception and abortifacients, and even offered to teach and pay for NFP. Although they recognized some of the risks, the bishops agreed to collaborate. They feared that if they did not, only BEMFAM would teach NFP, and bastardize it with use of the condom during the fertile time. The latter is actually written into the government plan, which, for those naive enough to believe it, incredibly claims it will give "preference" to NFP!

WARNING THE BISHOPS

I am afraid too many bishops fail to see these dangers. About 15 years ago the Filipino hierarchy fell into such a trap, only to learn later they were being used. Several

Billings (ovulation method) groups have likewise gone with the treacherous government program that also involves micro-abortions via Pills and IUDs, plus dangerous Depo-Provera injections.

The result has been the formation of a new and independent organization called *Açao Familiar*, which will teach the S-T (sympto-thermal) method of NFP with our help. Nationwide, NFP in Brazil is spotty; again, it is too little, too late. Brazilian intellectuals are quoted as saying, "NFP is for priests and religious."

Legalized abortion is inevitable in Brazil, because massive contraceptive/abortifacient programs are already in place, generously funded with your tax money (mostly), through USAID, IPPF and the rest. I told Brazil's bishops, priests and people this repeatedly, but most of them seem to have little awareness of the abortionists' devilish tricks. Even worse, perhaps, most politicians now running for office entertain the myth that they can contain or control abortion. These people will draw up Brazil's forthcoming new constitution.

Obviously, the people who are least aware are for legalizing abortion—especially the rich five percent who often have more maids than children. These want legal abortion to remedy their contraceptive failures and the unwanted pregnancies of their fornicating daughters.

I suggested to a high-ranking prelate that within perhaps three years Brazil will have legal abortion. He did not think so. "Were that to happen," he observed, "the Church would make a lot of fuss." I responded gently, "The time to make a fuss is *now*." He did not seem to catch the point.

In April 1986 the Brazilian National Bishops' Conference issued an excellent pastoral to guide those who will draft their country's new constitution, which is due next year. But in eloquently insisting on the inclusion of individual, human, parental and family rights, they failed to state unequivocally that *all* human life must be protected from conception/fertilization—as the Irish did in their constitutional referendum and as the Filipinos are now doing in their proposed new constitution. Such a clear declaration could head off the abortionists at the pass, as I tried to explain to every Brazilian bishop and leader I met.

In the Philippines the baby-killers and population controllers fought such a declaration, saying that people do not agree when life begins, a woman has a right over her body, and so on. Thank God, the authors of the proposed constitution (helped by HLI) wrote in protection of every human life from the moment of conception, by a vote of 44 to 2 (with one abstention).

The Brazilian hierarchy is in a state of considerable tension. The bishops are very much divided in their attempts to handle the Church's many enormous problems, not the least of which is liberation theology. In his powerful letter to them last March, the Pope begged the bishops to maintain honest dialogue about their differences, with a view to promoting unity and authentic doctrine.

At the Medellin Conference in Colombia in 1968, Latin America's bishops solemnly resolved to take up the cause of the poor. Many thinking, apostolic Catholics believe that, in their preoccupation with the poor and with liberation theology, the Brazilian hierarchy has neglected basic morality, sound doctrine and effective catechesis.

I asked at least 20 Catholic adults whether they had ever head a sermon on chastity, contraception, sterilization, abortion, *Humanae Vitae* and the like; none had. What *did* priests preach on, I wanted to know. The answers: "Liturgy, justice and peace, love, be nice to each other, human rights, liberation theology."

The lack of discipline, the doctrinal confusion and the false ecumenism which cropped up after Vatican II set the stage for a massive influx of U.S. money and Protestant sects, especially fundamentalists and Pentecostals, whose brightly lit and often large churches are very evident on Sunday nights.

After Vatican II, one bishop spoke carelessly about Brazil's being a pluralistic society. The government obliged by legalizing divorce in 1979. Asking about the number of divorces, I was told that divorce is of little concern because desertion and the shedding of spouses are so common. Seventeen busloads of feminists packed the galleries of the national congress in Brasilia to shout down any deputy who tried to oppose divorce.

Ninety percent of Brazil's people are baptized Catholics, but most are uncatechized. Of the 120 million who are nominally Catholic, only about 12 million practice their Faith regularly, but the number of serious Catholics is increasing. Many others are leaving the Church, though. Protestants number about five percent, but they are growing fast because of their explicit Biblical teachings.

Besides the doctrinal confusion over liberation theology, the false ecumenism and the abandonment of traditional devotions, there is a perennial shortage of clergy and religious. Brazil has only 13,000 priests (of whom 5,500 are foreign missionaries), 40,000 nuns and 7,000 brothers. The more than 200 minor and 100 major seminaries, however, are experiencing an increase in vocations—more than the convents, strangely.

Right now, because the bishops support agrarian reform, the rich and the government consider the Church subversive. In the last six months at least 100 lay people, two priests and a nun have been shot by wealthy landowners. The visas of some 200 missionaries are hanging.

BASE COMMUNITIES, LIBERATION THEOLOGY

Unique to the Church in Brazil are her approximately 100,000 Christian "base communities." Some 1,650 carefully chosen delegates attended their Sixth Interecclesial Assembly recently; most were under 35, married, employed as land, factory or service workers, and had a primary level of schooling.

They represented the whole political spectrum and every one of the 22 states, four territories, 204 dioceses and nine Indian nations. Joining 51 Catholic bishops, observers came from 15 Latin American countries, seven European countries and one African country, representing Pentecostal churches, six mainline Protestant denominations and the World Council of Churches. Even the Primate of Holland, Adrianus Cardinal Simonis, came, to seek hints on how to un-paralyze the Dutch Catholic Church. The Pope sent his blessing.

The topics discussed were faith, friendship, simplicity and a restless quest for a better world—one in which the poor can own land and make a living despite the exploiting rich (who also control the national government, in which 80 percent of the people have no effective voice). What these base communities work for (and sometimes produce martyrs for) is clearly sanctioned in Catholic social teaching.

But the dangers are formidable. The best of liberation theology serves and inspires those communities, but the worst of it easily leads to the false conclusion that socio-economic freedom, human rights and welfare can be a-chieved for sinful humanity without spiritual, sacramental means—without converting souls. Nonetheless, the 100,000 base communities may be little drops that will someday join together to make a roaring river. If that happens, woe to the exploiting rich!

In the base communities, liberation theology may have reached its zenith after Rome's gentle warning to Franciscan Leonardo Boff. His liberation theology has had an enormous but questionable influence, especially among the young clergy and religious and among some veteran American missionaries. The head of the Church's worldwide mission effort, Jozef Cardinal Tomko, recently warned that the use of liberation theology by missionaries risks reducing the Church's task of conversion to mere "human or social development" and to "the social-political liberation of man."

Faced with so much painful poverty, American missionaries told me, "We attempt to change social structures." But so did Karl Marx. What about changing hearts, souls, sinful lives, greed and the injustice in the malformed consciences of fallen human beings? As a sociologist, I can tell you that "society" as such does not exist—except as an interacting group of *individual persons* who can only be liberated from their destructive selfishness by the authentic Christian message. To improve society we must first convert people.

It was Lenin who predicted, "We will find our greatest success to the extent that we inculcate Marxism as a kind of religion: Religious men and women are easy to convert and win, and so will easily accept our thinking if we wrap it up in a kind of religious terminology."

Is this what happened to Boff and his followers? Is this what the Pope meant when he told the Brazilian bishops that, if Marxist Communism comes to their country, it will come through the clergy? Two old Brazilian Jesuits told me that "only" 20–30 bishops promote the worst of liberation theology, but that liberation theology of a kind is here to stay.

It is hard to assess Boff's teaching and influence. It seems that the best of Boff's theology is already included in the Church's splendid social teachings, all too little taught and practiced these days. Brazilian critics say that Boff (who rejected *Humanae Vitae*) wants to radically change the Church's authority, structure and even teachings to respond more effectively to modern problems, especially those involving human rights and poverty.

Thus, Boffian theology borders on being a glorified humanism which embodies ever so subtly the Marxist class struggle, while overlooking man's sinful nature as the source of all social and economic injustice. It also seems to overlook the remedy for the evil in human nature: the Church's spiritual, supernatural and sacramental means.

It is also strange how Boff can live in the midst of mass murder (via abortion) and rampant sexual immorality and never comment directly on these horribly exploitative problems. In one of his books he speaks of the "Mother-God," esoterically complicating the relationship between the Divine Persons and that between Jesus and Mary. In another book he staunchly defends radical feminism; he has openly supported radical feminist political candidates.

Although not invited, two sympathetic Brazilian cardinals accompanied Boff when he was summoned to Rome, allegedly undermining Cardinal Ratzinger by appealing to Cardinal Casaroli. Boff's theology has not been fully cleared, but when his year of imposed silence was over, he wrote insultingly to Ratzinger to thank him for approving liberation theology.

With his brother and sister theologians, he also published a bold statement in a Rio metropolitan paper asserting that the Holy See had fully approved and accepted his theology. His Brazilian critics accuse him of conducting secret courses to undermine Church authority. At the headquarters of the bishops' national headquarters in Brasilia, the staff is optimistically pro-Boff.

On birth control, a high-ranking prelate and fan of Boff remarked to me, "That's a very sensitive subject. I always emphasize that children should be the fruit of true love; I often stress responsible parenthood. I never get into methods; that is dicey." I found no prolife activity, a little NFP and lots of liberation theology in his archdiocese.

To save their seminarians from Boff, the Eugenio Cardinal Sales of Rio and other bishops have withdrawn them from the Pontifical Catholic University of Rio, where Boff teaches; the bishops set up their own theological institutes. To counter Boffian feminism, the Cardinal Sales was sponsoring his second national conference on Christian feminism, with an international faculty, while I was in Brazil.

After Vatican II many Brazilian nuns discarded their religious habits. They also gave up their schools, saying the rich did not need them and they would do social work in the slums instead. Some have come back to reality and recovered their truly religious vocations. There are six pontifical Catholic universities in Brazil, but the Catholic school system and the status of theology seem worse than in the USA. Brazil's future is hard to predict; the whole situation is difficult to assess.

THE SILENT SCREAM ROCKS BRAZIL

After seeing *The Silent Scream* (provided by HLI), Cardinal Sales wrote an article on it for a metropolitan paper. Then he put the film on national TV on Sunday, 28 September. At least 10 million people saw it; the reaction was enormous and loud. The feminists howled the loudest and condemned Sales. Archbishop Pedro Fedeldo of Curbitiba in the state of Parana promised to put *The Silent Scream* on regional TV later, to be seen by five million more, including some in Paraguay.

If we had done nothing else but help get this film on TV as we did, our three weeks in Brazil would have been worth it. But this is only the beginning.

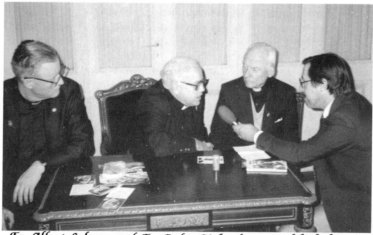

Fr. Albert Salmon and Fr. Pedro Richards are prolife fighters working in Latin America.

ARGENTINA: CHURCH BATTLES STATE

(No. 27—January 1987)

Directed by HLI's flourishing branch in Buenos Aires, I gave 19 lectures in seven cities, took part in four news conferences, did three TV programs and gave five radio interviews over a nine-day period. Our Latin American coordinator, New York's Fr. Albert Salmon, accompanied me and did just as much. They say that a noose around the neck concentrates your attention exceedingly; I can attest that flying in Argentine private planes concentrated my attention in saying my breviary!

When you visit Argentina, you are struck at once by the great differences between Brazil and Argentina. The latter is an educated nation with a European culture engendered by the Spaniards, the Italians, some Irish and some Germans. A huge country of one-and-one-half million square miles, Argentina is very rich in resources but is undeveloped, urban and empty. She has only 30 million people, one-third of whom are concentrated in metropolitan Buenos Aires. The nation includes almost half a million Indians and two-and-one-half million Jews.

Of the 10 million souls dwelling in Buenos Aires, at least three million live in poverty. The country is going through extremely trying times economically, having a $48 billion foreign debt, a six percent monthly inflation rate and high unemployment. As of October 1 the government of Socialist President Raul Alfonsin had set the minimum monthly wage at 110 australs (about $140), daily wages at 4.4 australs and hourly wages at 0.55 australs, excluding household helpers.

The Argentines have a nonreproductive birthrate of only two children per completed family, and an estimated 300,000 illegal abortions annually. The Pill, the IUD, sterilization, the diaphragm and the condom are the other birth control methods used, in that order. NFP has hardly started.

Ninety-five percent of the Argentines are baptized Roman Catholics, but there are 500–600 fast-growing Protestant groups, as in Brazil. In Buenos Aires, about five percent attend Mass regularly. As in all Latin American countries, priests and nuns are in very short supply, although vocations have increased lately.

Unfortunately, after Vatican II the nuns abandoned some of their schools, which they claim were run for the rich who did not need them; these nuns were going to work with the poor and do "social work." Most people in Argentina never really learned their Faith and are poorly catechized. Now religious instruction seems to be in crisis. The independent and conservative Argentines have been little affected by liberation theology, so far.

While I was in Argentina, a Senate committee was debating the legalization of divorce. The Chamber of Deputies had already passed the measure overwhelmingly, which brought a strong condemnation from the Permanent Commission of the Argentine hierarchy. The Commission reminded the Catholics who voted for divorce of the great scandal they had given; that the harm would be irreparable if the Senate voted as they had; that no Catholic worthy of the name could vote for divorce; that no Catholic deputy who did so should go to Communion until he had publicly acknowledged his mistake and atoned for giving serious scandal.

The bishops had generated large public demonstrations in Buenos Aires and other cities, to no avail. Many Catholics favored legalizing divorce, not realizing its consequences and hoping to legitimize those many living in bad marriages. At this time, Senate opponents of liberalization are bottling up the issue in committee; it may not pass, despite the 15-day extension of Alfonsin.

According to the present constitution (which will be amended next year, most likely deleting all references to Catholicism and the Church), Argentina's president must be a Catholic. Alfonsin is Catholic in name, but he is also allegedly a Mason. In any case, he is a Socialist ideologue as well as a subtle underminer of religion and the Church.

For example, he has proposed starting formal schooling at age four. In some countries they do this to keep more teachers employed, given dwindling birthrates. But Alfonsin is accused of more sinister aims; the Socialists always brainwash students as soon as possible.

The Cardinal Archbishop of Cordoba told me that with the present government it is a matter of "divorce today and abortion tomorrow." I found out that two proposals to legalize abortion have already been worked out for presentation next year. The present law authorizes abortion only in the case of a proven danger to the mother's life and in the case of a pregnancy resulting from the rape of a retarded woman. But doctors, midwives and nurses commit many illegal abortions.

Unmarried couples have most of the abortions; there is a considerable rise in teen abortions reflecting the increasing sex education in the schools. There are comparatively few radical feminists in this, the most conservative country in Latin America, but the Family Planning Association (Planned Parenthood) has promoted contraception/sterilization/abortion actively for years. Virtually every day, garbage collectors find aborted babies.

Last year, 1.3 million Argentines saw the TV program on abortion that HLI did. It received the top rating, the one that major athletic events get. Part of the program was *The Silent Scream*, which has been on Argentine TV so often that well over seven million people have seen it. Also, I did a 12-minute interview explaining the worldwide abortion situation on another Buenos Aires channel, preceding a showing of *The Silent Scream*. Argentina is one of very few foreign countries where I have met true-blue Catholics in high TV positions.

With the Pope coming to Argentina next year, the Alfonsin government may not want to discuss divorce, abortion and a Socialist constitution, and so HLI may have some time to further educate the nation. Our flourishing branch in Buenos Aires is led by a great priest, Fr. Angel Armelin, and by Victor Taussig, a holy, experienced, retired businessman. Acting wisely, they are now organizing a prolife movement throughout the country. Fr. Salmon and I visited 13 Argentine cities, lecturing, showing films, doing radio and TV programs and holding news conferences. The effort is already bearing fruit: an evening with doctors in Parana helped lead to the founding of *Consorcio de Medicos Catolicos*.

In Argentina, for the first time in years, I met a young archbishop and a bishop who really understood what was happening to the nation and Church and who want full collaboration with us. We must pull out all the stops and send them at least 50 films, as well as Spanish-language literature, most of which we can print more cheaply in Argentina. Our branch there has already distributed more than 25,000 *Life and Death* brochures.

In this Catholic nation the Mormons now have temples in several cities. The Catholic Church in Argentina has

3,000 secular priests and 2,000 religious priests, many of them foreign. There are 15,000 nuns and 3,000 brothers. Not a single bishop has ever spoken out against *Humanae Vitae*, nor has any prominent theologian! In the last six years there has been a noticeable increase in the number of religious and priestly vocations. For a time many nuns were giving up their religious habits, but, happily, that trend has been halted, and the sisters have more or less returned to their full religious ideals.

Five medical centers recently introduced a proposal in congress to permit teaching sex education in elementary schools, which would instruct six- to eight-year-olds on "the harmlessness of masturbation." I am glad to report that two groups to whom we have been sending literature were able to stop the measure.

About two years ago the Argentine Family Planning Association (PP) started promoting contraceptives and abortifacients in the schools. As elsewhere, they have twisted the Pope's messages to make him sound as if he favors contraception and small families. Recently PP's devilishly subtle 1976 plan to bring sex education into all the schools in Latin America fell into our hands.

Resources-rich Argentina is seriously distressed economically. The people are suffering, and the future is decidedly uncertain. I spoke to several bankers here and in Brazil, all of whom told me that paying their foreign debt was impossible because it would only worsen the plight of the poor. They hesitated to predict the future except that they were not very optimistic. A few rich, capitalist nations had the rest of the world by the throat, they said.

Our nine days in Argentina were very profitable. I never spoke to more bishops. Also, I addressed 50 law professors and legal experts, plus university, seminary and high school students, and priests and nuns. I stunned large audiences with *The Silent Scream*. Many people commented, "I had no idea what abortion really was."

At St. Nicholas, a small city of 120,000, the Blessed Virgin allegedly appears periodically to a barely literate woman. The seer writes out Mary's messages in perfect Spanish: prayer (the Rosary), penance, fasting, faith and adherence to religious duties. Many thousands are now praying the Rosary; cures and other miraculous events are reported. The local bishop is favorable. A shrine is now being built to house thousands. Ninety thousand marched recently in a commemorative procession. We have read

virtually nothing about this in our Catholic press, perhaps
because the Argentine bishops are very low key on it.

In a test case November 29, Argentina's supreme court
declared the 98-year-old law barring divorce unconstitutional. The rationale: The law relegated divorced (separ-
ated) remarried people to the second-class status of "con-
cubinage" and penalized the children of illegal marriages
after separation.

AUSTRIA: PROLIFERS vs. THEOLOGIANS

In August, Justice Minister Dr. Harold Ofner sounded
the alarm over the sinking Austrian birthrate and its
future consequences. Austria's bishops and her wild moral
theologians seem to have no such worries, even though
they are mostly responsible for the disappearance of the
Austrian family, because of their strong dissent to *Humanae Vitae* in 1968.

Today this "Catholic" country of seven million has more
abortions than births, 1.4 children per completed family,
20,000 registered prostitutes, ever more shacking up, relatively empty seminaries, and more closed kindergartens
and dying religious orders each year. This year Austria
ordained only 14 men to the priesthood.

The justice minister went so far as to say that "it has
even become a fashion not to found a family because raising children to adulthood means sacrifice." He asked,
"Who will support the growing layers of old people?" His
solution: larger family allowances and tax breaks.

He stressed that young people must learn that they do
not just have rights in society, but duties toward it as
well. Incidentally, Austria now has 200,000 foreigners,
many of them Moslems. Meanwhile, more die than are
born in this fast-aging nation.

Astonishingly, it never seems to occur to the godless
Socialists that the underlying causes of the developing
demographic disaster are abortion on demand, massive use
of the abortifacient Pill, increasing sterilization, rampant
and sickening pornography (imported mostly from West
Germany) and gross abuse of sex, which always strikes at
the heart of the family.

But then, the bishops, the moral theologians and most
Austrian priests do not seem to understand this either.
The official Austrian Catholic premarital program, *Ehe und
Familie*, teaches NFP on an equal basis with contracep-
tives and abortifacients. The Austrian hierarchy has also

Confessions of a Prolife Missionary

approved the test-tube-baby procedure, despite its condemnation by the Church.

The Pope is aware of the situation, though. For a full year he searched for someone to replace the retiring Francis Cardinal König. He finally chose a simple, more or less unknown, 67-year-old Benedictine, Fr. Hermann Groer. Fr. Groer was national head of the Legion of Mary and a great promoter of Marian devotion.

At his first news conference, the mostly anti-Catholic reporters were shocked when the newly appointed archbishop began by saying the "Our Father." They did not learn much, but their gut feeling was that Groer was "conservative," even "reactionary."

Later, a seemingly friendly reporter tricked Groer into a frank conversation. Carrying a hidden recorder, she had first appeared as a penitent. To the consternation of the Austrians and the embarrassment of the archbishop, she published his confidential remarks in the anti-clerical publication *Basta*. Actually, the new archbishop sounded rather orthodox despite her efforts to trip him up.

Nonetheless, Austrian Catholic papers have reported, and liberal Catholics keep saying, that Groer is on record as agreeing with the Austrian bishops' strong dissent from *Humanae Vitae*. He supposedly said Catholics must form their own consciences, whatever that means in the context.

The Austrian theologians have been writing, saying and teaching all of those things—and none more than the Jesuit Fr. Hans Rotter, the University of Innsbruck's Charles Curran. Rotter has weakly and pathetically defended Curran against the Vatican on TV and in the Catholic press. He has also attacked me several times.

This fall he will give three conferences on sexual morality to the Vienna clergy. Judging from his past writings, wherein he espoused Curran's condemned views even more boldly, he will proclaim the same errors for which Curran was declared unfit to teach as a Catholic theologian. Like Curran, Rotter cites the Austrian episcopal dissent when cornered.

Rotter is in good company with the Jesuit Scripture scholar Fr. Jacob Kremer, who also teaches at the university and seminary in Innsbruck. In a book on Lazarus, Kremer ever so subtly denies that Our Lord raised Lazarus from the dead. Then, even more insidiously, he denies the resurrection of Christ—while protesting his Catholicism and orthodoxy.

About 10 years ago Kremer gave a conference to the Viennese clergy. Afterward they broke into two groups, one accepting his strange views and the other rejecting them. When the aloof Cardinal König happened to drop in on the non-acceptors, they asked him where he stood on the matter. He gave them a non-answer by immediately condemning Archbishop Marcel Lefebvre. (Solid Catholics in Vienna keep asking me, "Does König believe?")

Austria's right to life movement is weak and divided. The one group with abundant financing, *Rettet das Leben*, pointedly refuses to condemn contraception. This is supposedly in deference to Austria's 100,000 or so Protestants. But mainly, people say, it is because most of its members practice contraception or use abortifacients, while others still believe that contraception is the remedy for abortion.

Director Ms. Grit Ebner refused to have her group show *The Silent Scream* until she could alter it; she was also instrumental in keeping it off national TV. *Burgerinitiative*, a totally prolife group under the courageous leadership of HLI's co-worker Martin Humer, is by far Austria's greatest defender of unborn babies, youth and the family.

Austria has a huge catechetical problem. An aggressive, anti-Catholic Socialist government is obviously out to destroy the family, with little opposition. To give you an idea of the religious situation, the abbot of famous Melk Abbey had parts of the Koran read in a pontifical High Mass instead of the Bible. Vienna's famous St. Stephen's Cathedral has a room set aside for all manner of other religions.

Austrian feminists talk loudly about women priests. Good priests are persecuted or neutralized by weak bishops who seem helpless before unorthodox theologians. With seminaries and religious novitiates almost empty and with more than 800 parishes without priests, the future looks bleak—like the Austrian apple trees dying from Chernobyl's fallout.

(According to reliable reports, Archbishop Groer has forbidden Fr. Rotter to lecture in Vienna. Also, Groer's handwritten responses to informed prolifers show he is thoroughly orthodox on contraception and totally prolife. Meanwhile, he is being attacked increasingly by the Modernists, who are also appealing to Austria's Apostolic Nuncio.)

HYPOCRISY IN THE LAND OF HIPPOCRATES

For condemning abortion and euthanasia 400 years before Christ, the Athenian doctor Hippocrates became known as "the Father of Modern Medicine." On one of her better days, the erratic anthropologist Margaret Mead wrote that he made the medical profession possible.

But on 3 July 1986, Hippocrates' descendants betrayed him by legalizing abortion on demand in Greece in the first 12 weeks of pregnancy, abortion for rape and incest up to 19 weeks, and abortion because of a defect up to 24 weeks—all paid for by the taxpayers. Both the Orthodox and Catholic Churches protested vehemently, but too late and in vain. For 10 years there had been threats of liberalization. In 1978 the Greek Jesuit publication *New Horizons* (formerly *Messenger of the Sacred Heart*) devoted a whole issue to the subject. Both churches had a decade to prepare their people and build a resistance, but the bishops did nothing, as in so many other countries.

In a bill outlining the State's duty to protect the citizens, the first section has five articles on "Protecting the Health of Women and Safeguarding Society." The second section has six articles on "Protecting the Environment." In Greece, as elsewhere, unborn babies are less important than ecology.

Any gynecologist may legally commit abortion in an approved hospital. The severe penalties for violation of the law are aimed only at the very many practitioners of clandestine baby-killing.

Four Roman Catholic bishops with whom I conversed agreed that some 1,000 babies are aborted daily, and surely well over 300,000 babies yearly in a nation of 10 million people. All of Greece's inhabitants are Orthodox Christians, as they call themselves, except for 45,000 Roman Catholics and thousands of American Catholic military personnel and their families (there are 50,000 Americans on Crete alone). Given estimated abortions and actual birthrates, there are at least two baby-murders for every live birth, with a nonreproductive birthrate of 1.9 children per completed family.

Neither the Orthodox Church nor the Roman Catholics have a single prolife film, slide or piece of literature with which to fight the abortionists. Bishops, priests and nuns were stunned by the films and literature I showed them. One bishop had already begun translating a piece I had sent in advance.

I left them $2,000 worth of the most persuasive audio-
visual aids, literature, etc., including 1,000 "Precious Feet"
lapel pins; and I promised much more. A Greek Jesuit
chaplain at an American military base promised to show
all of the films at all of the bases and to his youth groups.
He told me HLI could not send enough English-language
literature for distribution among U.S. servicemen and their
families.

NFP is unheard of among Greek Roman Catholics and
seemingly among the world's 400 million Orthodox, who
strongly condemn contraception. But Orthodox bishops
often imitate what the Catholic bishops suggest or start;
and the latter were most cooperative and eager to launch
prolife education despite their poverty. The only Catholic
weekly newspaper in Greece published my whole lecture.

The bishops begged me to return. I promised to raise
money for dubbing films such as *The Silent Scream* in
Greek.

With the cooperation of the bishops, we now have a
branch in Athens, run by a holy Franciscan, Fr. Dennis
Lambiris.

Only 10 percent of the Orthodox go to church regularly.
They are poorly catechized and at best are taught only a
vague, general morality. Married Orthodox priests tend to
have larger families than other Greeks. Being a married
priest in Greece seems to have one special disadvantage:
on the many islands (the country has 169 inhabited ones)
Orthodox Christians are often afraid to go to confession for
fear the priest's wife may find out their sins.

THE GROWING EUTHANASIA LOBBY

The World Federation of Right-to-Die Societies just met
in Bombay. Delegates came from most of the world's
nations. Today more than 60 nations have euthanasia
organizations. The USA alone has three such groups.

Death promotion always follows the legalization of
abortion and often involves the same godless people. Make
no mistake, euthanasia is already here, in the form of
medical neglect. And infanticide goes on daily, starving
babies who have handicaps. Holland and West Germany
are the countries closest to legalizing outright "mercy"
killing, euphemized as "death with dignity" or "merciful
self-release" or the "last right."

How well I remember saying "abortion today, euthanasia tomorrow" in my debates with pro-abortionists 25

years ago. My dishonest adversaries would always tell me and the audience that the idea was preposterous.

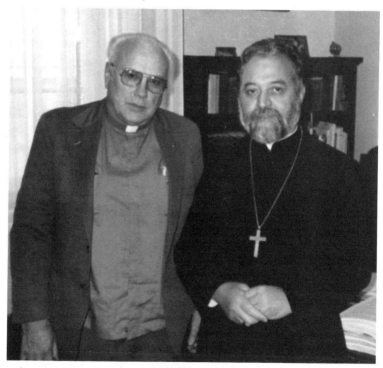

The Byzantine bishop of Athens (united with Rome) knows of Planned Parenthood's savagery.

UGLY AMERICANS TRAIN
MEXICANS TO KILL BABIES

(No. 28—February 1987)

Recently I spent five days in sprawling, fascinating Mexico City, making arrangements for our Third International Symposium. We hope that out of our historic Mexican symposium will come a new organization, the Latin American Alliance for the Family, to oppose the unscrupulous population controllers who were unleashed at the second World Population Conference in Mexico City in 1984. They are now wreaking great havoc on the people of this Catholic continent with massive, sometimes forced, sterilization programs and with abortifacient Pills, IUDs, injectables (Depo-Provera) and implants, while satanically propagandizing for legal abortion.

Mexico has enough economic, political and social problems without adding legalized child-murder. An informed Mexican quipped that so many abortions are already being committed in government hospitals and by *coma drona* (untrained midwives) that a law is not needed. And indeed it is not! Here, in the world's second-largest Catholic nation (82 million people), at least one million babies are killed annually.

Forced sterilization is another horror story. In government "Social Security" hospitals, doctors give you anesthesia for labor pains only if it is your first pregnancy—if it is your second, third, etc., you are on your own! Usually six birthing women are herded into one room; when they start moaning and screaming from birth pangs, they are faced with official forms to sign, allowing their sterilization. Many give in. Those who refuse will have another horrible experience to look forward to in their next pregnancy. The poor have no choice but these government hospitals.

I had a long discussion with five of the 10 medical students who came to my lecture at the archdiocesan center in San Jacinto. They assured me of a large audience of medical students if I did a future seminar for them on medical ethics—an opportunity I shall take. All of them were aware of many abortions' being committed.

In their training they are not forced to learn how to commit abortions; nor, to my surprise, are they asked to learn how to sterilize. But their many godless professors, mostly trained in the USA, make fun of the Catholic Church's prolife teachings by using word games and inaccurate pictures of unborn babies.

Not a few of these professors have taken month-long, condom-to-abortion anti-baby courses taught at four U.S. medical schools and paid for with your tax money by USAID (Agency for International Development). Over a long dinner, a good Catholic doctor who works for the government described in detail such a course he took in Denver. Flown in first class, wined and dined in the best hotel, these fledgling gynecologists were taught the latest techniques of artificial birth prevention. Natural family planning was laughed out of court.

I shall never forget how this young doctor angrily told me, "Your country pays our way to learn all about comprehensive birth control. In the end, you load us down with Pills, IUDs and what-not, including the equipment for menstrual extraction [early abortion], with assurances of more as needed, to do abortions in my country where they are forbidden." One can only hang one's head in shame. (Johns Hopkins Medical School conducts such programs in African cities, again with your tax dollars via USAID.)

Our three-person branch in Mexico City is working out of a one-room office in an archdiocesan complex next door to Auxiliary Bishop Francisco Aguilera. Cardinal Corripio-Ahumada and his eight auxiliaries have welcomed and encouraged HLI. Rent, equipment, audiovisual aids, literature, etc., cost HLI about $2,000 monthly.

Heading the office is the incomparable Mrs. Angelina Muñiz, who teaches NFP courses, coordinates youth-seminarian programs, and right now is translating Coleen Kelly Mast's pro-chastity books and adapting them to Latin America. People there have virtually nothing with which to combat the horrendous, mandatory Planned Parenthood-type sex education books being produced by governments victimized by fanatical foreign population controllers.

TACKLING EVERY PROBLEM BUT SIN

While I was in Mexico City, 70 liberation theologians, including 25 women from Latin America, Asia and Africa,

met for a week in their eighth annual closed gathering.
(The Ecumenical Association of Third World Theologians,
with a total worldwide membership of 111, was founded 10
years ago in Tanzania.)

Several theologians gave nightly open seminars to
mostly female audiences. These evening sessions were
hosted by the Dominicans at the leftist National Autonomous University of Mexico, where they have a center.
Addressing the overflow crowd of 500 were all the big guns
of liberation theology, such as Brazil's Fr. Leonardo Boff;
Peru's Fr. Gustavo Gutierrez; the best-known Protestant
exponent of liberation theology, José Miguez Bonino of
Argentina; an ex-nun and disciple of the Dominican Fr.
Edward Schillebeeckx, both of whom I once saw flailing the
Church and the Pope on Dutch TV; a nun from Zaire; a
wild Catholic bishop from Sri Lanka; and others. No one
seemed to know who paid the huge bills.

On the first evening a fight—almost a riot—broke out
between right-wingers in the audience and the libera-
tionists. Mexican Church officials immediately disowned
both. Thereafter the police were able to keep the theologians and the avid participants (who totalled 5,000 for the
week) from harassing each other.

Here are some samples of the theology: Brazilian
Dominican Frei Betto, organizer of a Christian "base community" and author of the notorious *Fidel and Religion*,
began his speech by saying, "All Christians were disciples
of a political prisoner who had been assassinated on the
cross." He then questioned the Pope's support for the
struggle of the oppressed. That is when the shoving and
shouting began.

But the police stepped in when Filipina Benedictine
nun Mary John Mananzar, focusing on the "oppression of
women in the world," offered: "The Pope told us when he
came to the Philippines that nuns and priests should not
involve themselves in politics. Yet he is the most political
pope we have ever seen." In a rather un-Benedictine way
she went on, "We don't just want women to get into the
hierarchy; we want the hierarchy dissolved to have a more
secular church." She reminded her audience that the early
Christians elected bishops.

Incidentally, when peace was restored, Betto, who had
for many hours sat at the feet of atheist Fidel Castro to
hear his "religious convictions," ventured grandly, "It is
impossible to live our faith in isolation."

A Catholic bishop from Sri Lanka, Tissa Balasurorya, advocated the ordination of women priests. Emphasizing this as an example of the direction the Church should take, he remarked triumphantly, "I do not see any reason why there can't be a brown, white or yellow woman pope." Quite a contrast to Pope John Paul II's insistence that women's ordination is contrary to Tradition, Scripture and common sense.

A leading Nicaraguan church activist gave the Sandinistas unequivocal support: "As a Nicaraguan and as a Christian," he intoned, "the first thing I must do is state my solidarity with my people in their struggle against aggression." Once known as the "Red Bishop of Cuernavaca," Mexico's retired Sergio Mendez Areo announced from the stage, "We on this platform wish to manifest our opposition to the Reagan intervention in Nicaragua."

"Theology and the Socioeconomic Crisis" was the theme of the Peruvian pioneer Fr. Gutierrez—who will teach this summer at the Jesuits' Boston College, along with the Church-despising, pro-abortion Rosemary Radford Ruether, ex-Jesuit priest Bernard Cooke, confused ex-Christian Brother Gabriel Moran and other dissidents.

Describing his work among the poor in the slums of Lima, Fr. Gutierrez remarked, "Poverty means both physical and cultural death. We have to look at the causes of a socioeconomic system that produces poor people." (For him and the other speakers, sin never seemed to be a cause of human misery.)

Fr. Gutierrez had come to terms with a Marxist critique of religion, using Marx (Karl, not Paul!) for his own economic analysis. He rejected "the fatalistic perspective of the orthodox Catholic Church, which promises a paradise after death." (Has he ever read the Church's social encyclicals?) Instead, he insists, religion should be concerned with the present world—which seems to be the preoccupation of the liberation theologians, who also seem strangely allied to the religion of radical feminism.

Marianne Katoppo, an Indonesian Protestant and author of the prize-winning book *Compassionate and Free*, chose to speak about the Virgin of Guadalupe, whose apparitions had been celebrated the day before. Katoppo accused the Catholic Church of not respecting the wishes of the Virgin, who asked that a temple be built where she appeared. "As the Lady appeared as a peasant on the hills and asked for a shrine to be built for her there,"

Katoppo asked, "would she really want this futuristic edifice that now exists?" (A new, modernistic shrine was built 10 years ago near the old one, which is crumbling due to unstable soil.) Why did Katoppo, who has no room for Mary in her life or her theology, even bother?

It is strange that in a meeting of mostly Catholic theologians who purportedly love and wish to foster Catholicism, nothing was said about sin, humanity's fall and proneness to evil, or our need of redeeming grace—not to mention prayer, penance, the sacraments, the corporal and spiritual works of mercy, the seven capital sins, the commandments, the magnificent social doctrine of the Church and other essentials.

The liberation theologians have an enormous confidence in our flawed human nature, in social action and in politics. But society is only an abstraction and does not exist. While "saving" this phantom, they neglect woefully the Church's mission of converting individual persons by spiritual/moral means.

And although they alleged that the Pope is a priest who engages in politics, politics is about all they talked about—coupled with a vague utopianism to be achieved by some indefinite sociopolitical, perhaps even revolutionary, means. That is why at our symposium we presented Cardinal Ratzinger–approved reconciliation theology versus liberation theology in talks by Peruvian authorities.

The theologians' meeting took place in an important but poor country of many contrasts and contradictions. Mexico has an anticlerical constitution and does not even allow the 11,000 priests (and more religious) to vote, own property or wear clerical dress in public. But the Church operates 8,000 Catholic schools anyway.

Meanwhile, a new clerical advocacy is establishing itself on the Mexican scene. Risking the dangerous charge of meddling in politics, six northern bishops in July issued an unusual pastoral letter condemning rigged elections. In the border state of Chihuahua, Archbishop Adalberto Almeida, to protest voting irregularities, suspended Mass for one Sunday. The Vatican overruled him when the government (!) appealed to Rome.

Atheism-promoting, government-sanctioned schoolbooks grudgingly admit that it was a village priest, the national hero Miguel Hidalgo, who ignited Mexico's 11-year struggle for independence from exploiting Spain. But anticlerical forces are angry at the Pope for announcing his intention of beatifying the beloved Fr. Miguel Pro, SJ, one of many Mexican priests martyred "in hatred of the Faith" in the 1920s.

HLI has an important mission in this fascinating and culturally rich country of 82 million, which will grow to 112 million by the year 2000. Our bilingual symposium will organize leaders from all over the restless Latin world and teach them how to resist the antilife/anti-family destroyers from the affluent and dying North, while shoring up their own Catholic family structure and culture. Please *pray*, and come help us!

CARDINAL BERNARDIN'S INCONSISTENCIES

U.S. bishops talk about a "consistent life ethic" but are consistently inconsistent in their own actions on life issues. A conspicuous example is Chicago's Joseph Cardinal Bernardin, who recently tried to save Fr. Charles Curran.

In 1984 Fr. Charles Fanelli, Chicago's archdiocesan prolife director, sponsored two well-attended Holy Hours and Masses of reparation for the sin of contraception. Cardinal Bernardin stopped these penance services and moved Fr. Fanelli to a distant parish.

Last year Bernardin incurred the wrath of Chicago's homosexuals when his commendable intervention prevented passage of a city "gay rights" ordinance. But in a subsequent pastoral on homosexuality the Cardinal chided certain Protestant ministers for saying AIDS is a divine punishment for the sin of Sodom. (How does he know it is not?) Recently he appointed a Loyola University professor as Church liaison to AIDS patients, a move greeted with more than skepticism by homosexual leaders.

As episcopal moderator of the Bishops' Committee for Pro-Life Activities, the Cardinal issued a good-sounding statement (also given at the last meeting of the American bishops) on the institutionalization-integration of NFP. He wrote:

1. NFP should be integrated into the mainstream of marriage and family life ministry. It should be seen as an inherent and indispensable part of this ministry, with positive support from all other marriage and family agencies.
2. All diocesan agencies should provide positive information and motivation in regard to NFP.

They should assist, collaborate with and recruit for
NFP instruction.
3. In the overall allocation of diocesan resources,
proportionate money, personnel and other resources
should be assigned to the NFP program.
4. The diocesan NFP program should be given
appropriate status and leadership. Other NFP
groups should collaborate with and be integrated
into the overall diocesan program, with the understanding that the diocesan program enjoys the
bishop's approval and support.

If these fine sentiments are Cardinal Bernardin's, why
has he allocated only $15,000 for the Chicago NFP project?
And what is the use of institutionalizing NFP into an
episcopal bureaucracy that is almost antilife?   I know
bishop-appointed lay persons in charge of diocesan NFP
programs who are semi-hostile to NFP or are themselves
sterilized. And the NCCB *apparat* certainly does not have
NFP talent, literature or experience, even though Pope
Pius XII called for NFP research and development twice in
1951, when he also warned prophetically about the consequences of contraception.

Might not the $300,000 that the Knights of Columbus
gave the bishops to promote NFP have been better spent
on loyal, orthodox NFP teacher-trainers such as the Couple
to Couple League and others who are the pioneers and
veterans?   Whatever he may think now, Msgr. George
Higgins told me years ago, "If you want to stifle or kill
something, bring it into the national bishops' conference."
Are we seeing episcopal tokenism again?

Last October the Cardinal addressed the Consistent
Ethic of Life Conference at the University of Portland in
Oregon. He spoke on the "seamless garment" concept of
prolife issues. When a gynecologist told him privately that
contraception and the contraceptive mentality should be
part of the "seamless garment," Cardinal Bernardin dis-
agreed defensively, saying that contraception was an altogether different and unrelated moral issue.

Later, in his address, he repeated this, saying that he
would issue a pastoral on sexual morality. What would
the Cardinal say if he knew that so-called contraceptive
birth control is abortifacient? And why does he not know?

OREGON CHURCH PROBLEMS

A recent conference on the "consistent life ethic" in Oregon revealed the serious problems facing the Church in the Northwest. This conference began each day not with the usual formal prayer but with liturgical dancing and meditation. The Oregon Catholic Bishops' Conference cosponsored it with the University of Portland. Its chief organizer was anti-*Humanae Vitae* Fr. Thomas Odo, CSC, president of the university and coauthor of a highly questionable handbook on homosexuality, *Homosexual Catholics: A New Primer for Discussion.*

(Fr. Odo was scheduled to offer the Mass and preach at the Dignity convention (homosexual Catholics) in the embattled Archbishop Hunthausen's cathedral in Seattle, until pressure from the University's Board of Regents caused him to decline. The Regents asked him not even to attend. He attended anyway and received a standing ovation for his contribution to Dignity.

(Also addressing the Dignity conference was the Dominican Fr. Matthew Fox, who said, among other things, "You cannot sin because you are god [God?]." (See Gen. 3:4–5.) His female witch colleague Starhawk did not accompany him. The Holy See is investigating Fr. Fox's writings again.)

Back to the Consistent Ethic Conference: Another speaker was the irrepressible Sidney Callahan, who dissented loudly to *Humanae Vitae*. Protesters picketed her (inside the hall) and finally forced her, in the question/answer period, to say whether she still espouses her sharp dissent. (Trying to keep the question from being asked were the Oregon bishops' legal counsel, Robert Castagna, and two ladies helping him to sift the questions.) Callahan boldly assured the audience that the encyclical was a colossal mistake and that it would fade away.

She also used the occasion to promote women's ordination; the audience, largely priests and religious men and women, applauded vigorously. At the end of the session Auxiliary Bishop Steiner praised her copiously. Does he know that "contraceptives" abort?

Oregon's Sen. Mark Hatfield, a Christian who has cast some crucial pro-abortion votes, addressed the group by videocassette. He said, "Those anti-abortionists exhibit a death-wish in certain pieces of legislation they try to pass." The senator, who is known as a vigorous promoter of PP, agreed with Cardinal Bernardin's "seamless garment" concept. Instead of refuting him, the supposed defenders of life applauded him.

Bill Olson, a young and magnificently prolife Protestant state senator from Medford, attended my recent seminar at Portland's Holy Rosary Parish. In the Q/A session he complained about how weak the churches were in helping the few legislators who are fighting the introduction of sex clinics in high schools. When I asked him whether the Catholic bishops did not have a lawyer to monitor things and fight their cause, Olson said they did indeed, but that he—Castagna—was totally ineffective.

At this conference the progressive Fr. Burton Griffin, pastor of Pius X Parish, spoke of "our martyred Hunthausen who is under unjust attack." The hall roared its approval, with Bishops Kenneth Steiner and Paul Waldschmidt applauding. Then he "deplored right-to-lifers for not having charity and compassion towards girls entering an abortion center." This, of course, did not set well with those in the audience who had just completed an all-night vigil at Holy Rosary Parish and who pray on Saturdays in front of the Lovejoy (!) Clinic, Portland's largest killing chamber.

The same Fr. Griffin obtained 101 signatures from the priests' senate on behalf of Hunthausen. He was going to announce it at a press conference, but was dissuaded from doing so by Portland's new Archbishop William Levada, who will have to stem the Hunthausen disease in the archdiocese. Archbishop Levada will no doubt also catch up with the archdiocesan education office's disastrous policy statement on sex education, which his predecessor approved on 24 March 86.

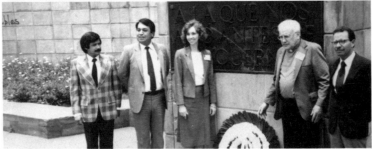

Prolifers presented a wreath at a plaza in Mexico City dedicated 'to her who loved us before she knew us'—to mothers.

CANADIAN BISHOPS WAFFLE IN FACE OF MODERN HORRORS

(No. 29—March 1987)

Truth raises against itself the storm that scatters its seeds broadcast. — Rabindranath Tagore, India's poet laureate and Nobel Prize winner.

I am just back from my latest missionary journey to Canada. I spent 17 days in six archdioceses giving pro-life/pro-family talks and doing 10 radio and TV programs—one for multiple showings on cable TV.

This French- and English-speaking country, 80 percent Christian and 47 percent Catholic, is a world of contradictions and contrasts. For example, Canada is the only country in which Catholic politicians engineered virtual abortion on demand. The culprits were the slippery "Catholic" Prime Minister Pierre Trudeau, who manipulated the bishops, and "Catholic" Member of Parliament John Turner. The latter may be the next premier of this huge, dying country, which has only 1.7 children per completed family. The birthrate in "Catholic" Quebec province matches West Germany's, which is the lowest in the world: 1.3 children.

According to the 1969 Canadian law, doctors may kill babies only in accredited hospitals after the approval of a medical committee. The decisions are always the same. The provinces of Prince Edward Island and Newfoundland are abortion-free. Saskatchewan has a prolife government and no legal abortions, but there are about 1,000 illegal ones annually among her one million citizens. Manitoba, with only two million people, has 3,400 teen pregnancies a year.

The highest abortion rates are in French Catholic Quebec, followed by Ontario and British Columbia. The prolife and Catholic premier of the latter has rejected "safe sex" education and has called for chastity education instead. The media are crucifying him.

In December 1986, Ontario passed a bill amending its civil rights code to include "homosexual orientation." Along

with this sin go horrendous medical consequences totally
covered up by the media.

The bishops of Ontario issued a heavily theological
statement opposing the "gay rights" bill. They failed,
however, to mention the gruesome medical/social results of
homosexual activity—the one thing that might have in-
fluenced the politicians. Other Canadian Catholics wondered with me whether the bishops really know how homosexuals destroy the family, the Church, society and each
other.

Ontario is now considering setting up free-standing
abortuaries that will be "legal" because they are near
hospitals. This is at the instigation of Marian Powell,
M.D., whom I debated on Montreal TV. The same province
is pioneering "safe sex" education for young teens, causing
a furor among believing Catholics. According to the Toronto *Star*, schools are already implementing programs teaching homosexual-relations-plus-condom.

Vancouver TV showed a classroom of children, 10–14
years old, playing with condoms and an erect plastic penis.
The teacher showed them how to use condoms to avoid
AIDS; the children blew them into balloons. Only a society that has become Sodom and Gomorrah allows such
things. Parents from a Quebec Catholic (separate) school
complained about a religion teacher who had his 15-year-
old boys and girls fondle contraceptives in class. The
godless Quebec government recommends this to health
nurses who speak to students.

Proportionally, Canada is second only to the USA in
number of AIDS victims, with almost 1,000 cases (according to Bishop Crowley's *Catholic Times*, Montreal's equivalent of the American *National Catholic Reporter*). Catholic
theologians at Montreal's St. Augustine's Seminary were
speculating whether using condoms would be moral for
"safe sex" because, after all, the Canadian hierarchy allowed contraception for hard cases.

Fr. Jack Gallagher, professor of moral theology at
Toronto's St. Michael's College, wrote a typically subtle,
waffling, almost naive policy statement for the archdiocese.
It was approved by Cardinal Carter and seen by all the
bishops of Toronto. Said Fr. Gallagher, "It seems that at
the appropriate grade level, one should include in the
program the technical information about the use of condoms . . . to avoid the disease," while also giving orthodox
moral teaching (by mostly contracepting teachers?). Their

dissent to *Humanae Vitae* (which they now deny) will haunt the Canadian bishops for ages to come.

Quite different is the approach of the Irish, English and German hierarchies. AIDS is epidemic in Ireland, but mostly due to drug abuse. The Irish bishops' recent statement begged people to pray for "a strong moral response." Offering condoms would only "give further encouragement to permissiveness," thus feeding the disease even more. They appealed urgently for faithful monogamy and chastity, and said the solution does not lie in "free needles or easy availability of condoms."

In AIDS-frantic England, George Basil Cardinal Hume wisely recommended "refusal to engage in extramarital sexual activity." He insisted that "promiscuity is the root cause of the present epidemic; it has always been sinful; it is rapidly becoming suicidal." The government's massively funded "solution" is condoms, even though the *British Medical Journal* declared the recent 2.5-million-pound ad campaign a failure (25 October 1986).

Dr. Rita Süssmuth is Germany's "Catholic" pro-abortion health minister and vice-president of the German Catholic Women. In a national advertising campaign, she recommends the condom when you have "intimate sexual intercourse with unknown or changing partners." The ads say, "Trust is good, but the condom is better. To die of AIDS is painful—condoms are not painful."

"Such conduct and such a 'solution' is unworthy of human beings," thundered the German bishops. "[T]he problem lies deeper," they added. "Human sexuality requires control by reason and morality, so that passion does not rule man but man passion." Alas, these same bishops forgot this in 1968 when they strongly dissented to *Humanae Vitae*, under the influence of Fr. Karl Rahner and similar theologians.

In a Sunday afternoon parish session for engaged couples in Manitoba (which I learned about), someone asked about the morality of contraception. The priest waffled, thus destroying in minutes what the couple teaching natural family planning (NFP) had tried to accomplish in two hours. Canadian priests are mired in contraception to an astonishing degree, because "they don't want to make waves," "they run popularity contests," "they fear losing parishioners and getting a smaller collection" or "they don't want to disturb anyone," as enlightened Catholics will tell you. Thank God, you also meet the courageous priest who stands up even if he is persecuted—as happens around the world.

Again and again women in prairie towns and cities asked me where they could get NFP information. In the village of Roblin, Manitoba, I conducted an afternoon NFP seminar for 14 people, after a morning address to 40 students in a minor seminary run by Ukrainian Redemptorists.

In a small city parish elsewhere in Canada, a layman conducts a morning Word Service every Sunday. People are led to believe this fulfills their Sunday obligation, even though there are Masses all around. When scandalized Catholics brought this to the archbishop's attention, he defended the pastor and refused to answer whether attending Sunday Mass was an obligation.

In a public school (which has mostly Catholic students) in Swan Lake, Manitoba, Protestant teachers stopped my showing of *The Silent Scream* (produced by a Jewish agnostic) because it is too "Catholic." I spoke in more than 20 Catholic schools, but in only one did the students know the meaning of chastity. In the presence of 16- and 17-year-old girls and boys, I asked one teaching nun whether it was true that nothing was taught on sexual morality. She said she had been there only one year, but that a priest comes in to teach something about the Sixth Commandment at the end of high school.

A Ukrainian bishop who heard my banquet address to 350 prolifers in Yorkton, Saskatchewan, agreed thoroughly with what I said in my talk. He told me that contrary to what I had believed, things were no better among the Ukrainians.

(This year his people celebrate the 1,000th anniversary of Christianity in their homeland, where a large portion of the 50 million Ukrainians still practice their faith, although underground.)

I had a very interesting closed session with 18 priests of one archdiocese. One can only sympathize and agonize with good priests who labor under weak bishops and face ultra-feminist nuns and contracepting teachers in "Catholic" schools and CCD classes. But most of these good priests seemed to have little understanding of how contraception is the gateway to teenage and other fornication, sterilization, runaway VD, abortions, low birthrates and other horrors. I urged them to promote NFP. These overworked priests were great.

Speaking of birthrates, I showed films and spoke to 18 enthusiastic Trappists in Manitoba. All studies, worldwide, show that priests and religious usually come from larger families. So I asked each one the size of his family; the average was 7.8 children! This highlights the importance of our *One More Child* booklet and the One More Child movement, which promotes larger families.

All the episcopal hand-wringing, all the work of vocation directors and, yes, all the prayers may be of little worth unless fervently Catholic couples learn once more that they beget children for God and Heaven. The future is empty until generous husbands and wives are motivated to oppose our affluent, sex-soaked society and have more children, who, raised by self-sacrificing parents, will again want to work for the Lord exclusively.

Unfortunately, Montreal's Auxiliary Bishop Leonard Crowley, who boycotted our international symposium in Montreal last April, has not accepted our public offer of space in our *Special Reports* and *HLI Reports* to prove his accusations against HLI. The recent instruction from the Holy See on homosexuality states that one should not give even the slightest hint that homosexual acts are justifiable. So we wonder whether Bishop Crowley will celebrate Mass for and preach to the homosexual Dignity convention again, as he did last year.

We congratulate him for taking the lead in organizing a treatment shelter for AIDS victims in Montreal. But we are astonished that he allowed psychiatrist Jack Dominian, Britain's most notorious dissenter to *Humanae Vitae*, to preach his errors to Montreal's English-speaking Catholics. The beleaguered Fr. Charles Curran embarrassed the Canadian bishops by saying his views on *Humanae Vitae* were no different from their dissenting statement.

The battle is raging over the Canadian bishops' radical-feminist "Green Kit" discussion packet, the errors of which have inspired the formation of no fewer than three orthodox women's groups, one ecumenical and two Catholic. The ecumenical one is REAL Women (Realistic, Equal, Active and for Life). The Catholic ones are the Canadian contingent of Women for Faith and Family and Women for Life, Faith and Family (WLFF). I taped a lecture, the "Differential Psychology of Man and Woman," for the latter group.

WLFF produced a "Blue Kit" of orthodox discussion guidelines. The bishops repudiated the Blue Kit, as they

did both Catholic groups, but WLFF has been accepted to
make a presentation in Rome at the Synod on the Laity
this year. The national Canadian Women's League seems
about as moribund as its American counterpart, the 14-
million-strong (weak?) National Council of Catholic Women.

It will be interesting to see what the American bishops
say about women in their 1988 statement. Given today's
theological and religious climate, they cannot win. As
Shakespeare warns us, "Hell hath no fury like a woman
scorned."

Thanks be to God, our Canadian branch in Montreal
and its subcenter in Ottawa are truly flourishing, distribut-
ing prolife/chastity materials throughout Canada and translating literature and audiovisual aids into French for Quebec and French-speaking African countries.

But we are still fighting to get the truth out. Archbishop Antoine Hacault of the Archdiocese of St. Augustine
in French Winnipeg is the first bishop in my 39 years of
priesthood to forbid me to speak in his archdiocese. Chancellor Fr. Rolland Belanger explained that I might be
"another Curran," I was "too radical," "I don't speak like
the Canadian bishops" and I am "a lone ranger." It was
sad to hear responsible Catholics observe that Archbishop
Hacault is "more French than Catholic" and surely not
very prolife.

STRUGGLES, VICTORIES IN THE PHILIPPINES

The judge and chairwoman of the Constitutional Commission (ConCom) which created the Philippines' new
anti-abortion constitution remarked that "no other issue
received as much support as the prolife and family issues"
(76 percent of the people voted for the new constitution).

In 1972 President Marcos issued an executive order
that established a huge population control program. In
poured American money. Now the offensive population
commission (POPCOM) is being reoriented from population
control to population care! USAID is stymied. They do
not know where to put your money because the new
POPCOM chairperson, a prolifer, refuses to sign all the
project proposals on sterilization, abortifacient IUDs and
Depo-Provera, etc.

Our people are working to get President Cory Aquino
to revise Marcos' executive order which called for a draco-
nian reduction of population to replacement level by 2010.
Our friend Bishop Jesus Varela, chairman of the Episcopal

Commission on Family Life, wrote an open letter on behalf of the Filipino hierarchy to the president, reminding her of three points raised in the constitutional debate:

1. A billion and a half pesos have been spent on population programs without any effect on alleviating mass poverty.

2. It is unjust to have such a policy imposed on our people by the World Bank and the IMF [International Monetary Fund], and

3. The creation of new life involves religious and spiritual values which public authorities should not interfere with. It is vitally linked to bodily integrity which is inherent in dignity and self-determination.

Bishop Varela pointed out how the commission "proved the population panic to be groundless and unjust," and observed, "Family Life workers across the country are indignant over the continuing violation of the human right [to] life and respect [for] individual consciences." He then insisted that the issue is not responsible parenthood or family planning methods. Instead, it is "whether . . . the State should make it a policy to curb the growth rate of our people—this is what the ConCom rejected."

Then he requested that the money formerly used for coercive sterilization and destruction of the family be used instead for family welfare and for socio-economic development involving value formation and the private sector. President Aquino has finally agreed to move against the population coercers and to channel their monies into all manner of family-support/welfare programs. We have been asked to help work out the details. But will USAID fund them? Its officials always proclaim they only support what governments want. We shall see.

One of the heroes in this battle was Fr. Al Schwartz, the generous genius of Korean Relief in Seoul, who contributed more than 200 copies of *The Silent Scream* for the prolife battle in Asia's only Catholic nation. This film has been on Filipino TV many times.

Our Filipino workers now have the Heaven-sent help of an ex-abortionist gynecologist who has come out strongly in giving testimony. Now he is helping to identify illegal abortion clinics. Our organizer on the scene, the resourceful Sr. Pilar Verzosa, RGS, writes that he needs many prayers, because he falls into depression and guilt over the babies he killed.

N.F.P. AND FAITH GO HAND IN HAND IN POLAND

A nation of 27 million when World War II began, Poland suffered six million deaths as Nazi Germany and then the USSR overran her. Despite all obstacles, or maybe because of them, the Church today truly flourishes in this Catholic nation, which now numbers 37 million, including a sprinkling of mostly German Protestants.

Some 90 percent of all Poles attend Sunday Mass, in 38 dioceses. All seminaries and novitiates are filled; the archdiocese of Krakow alone has 10 major seminaries, and last June ordained 77 priests. Poland today is the chief Western source of vocations, sending hundreds of priests and religious into the foreign missions yearly. Hundreds of Polish priests have gone to Canada and the USA, now that these countries have become mission lands once again.

At this moment Poland is building 1,000 new churches. Because there are no Catholic schools, hospitals or other institutions (apart from Europe's only two pontifical universities, at Lublin and Warsaw), life centers around the parish, where intensive religious instruction takes place. Every priest and nun attached to a parish teaches six to seven hours of religion daily!

Today Ireland and Poland are the only developed countries still reproducing themselves. One out of five children in Western Europe today is Polish. More than 40 percent of all Polish married couples practice NFP, learned before marriage in some 3,000 NFP teaching centers in a country the size of New Mexico.

When he was Cardinal Archbishop of Krakow, Pope John Paul II urged his priests to try never to marry a couple who had not learned God's built-in way of natural fertility control. For this purpose, he set up a comprehensive premarriage course. This program eventually spread through the whole of Poland. I remember sending him natural family planning materials when he was Professor of Philosophy at Lublin.

The government does not want women to be pregnant, because they drop out of the work force. Because housing is short (and also to embarrass the Church), the government fosters and pays for abortions, of which there are an estimated 200,000 each year (not 800,000 as Planned Parenthood falsely reports).

The Polish situation has its oddities. As a youth, Premier Wojciech Jaruzelski served Mass in Stefan Cardinal Wyszynski's private chapel. They say the premier's wife is a fervent Catholic. One million Soviet soldiers "keep order." It was Soviet soldiers in Polish uniforms who imposed martial law. Like most non-Soviet soldiers behind the Iron Curtain, Polish soldiers are not entrusted with the most powerful weapons.

All things considered, Catholicism flourishes more in beleaguered Poland than in any Western country. Affluence is unknown, and the Faith is nourished and tempered by hardship. Except for the Philippines, we have poured more prolife materials into Poland than into any other country.

STERILIZATION RAVAGES PUERTO RICO

A film shown at the San Antonio Latin American Film Festival last November was dynamite for prolifers: *La Operación* (The Operation). This film documents the genocidal sterilization of Puerto Rican women through a government-imposed, island-wide campaign using tubal ligation for population control. The anti-child forces have neutered an estimated 35–40 percent of Puerto Rican women with this barnyard, veterinarian approach to birth control.

The film has received several awards. Incredibly, it was produced and sponsored by feminist organizations and financed in part by the Playboy Foundation.

Given the influx of Protestant ministers, this Caribbean nation may be the first in Latin America to go Protestant.

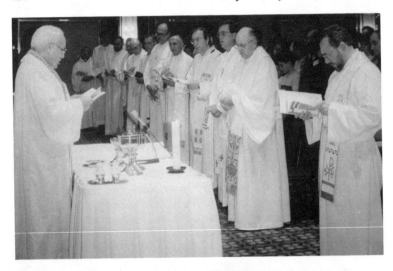

Mass at HLI conferences are usually concelebrated.

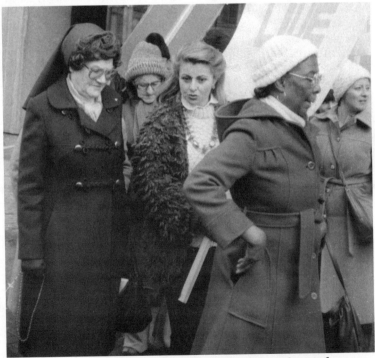

Sister Lucille Durocher prays with picketers in Montreal.

DAVID AND GOLIATH
at the AIR FORCE ACADEMY

(No. 30—April 1987)

Out of the wild blue came an invitation to moderate a roundtable conference at the U.S. Air Force Academy. Each year the American Assembly of Columbia University sponsors a foundation-funded "Academy Assembly." Prominent government officials, military officers, businessmen and educators discuss important national issues with undergraduate delegates from major universities and then make recommendations in a final consensus and summary paper.

At this, the 29th Academy Assembly, the topic was the USA's overseas population control policy. But the cards were stacked: almost everyone took it for granted that obviously there is dangerous overpopulation (even though the world's population growth rate has been declining since 1971), and that contraception, sterilization and abortion are absolutely necessary. Virtually nothing was said about economic development, just distribution of goods, and fair trade laws; nor did anyone mention that the West is dying because of low birthrates. The extensive bibliography was woefully one-sided.

The scheduled keynote speaker was to be Rafael Salas, the notorious Filipino "Catholic" who headed the United Nations Fund for Population Activities (UNFPA). But Salas had died suddenly in a Washington hotel room a few days earlier. The present pope once gave him a dressing down when Salas went to Rome seeking a blessing for his enormously wicked worldwide population control efforts. It was Salas' UNFPA (along with IPPF) that gave Red China special honors for its hideous forced-abortion campaign.

Taking Salas' place was Dr. Duff G. Gillespie from USAID. The student participants, official observers and faculty came largely from antilife organizations such as PP, USAID, the Ford Foundation and the Population Council. Gillespie moaned that less than one percent of our GNP and only two percent of U.S. foreign aid money is spent on birth control.

He asserted falsely that Buddhism and Hinduism do not object to Western forms of fertility control, said nothing about Moslem objections, and boasted that even in Catholic Brazil "60 percent of Catholics practice contraception" (where did he get that statistic?). Gillespie said nothing of the dying West. By the year 2000, he hoped, four billion dollars would be spent annually to reduce world population, with the World Bank being the chief source of funds.

Astonishingly, Gillespie revealed that the USAID bought more Pills and IUDs for distribution to the world's poor in a year than are used in the USA in one year. Like PP's foundress Margaret Sanger, Gillespie loves humanity but cannot stand people.

In a question-and-answer period I presented barbed questions and pointed observations until Gillespie got himself off the hook by saying, "Others want to ask questions." It is astonishing how much fiction and even falsehood is given out and accepted as fact today by "intellectuals" and "authorities" in high places.

I experienced that painfully the next evening. As a guest panelist, I tangled with a vice president of the notorious Population Council and a Chinese population "expert" who advises Red China's UN delegation.

After admitting that I practiced birth control all the time, I gave a 15-minute lecture explaining how the authentic Catholic Church *does* believe in birth control: it forbids fornication and adultery and, ideally, recommends a thorough course of marriage preparation, with responsible family planning by NFP when necessary. I reminded the audience that some 80 percent of doctor-done abortions last year were committed on babies conceived through unmarried sex. I also pointed out that the Catholic Church had the perfect and only solution to the VD plague and the spread of AIDS: chastity before marriage and then faithful monogamy.

We must not, I insisted, treat our young as if they were animals, as does PP. (Arguing for contraceptive advertising on TV, PP President Faye Wattleton said to the *Los Angeles Times*, "They advertise for [cock]roach birth controls. Manufacturers of [contraceptive] products ought to have the same access.") Knowing the abysmal ignorance of NFP even among Catholics, I explained that way of life briefly.

I then cited evidence from ruthless and notorious population controllers such as PP's Malcolm Potts that contraception increases the abortion rate, and that those two evils feed each other. It is the Catholic Church, I showed, that fosters true sexual freedom, self-control and genuine love.

I also cited the coercive population control measures recommended for U.S. population programs by PP's Frederick S. Jaffe. The vice president of the Population Council, Paul Domeny, a native Hungarian fallen-away Catholic, came back with a typical PP pitch. He claimed his friend Jaffe was for voluntarism. I replied that I could only go by what Jaffe had written and circulated widely.

To my amazement the Chinese expert denied my charge that there was forced abortion in Red China! In any case, he said, China had no choice but to reduce radically its population growth. He contradicted himself again and again. He claimed he had never heard of Steven Mosher's two books exposing the brutality (summarized in the lead story of the February 1987 *Reader's Digest*) and other evidence from reputable investigators.

Nor was he happy with my informing the audience that Red China, because it allows only one child and boys are preferred to girls, has some 500,000 female infanticides yearly, according to reliable reports. But the audience was delighted with the two-against-one debate. I left them with HLI literature proving what I said. Several people told me privately, "It's good you were here; otherwise it would have been a typical one-sided affair," as are all of these population conferences, which are widely reported in the press.

The roundtable discussion of bright political science university students went well; they seemed much more moderate in their views and sensitive to the freedom/coercion issue than the high-powered faculty. Surprisingly, only a few realized that minors in the USA can abort their babies without parental consent or knowledge.

The Air Force Academy is a fascinating institution. Forty-two percent of the cadets are Catholic, and 12 percent women. Some 80 go to Mass daily. During Lent, some 200 attend Mass daily at the unique and beautiful chapel, Colorado's chief sightseeing attraction. Academic standards are high. Celibacy is insisted upon and mostly observed. As you enter the grounds, the words "We Seek Men," carved in stone, stare at you.

I asked why the Catholic percentages at this academy and at West Point (52 percent) are more than double that

in the U.S. population. The answers: Catholic parents
still insist on more discipline; Catholics are more conservative politically; geography plays a part, as there are seven
times more Mormons at Colorado's Air Force Academy than
at heavily Catholic New York's West Point. Will these
Catholic majorities be found in future service academies,
now that the Catholic birthrate (minus Hispanics) is lower
than the national average?

SINGAPORE FRANTIC FOR MORE BABIES

With the "help" of PP, this island city-state of 2.5
million people on 618 square kilometers began a population
control program in 1966. In 1970 Singapore allowed abortion on demand, and 1,913 babies were legally aborted; in
1985, doctors killed 23,512 babies, putting the nation
15,000 babies below the number needed for replacement.
Today the government openly admits that abortion has
become a primary means of birth control, as it always does
wherever it is legalized.

In the early 1970s the government strongly recommended a maximum of two children. "Stop at Two" was
the slogan. The State penalized parents with three or
more children; it pressured those with two children to
submit to sterilization.

The campaign succeeded so well that the government
has now thrown PP out. To remedy "the procreation problem," it has begun to promote births and discourage abortion. Astonishingly, the desperate government, citing
Eastern European experience, has revealed a fact that an
international conspiracy of silence has suppressed for
years: a nation with a high abortion rate suffers an alarm-
ing increase in miscarriages and underweight, stillborn and
premature babies. Prematurity is the chief cause of mental retardation (that is why you should never give a nickel
to the March of Dimes, which is up to its ears in amniocentesis leading to abortions).

The health department has made pre- and post-abor-
tion counseling mandatory. It has produced two videocassettes discouraging abortion, "Decide with Care" and "Abortion Is Not a Method of Birth Control," to be shown before
and after the "procedure," respectively. Also required is a
14-day training program for counselors.

To commit a legal baby-killing, the killer-doctor must
now have a registered nurse trained in counseling, provide
a private area for counseling, and have a TV set and

videocassette player to show the two rather gruesome gov-
ernment-produced videos. So loud was the howl over
showing the "gory" aspects of an actual abortion that the
government has agreed to replace them with diagrams.
The politicians have installed a whole battery of positive "procreation" incentives, from tax-relief to full, paid
maternity leave.   "Stop at Two" has become "Three Is
Better."
Will it work? No. It has not worked anywhere else.
That is why the legalization of abortion is the start of
national suicide and is always a nation's greatest tragedy.
Permissive abortion is the point of no return. Prime Minister Lee Kuan Yew, who engineered permissive abortion
and is now desperately trying to recover, is frantic. He is
accused of "hounding" female college graduates to have
children; he has actually sponsored (unsuccessful) "love
boat" moonlight cruises for singles, as well as tea dances
and dinner parties to bring professional young people
together in hopes of marriage and babies.
So the government plays Cupid and becomes a match-
maker in Singapore, whose only natural resource is people.
The newest slogan is, "Have three, or more if you can
afford it." The better-off Singaporeans are paid lavishly to
reproduce, like manipulated animals, while the illiterate or
poorly educated woman is still paid $10,000 (Singaporean)
if she submits to sterilization after her first or second
child.
Meanwhile, the godless Yew fears a radical new trend:
educated but unmarried women having children and raising them as single parents. He has rightly called this "the
next step down the road that the Western woman has
taken." Singapore's well organized feminists fear he will
restore polygamy. Even brilliant law professors like Yew
get "too late smart."
Yew would welcome the USA's Pearson Institute, which
has more than 100 very successful baby-saving centers
(now under fierce attack in the courts by PP and NOW,
who conducted a joint seminar on how to close them
down).
Meanwhile, HLI's Singapore branch flourishes, saving
babies, educating the young in chastity and teaching NFP
to the engaged—all with the consistent support of their
great archbishop, Gregory Yong, who could tell Yew, "I told
you so."

CHURCH vs. THEOLOGIANS IN BRAZIL

The Silent Scream was shown nationwide twice on two TV channels, prefaced by strong comments from Rio de Janeiro's Eugenio Cardinal Sales (whom liberation theologian Fr. Leonardo Boff attacked fiercely when the Cardinal removed Marxist teachers from the Pontifical Catholic University of Rio).

Last fall letters from Cardinals Ratzinger and Hamer to Franciscan superiors in Rome and Brazil appeared in Brazilian and Italian newspapers. The letters asked the American Superior General in Rome, Fr. John Vaughn, and other responsible Franciscan officials in Brazil to insist on theological orthodoxy and to discipline dissident theologians. It was to no avail.

However, the whole editorial board of the huge Franciscan publishing house in Petropolis has been replaced, including Fr. Boff; publication of its collection of 40 volumes on liberation theology is suspended. A frustrated orthodox bishop, summarizing Brazil's National Congress of Base Communities, closes his article with, "Ad quem ibimus, Domine?" (Jn. 6:69)

Fr. Boff has subtly criticized the two papal documents on "Christian Freedom and Liberation." He preaches land-seizing by landworkers during the ongoing rural reform. Now the rambunctious, unchecked Franciscan is supporting (on TV) pro-abortion and feminist candidates for the November elections.

He recently published a new book on the Trinity, his second book since he was "liberated" from silence last Easter night, the time deliberately chosen by his rebellious superior. The volume's *imprimatur* is not genuine. In this new work Fr. Boff pushes feminist theology so far that he asserts that the Virgin Mary is God (p. 257); he says the Holy Spirit is hypostatically united to her as the Son of God is hypostatically united to the humanity of Christ (p. 256).

The book is all the more dangerous because of its mild tone and the mix of faint praise and subtle attack with which Fr. Boff criticizes the Magisterium and Tradition of the Church. Fortunately, Rio's Archdiocesan Commission for the Doctrine of the Faith has issued a 27-page refutation of the book's errors. The critique will appear in several languages, including English.

The familiar, satanic pro-abortion disinformation and maneuvering has begun in Brazil. At the First Women's

National Health Conference, feminists failed to pass a pro-abortion resolution. Even so, such a resolution appeared in the final document! (Honesty is no virtue for "pro-choice" killers.) An administrative directive forcing public hospitals to murder babies in cases of rape is imminent.

The bishops' lobby at the national conference that is building a new constitution does not want the Church to seem intolerant on abortion. In a newspaper interview last November, Paolo Avaristo Cardinal Arns (who defends Boff) said "it is not worthwhile troubling our unity with discussing such a problem [abortion]; people have already made up their minds and will not change." At a recent conference at the Brazilian Pontifical College in Rome, a Brazilian theologian told me that whatever one may think of liberation theology, the Church is less and less identified with the rich and more and more as the defender of the poor.

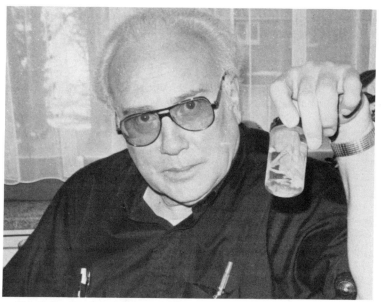

Who defends the poorest of the poor?

WILL A.I.D.S. KILL MILLIONS OR BILLIONS?

(No. 31—May 1987)

President Reagan says AIDS is our number-one health problem. (Dr. Paul Cameron says homosexuality is.) This disease is now the world's worst medical nightmare, because it is fully capable of destroying humanity. "Yes," says Harvard's learned biologist S. Jay Gould, "AIDS may run through the entire population, and may carry off a quarter or more of us." Dr. William Haseltine of the Harvard Medical School warns that AIDS is "species-threatening." Cases have now been reported in 98 countries.

But our politicians are treating AIDS as if it were bad breath instead of a monstrous public health problem. Why? Because of pressure from homosexuals and their sympathizers in the media, medicine and the bureaucracy. People who reject God and His plan for sex naturally do not want you to know the truth about AIDS.

AIDS stems from one thing and one thing only: the abuse of God's powerful gift of human sexuality. Once you abuse it, sexuality always strikes back. Nature is jealous of her fertility! As the old saying goes, God always forgives, men sometimes, nature never. Even the pagan Freud wrote that the abuse of sex always leads to violence.

Like the USA, European nations are scrambling madly to contain or cure the disease with research and public education programs. Our Surgeon General Koop and Planned Parenthood have only "safe sex" education (from the third grade on) and condoms to offer. It is strictly a matter of health, Koop says, and so he recommends condomized intercourse (homo or hetero), as if morality had nothing to do with health!

With typical hypocrisy, PP is hiding away condoms' often-published 15–20 percent failure rate for heterosexual adults (condoms break about 50 percent of the time when used by homosexuals). "Explicit safe sex education, including promotion of the use of condoms everywhere" is the only way to go, moralizes the *New York Times*, "since about 40 percent of American adults are unmarried."

Some Catholic priests, such as Fr. Steve Manning of Montreal's AIDS Committee, agree. "The issue of condoms is secondary," he insists. "What's primary is saving people's lives." Don't look now, Father, but your own Catholic Church has the only sure preventative: the forgotten virtue of loving chastity before marriage and faithful monogamy within it.

Where are the dissenting theologians, bishops and teachers who unleashed the sexual instinct by rejecting *Humanae Vitae?* When will they shout the true solution from the rooftops?

Biological sex education to try to prevent the disease is the solution for many school and health officials. But they are only repeating the ancient Socratic error that mere knowledge is sufficient to be virtuous, or at least to prevent the hideous consequences of evil—in this case, sexual sin, even sexual perversion.

"Man is prone to evil from the very beginning," the Bible says, proclaiming a profound, seminal truth about human behavior. Too many Catholic theologians and bishops overlook this truth in approaching the AIDS disaster. NO ONE can be chaste without God's grace; when will they remind us of this again?

Humanae Vitae, which shone forth a truly human love and God's norms for birth regulation, should now be read, taught and preached as never before—as should that magnificent manual for Catholic marriage preparation and married life, the virtually unknown *Familiaris Consortio.*

It is great to be a Catholic today if you know your Faith and the kind of world you are living in! For you, the solution seems so obvious. As Pope Leo XIII wrote long ago, "We must look at the world as it really exists and then look elsewhere for the solace of its troubles." So many TV-addicted Catholics have no idea what is happening and what needs to be done—or do not even care, I am afraid.

Meanwhile, the Benedictine Archbishop of Milwaukee finds that racism and sexism, not rampant disloyalty or doctrinal chaos, are the most urgent Church problems to be discussed in the forthcoming Synod on the Laity. He would be much more credible and would do everyone a great favor if he would invoke Canon 812 and remove Daniel Maguire, the married ex-priest who teaches theology at "Catholic" Marquette University in Milwaukee. And will the bishop of Fort Wayne–South Bend have the courage to invoke the same canon and prevent Fr. Charles Curran from lecturing at "Catholic" Notre Dame this summer?

CATHOLICS FIGHT THE GOOD FIGHT IN AUSTRIA

When Franz Cardinal König resigned as Archbishop of Vienna two years ago, he left the archdiocese and the Church in Austria in a theological mess, much as did Cardinal Alfrink in Holland earlier.

Among other enormities, the "progressive" Cardinal König had led the Austrian hierarchy's strong and repeated dissent to *Humanae Vitae* and had approved test-tube conceptions, along with other Austrian bishops, before Rome acted. Between 1971 and 1981 some 200,000 Austrian Catholics left the Church; more have left since then. In the last decade an average of eight secular priests were ordained per year in this "Catholic" country of seven million.

Austria has more abortions than births and therefore a very low birthrate. According to the government's chief statistician, for upper Austria to have a reproductive birthrate, every woman who is in a fertile marriage would have to have four children. Today, 30 percent of Austrian women have no children at all: 10 percent because they do not want to and 20 percent because they cannot. Such have been the ravages of sex-abuse, the fruit of rejecting *Humanae Vitae*.

Because of the shortage of priests, a burgeoning and stifling Church bureaucracy of 24,000 sprang up in Vienna and Austria under Cardinal König, according to the ultraliberal magazine *Profil*. Pope John Paul II took a year to find a suitable replacement for him. Bypassing all of the Austrian bishops, the Holy Father chose a simple, orthodox Benedictine monk, Fr. Hermann Groer, a retreat master who was head of the 30,000-member national Legion of Mary.

The complaints from the liberal church and the secular menagerie were swift and loud. But all hell broke loose recently when Rome appointed as auxiliary bishop of Vienna the actively prolife, learned, orthodox, Regensburg theology professor Fr. Kurt Krenn (with whom I once had a great afternoon's discussion and who is an admirer of Opus Dei).

To make matters worse, the gentle Archbishop Groer put Bishop Krenn in charge of culture, science and art in this cultured city. "We're going back to the Middle Ages and the Inquisition!" complained the dissenting intellectuals whom Cardinal König had cuddled up with. So loud was the protest from so many quarters, including 17 of the

20 archdiocesan deans, that the Pope telephoned Archbishop Groer to instruct him not to withdraw Bishop Krenn's appointment under any circumstances. As in Holland and elsewhere, the Pope is trying to straighten out the hierarchy and bring Austria back to its truly Catholic tradition.

The widely read *Profil* (30 March 1987) was furious over Bishop Krenn's appointment; it condemned his relations with America's "fundamentalist Human Life International," whose leaders the author called "US-Ayatollahs"— after misquoting a lengthy passage from one of my *Special Reports*.

What *Profil*'s editor perhaps does not know is that we furnished *The Silent Scream* films and other potent items to Austria's best prolife group. These eight films are shown virtually every day or night countrywide, thanks to the indefatigable Martin Humer and Fr. Hans Gruner (whom Cardinal König deprived of his parish because of his orthodoxy). They have made an enormous impression on the Austrians. Now we will send Austria 10 copies of Dr. Nathanson's latest abortion film, *Eclipse of Reason*, which I think will be even more effective.

Incidentally, what the "progressive," pick-and-choose Austrian Catholics fear most of all is that the orthodox Archbishop Groer will insist on sexual moral orthodoxy, including *Humanae Vitae*. The Benedictine archbishop has already silenced Austria's loud Jesuit counterpart of Fr. Charles Curran. Our friend and colleague, the well-known Salzburg law professor Dr. Wolfgang Waldstein, described the current situation this way: "In Austria no one knows anymore what the true teachings of the Catholic Church are." Archbishop Groer and Bishop Krenn have a gigantic task before them.

SWEDEN: NEW ASSAULTS ON THE FAMILY

If there is one common feature of Socialism, it is to modify, neutralize or even destroy the family and the roles of parents. It is also PP's hidden strategy. If you travel the world, you see it everywhere. Sweden is the classic example, though.

The Soviet Union was the first country in modern history to permit abortion on demand (1918), but Sweden was one of the first in Western Europe to start down the slippery slope by allowing abortion for hard cases in the late 1930s. Today this Scandinavian country has had to import more than one million people from 29 countries to maintain its national existence.

Having the longest experience, Sweden has proven that so-called value-free sex education does not work; it only worsens the problems it is supposed to solve. In 1956 the Swedish government mandated explicit, biological/anatomical sex education from kindergarten through 12th grade. It was a total disaster, as proven by ever more fornication, VD, divorce, shacking-up, abortions, etc., etc.

Today, 40 percent of the Swedish babies who are allowed to escape from the womb alive are born to unwed girls. The hopeless State (Lutheran) Church functions mostly as a kind of government agency. Fewer than three percent of its members attend services. All but one Lutheran bishop (Pere Lonning) in the parliament voted for abortion in the 1970s. At one time 400 Swedish doctors begged the government to stop the destructive sex education program because it was destroying the nation.

Currently a standing parliamentary commission, which outlawed parental "tactile discipline" (spanking), has proposed that children over the age of 12 be allowed to appear personally in divorce and custody cases. If the child is not able or willing to argue in court, the State would pay a lawyer to represent him. The child's position would have as much weight as the parents'.

The commission has also suggested making social security payments to children as young as 12 who want to leave home without parental consent. Children 12 and older would also gain the "right" to hide from their parents vital information such as VD, sterilization and abortion experience. What is more, young Swedes would start voting at 12.

The insane idea of "equal rights" between parents and children will put the Swedish family in an even worse shambles and will weaken even more the already precarious position of the parents. But that is what the Socialists want. In their godless ideology, strong family life and parental roles obstruct "progress" toward an atheistic, semi-totalitarian welfare state. The State is not only Big Brother but also Big Parent.

That is why PP, too, whenever it can, bypasses or neutralizes the parents; if they knew PP's plans to destroy their families, they would resist. The family is a microcosm of society; it is the generator and instiller of moral values. As such, it is the mortal enemy of the Socialist state.

CANADIAN BISHOPS LET BABIES DOWN AGAIN

In past *Special Reports* I have told you how this is the only country in the world where Catholics legalized abortion (1969), thanks to the machinations of the treacherous "Catholic" Prime Minister Pierre Trudeau and the incompetence of the bishops.

Now Member of Parliament Gus Mitges has proposed a private member's bill (Motion M37) which calls for amending the constitution to include protection of unborn children. Furthermore, it would amend Section 7 of the Canadian Charter of Rights and Freedoms to guarantee the right to life of preborn babies.

On 18 February 1987, the general secretaries of the English and French hierarchies, the Jesuit William F. Ryan and Msgr. Denis Robitaille, wrote to all members of parliament, citing the unequivocal position of the bishops on abortion. The priests included the prelates' last two statements on abortion. Then they concluded, astonishingly: "However, they [the bishops] do not want their position to be understood as necessarily endorsing the constitutional amendment recommended by Mr. Mitges as the most suitable means to implement this right to life of the fetus."

HLI-Canada contacted several bishops, who claimed they knew nothing of the priests' letter. But HLI-Canada has letters and communications from waffling members of parliament who took the priests' letter seriously, even sending us copies of it to justify their positions! Who is running the Catholic Church in Canada, the bishops or their bureaucracy in Ottawa?

We commend Ottawa's Archbishop Joseph Aurele Plourde for making perfectly clear where he stands. In a news release of 6 March 1987, he not only urges passage of Mitges' bill but also condemns Dr. Marian Powell for recommending to the provincial government of Ontario that it make abortion more available. He also urged a letter-writing campaign in support of Mitges' bill.

Meanwhile, according to the 1986 census figures, Canada last year experienced its lowest population growth rate in the last quarter-century: 4.1 percent. "Catholic" Quebec had the least growth, 1.6 percent. Quebec women bear an average of 1.3 children, one of the lowest birthrates in the world. Canada's bishops have nothing to say, but the

Montreal *Gazette* editorially referred to Quebec province as "an incredible shrinking society" and pointed out the dire consequences for the future. An eminent German doctor lays the blame for low birthrates largely on the bishops and theologians who dissented to *Humanae Vitae*. I agree.

So often I am told that the real problem in the Church is that of weak and disloyal bishops and priests. There is a growing consensus that the laity will have to save the Church. This was obvious in Toronto recently, where the trustees of the Catholic school system voted overwhelmingly (only three against) to teach the use of condoms to limit the spread of AIDS.

Theologian Fr. Jack Gallagher wrote guidelines for the bishops in which he recommended moral education, but also advised teaching children to use condoms. Lines of parents, doctors, educators and others appeared before the board to insist that under no circumstances should the teaching of condoms be introduced in the Catholic school system. What has happened that the laity and parents see the immorality of teaching kids to use condoms, but the clergy and Catholic school authorities do not?

Last month 12 French parishes in Montreal published an ad for a local "family planning" center that commits abortions. When alert Catholics called their pastors' attention to this enormity, the latter made light of it. The ads were stopped only when a truly prolife doctor (an HLI co-worker) complained to the archbishop.

Another case: 19 prominent faculty members of Canada's leading theological institution, St. Michael's in Toronto, put out a statement defending Fr. Charles Curran, whom the Holy See declared unfit and ineligible to teach Catholic theology. According to Fr. Curran, you may sometimes murder your unborn child, fornicate, divorce, masturbate, sterilize, murder terminally ill people and engage in homosexual acts "under carefully nuanced circumstances." What will Cardinal Carter say or do as the official teacher and guarantor of theological orthodoxy in the Archdiocese of Toronto?

Meanwhile Fr. Curran, who will teach his errors from Cornell University next fall, told an awards evening of the Women's Ordination Conference that the question of women's equality in the Catholic Church is "the most pressing internal issue" facing the Church today.

THE POPE'S WORDS TO FRANCE

The Pope has asked the bishops of France to start a right-to-life movement. You can be sure he told them to fight contraception, too, as he did Dr. Jack Willke and other prolifers in Rome last year (an admonition deliberately left out when Willke's *National Right to Life News* reprinted the Pope's remarks).

A CONDOMIZED WORLD

Last December the United States Agency for International Development (USAID) airlifted two million condoms to Uganda "to slow AIDS and to prevent abortion."

Homosexuality is a big problem in our seminaries, but it is much worse in our jails. Sodomy seems to plague prisons worldwide, especially in Brazil. Condoms are available routinely in New York State jails for conjugal visits; soon the authorities will issue them to all inmates. New York City now segregates homosexual inmates (I predict the ACLU will sue the city for discriminating). The city also gives condoms to every inmate upon release. In March, correctional officials in Vermont began making condoms available throughout the state's jail system.

BISHOPS CONDEMN GENOCIDAL BIRTH CONTROL

The Administrative Board of the U.S. Catholic Conference has condemned Indonesia's genocidal forced birth control campaign in heavily Catholic East Timor. The Moslems there give the Pill to the poor and illiterate only; they inject the abortifacient Depo-Provera (made in the USA but forbidden to American women by the U.S. government) into these women, who are unaware of what is actually being done.

GOING DUTCH

Dutch government and medical officials are worried that the nation may become known worldwide as a giant AIDS hospice, especially since the Netherlands has always been rather tolerant of homosexuals. Several AIDS victims have been murdered through euthanasia in Holland. This nation of 14.5 million people has an estimated 250,000 homosexuals. It has 260 known AIDS sufferers; they are expected to grow to an estimated 4,500 active cases and 150,000 virus carriers in four years.

One of the largest red-light districts in Europe is in Amsterdam. Because sexual intercourse is one of Holland's favorite indoor sports, the government is much concerned about the hundreds of heroin-addicted ladies of the night. An estimated 30 percent carry the AIDS virus and can spread it to the general public. The government's answer? Condoms, passed out literally by the truckload on the public streets. They are also passing out 400,000 clean hypodermic syringes this year to some 8,000 drug addicts. In more ways than one, sin is very expensive. Chastity is so much cheaper and more healthful, and good for you in so many ways! And there are no known cases of people dying for lack of sex!

GROWTH IN KOREAN CHURCH
Nowhere is the Catholic Church growing faster than in South Korea: eight percent yearly. With slightly fewer than two million Catholics, the Republic of Korea has more converts every year than the USA with 53 million! In this nation of 41 million people, the Catholics are growing five times faster than the general population.

Korean parishes have convert instructions five nights a week; on the sixth night they baptize, with huge crowds on hand. (On the seventh night they rest, I guess!) The four seminaries are filled, with the archdiocesan seminary in Seoul having more than 500 major seminarians.

ABORTION-FREE ZONES FOR POPE'S VISIT
When he spoke in Washington in 1979, Pope John Paul II declared (with then-Chief Justice Warren Burger right in front of him), "When life before birth is attacked, we will stand up. No one ever has the authority to destroy unborn human life!"

Our courageous John Cavanaugh-O'Keefe, who edits *HLI Reports* and who prepared the "Dumpster Babies of Washington" pamphlet, is determined to answer His Holiness' call. John and his fellow heroes in the Prolife Nonviolent Action Project (PNAP) are working to turn all nine cities which the Pope visits into "abortion-free zones" for as long as he is there. Their goal is to close down all abortion mills in all nine cities by nonviolent action and picketing.

Why don't you join them? You can at least exercise your constitutional right to picket or pray outside the mill for an hour or so. If you have never done it, it will change you forever.

ONE MORE CHILD

I had an astonishing call from California recently. A happy young wife told me, "You're the only priest in the world who can get a woman pregnant, not have to go to Confession, and offer Mass the next morning. I'm pregnant." She was referring to our booklet *Eight Reasons You Should Consider Having One More Child*, which inspired her and her husband to become parents.

The demand for *One More Child* has been excellent. It is being translated into French, Spanish and Dutch. We also have a German translation ready, with a publisher in Switzerland. What a healthy reminder this could be for dying Germany, Austria and Switzerland.

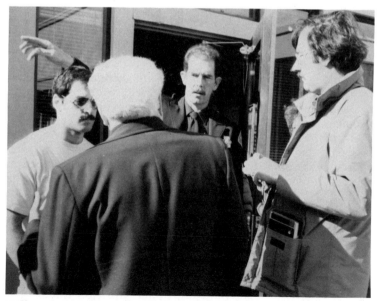

Killers do not want the services of a chaplain.

SYMPOSIUM MOBILIZES LATIN AMERICANS

(No. 32—June 1987)

More than 1,300 people from 32 countries came to the world's largest city for our Third Annual International Symposium on Human Sexuality. During the symposium, on Friday afternoon and evening from 2:00 to 9:00 p.m., while the adult participants visited the Shrine of Our Lady of Guadalupe and the famous pyramids, we met with 1,500 lively teenagers. (This young nation's population averages 15 years of age because of high birthrates.)

The young Mexicans heard a dozen short talks, saw two prolife films, discussed the issues in small groups for an hour, and reported back. Then they heard the final renditions of winners of various prolife song festivals previously held around the city. In every festival, each group had to produce a prolife/pro-family song or musical piece. In this way the dynamic head of our branch in Mexico City, Angelina Muñiz, involved thousands of parents and teens in the prolife movement.

After the awards were given, a young concertmaster performed three piano masterpieces brilliantly. This young man was so crippled by cerebral palsy that he had to be helped on stage. The tearful audience knew he was to have been aborted.

Among the very many interesting comments delivered to the youth by speakers from several countries was an unusual observation by a Mexican priest adept at helping people, including AIDS victims, to die. After describing their pained and prolonged dying, he told the teens, "God is really being very good to these severely suffering victims. According to Old Testament and other scriptural sources, homosexual acts are always seriously wrong," he explained to the totally alert young people. "God, without warning, burned the cities of Sodom and Gomorrah because of their unnatural vice. Today the Lord allows the victims of AIDS, caused mostly by the perversion of homosexual activity, to do penance, to make numerous acts of contrition and Confession while they slowly die a painful death." (For U.S. bishops who talk as if they had a divine revelation that AIDS is not punishment for sin, this would be a striking statement; the Mexican youth took it quite in stride.) The topic of AIDS intrigued teens and adults alike.

It is difficult to summarize 51 talks of lecturers from 18 countries. The Cardinal Archbishop of Mexico City, Ernesto Corripio-Ahumada, and four of his eight auxiliary bishops opened the conference with a pontifical Mass. His Eminence preached a magnificent, pertinent sermon. During the symposium three theologians from Peru discussed how to assess and handle the dangerous liberation theology and were universally appreciated.

Our own John Cavanaugh-O'Keefe and Dr. Paul Cameron fascinated the audience with the latest factual information on homosexuality and AIDS. Cameron eloquently pointed out the lies in the Koop Report on AIDS, the dangers of AIDS to humanity, and the flagrant dishonesties and evil motivations in the 1948 Kinsey Report. AIDS, Cameron said, is history's most dangerous and complicated plague, and its chief source is sexual abuse.

Besides the homosexuality/AIDS presentations, no lectures were more appreciated than the four by the spirited Coleen Mast, whose lucid, orthodox and thoroughly Catholic manuals for parents, teachers and teens on sexual education are without question the very best in the USA. We recommend them totally. There are two versions: *Love and Life* for Catholic schools and *Sex Respect* for public schools. For each there is a manual for parents, teachers and students. Holland's great prolife priest Fr. Joannis Koopman was so impressed that he took home a copy of the Catholic version to translate for the Dutch.

Both Dr. José Espinosa and Fr. Denis St. Marie regaled their large audiences with wisdom and humor while instructing them insightfully with Catholic views on sex and love, marriage and family life, NFP vs. contraception/-sterilization/abortion, euthanasia and allied subjects. No one who heard the incomparable Valerie Riches of England will forget her revealing picture of how our enemies have infiltrated and networked worldwide to bring down the family with the most devilish means, particularly pornographic sex education, often deceiving both religious and secular leaders.

Paris's Fr. René Bel explained the motivations and plans of the population controllers as well as the myths and realities of the so-called overpopulation problem. The Archbishop of Guatemala City, Prospero Penados del Barrio, brought along two doctors who proved that the United

States Agency for International Development (USAID) does sterilize people forcibly, as he had complained to President Reagan in a celebrated letter last year.

Dr. Bernard Nathanson fenced fiercely with reporters in a news conference. Then stunned everybody at our banquet by reminding them of *Humanae Vitae* when he said the heart of the problem is the separation of sexual activity from procreation and the family, creating a society that seeks only sexual pleasure without duty and responsibility, to a point where we are now fast destroying ourselves. He publicly pledged his work, his life, even his death, to end the monstrosity of abortion and then ended his speech with a ringing "God bless you." Never had this fallen-away atheist spoken so, said his tearful wife, Adelle. He deserved the standing ovation he received.

The six Mexico City daily papers gave the symposium much press coverage, several times even headlines. Every day the key events were telexed to the international media. Three weeks later the papers were still publishing symposium news stories. But one of the greatest gains of all, perhaps, was the professional Mexican news company (like the U.S. program *60 Minutes*) that gathered documentation on various vital subjects to be distributed and shown throughout Latin America. They had a field day, because virtually all the speakers were authorities of some kind; the newsmen quickly sensed that the topics were entirely up-to-date and that they were dealing with experts in various fields. As a result, they interviewed more than half of the 51 speakers!

Thanks to the genius of our Latin American coordinator Magaly Llaguno, the symposium in Mexico City also gave rise to the Alliance for the Family (ALFA), an organization to oppose the population controllers in Latin America. The board of directors met, the bylaws have been accepted, tax exemption has been secured, and the word is *go*. In every way possible, this organization will resist and counter that great destroyer of youth, family, Church and society, namely, Planned Parenthood (and its cohorts), which works with foreign money under various seemingly prolife titles throughout Central and South America. Once this is launched successfully, the idea is to organize a similar alliance for the family on every continent to oppose the worldwide International Planned Parenthood Federation (IPPF).

Not the least fruit of the symposium was our "Urgent Appeal" about AIDS, a public declaration released to the international media as well as to President Reagan, Dr. Otis Bowen, Dr. C. Everett Koop, selected prelates of the Church, various congressmen and other key persons. The Appeal spells out the inadequacies of the Koop Report on AIDS, and explains the AIDS cover-up and the danger of AIDS to mankind. Finally, it calls for "Condom Koop's" resignation.

We came back from Mexico exhausted but joyful that so much had been accomplished. We are already planning for next year's international conference in Irvine, California.

While we were in Mexico two federal deputies in parliament asked that people with AIDS be killed because their care "costs too much." The government admits to some 500 cases in this nation of 80 million.

Sterilization without informed consent is common in Mexico. Upjohn's dangerous injectable abortifacient, Depo-Provera, forbidden to American women, is very used widely, and Norplant (an abortifacient capsule buried in the flesh) is used increasingly.

You would not believe the gruesome accounts of American Catholic medical missionaries in Mexico who described at length what is going on even in the hinterlands in the drive to curb births at any cost.

Indeed, all is not well in resource-rich Mexico, with perhaps the world's worst, most incompetent and corruption-plagued government. The value of the dollar has soared by 5,000 percent against the peso since 1982; inflation is currently running at an all-time high of 120.8 percent; the foreign debt has climbed to more than $100 billion, and the country's gross domestic product shrank by 3.7 percent last year. Again, Mexico's problems are manmade.

As we left Mexico City, there began an International Forum on Population Policies in Development Planning sponsored by the United Nations Fund for Population Activities. Virtually all the worst people-destroyers were present, including IPPF.

THE CHURCH'S SOLUTION, THE ONLY SOLUTION

Chastity before marriage and chaste and faithful monogamy within— why do our theologians, religious teachers and bishops not exploit these as the only solutions? The

distinction between sin and sinner, yes; truly Christian
compassion, yes—but not at the expense of others' well-
being and rights. Here we cannot afford to be wimpy.
The AIDS epidemic is a health problem, not primarily a
civil rights issue. It is a problem that can be solved by
behavioral change, which is above all the business of religion and religious leaders to effect. AIDS is the only
politically protected plague in history—eloquent witness to
the moral bankruptcy of our time.

Eleven bishops have stopped having special Masses for
the homosexual group Dignity, not including the Cardinal
Archbishop of Chicago or the maverick Benedictine Archbishop of Milwaukee. Bernardin says the Holy See's recent
document is not clear on this point. And so a Mass for
Dignity goes on at Chicago's St. Sebastian's Parish.
Preaching on the 75th anniversary of this parish, the
Cardinal told the congregation, "You all have dignity," to
the delight of some 50 members of Dignity who were
present.

At the University of Chicago, he told students he accepts (!) the recent papal statement on biomedical ethics,
but Catholics will know what to do and how to decide. Is
that not a dangerous declaration from a Prince of the
Church, who should be the acme of loyalty to the Holy
Father? Fr. Richard McCormick, the "progressive" Jesuit
moral theologian now ensconced fittingly at Notre Dame,
backed the cardinal. Did McCormick write the prelate's
otherwise good lecture? This Jesuit dissenter to *Humanae
Vitae* made the same observation to the press when the
papal guidelines first appeared.

Our times cry out for vigorous, moral, realistic episcopal leadership. The best and kindest thing one can say
about the California bishops' recent pastoral on AIDS ("A
Call to Compassion") is that one hopes they did not read it
before signing it, that a fantasy-land, underling bureaucrat
composed it. Let a great Jesuit, Fr. Francis Canavan
(writing in *Catholic Eye*, 15 May 1987), tell you about this
curious episcopal document:

> If you don't think "compassion" can cover a multi-
> tude of sins, you should read the "Pastoral Letter
> on AIDS" just issued by the California Catholic
> Conference. It's an amazing document. Little or
> nothing in its dozen pages will remind you of
> church teaching on homosexuality. Rather, it's a

highly emotional hymn of "compassion" *to* homosexuals, beginning with the totally irrelevant fact
(described as a kind of *honor*) that Californians
were the first to get AIDS. It highly recommends
Dr. Koop's *Surgeon General's Report*—thus tacitly
backing Koop's condommania as well—supports
"strict confidentiality" for the infected (which *doctors* oppose—they can't inform the endangered!),
jargonizes about "interdisciplinary programs"
and . . . naturally, compares AIDS "anxiety" to "the
specter of possible nuclear destruction." God only
knows what the faithful will make of it all, but the
document should be a best-seller in the Gay Community.

It's hard to believe that the Bishops really support such stuff (surely LA's Archbishop Roger Mahony doesn't?—*eye*'d love to know), but it is being
issued in their names. And it hurts: the extrava-
gant support of Koop sends an unmistakable message that cannot be gainsaid by the short 10-line
paragraph (p. 5) that allows as how "sexual abstinence" and "monogamous fidelity" now recommend
themselves as "medically necessary as well as morally responsible." The strongest line in the document uses the *subjunctive*: "The recovery of the
virtue of chastity *may* [*eye*'s emphasis] be one of
the most urgent needs of contemporary society."

That of course is the trouble with the Bishops'
standard "Seamless Garment" rhetoric. "Contemporary society"—like every society in history—suffers a multitude of problems—it's crazy to keep
insisting that you've got to solve 'em *all* before you
can focus on *one*. Yet that's precisely the position
to which the Bishops have retreated on the other
great "single issue"—abortion. And if the apoca-
lyptic predictions about AIDS are true, *it* may
"solve" our society's problems by wiping us out.
That's why it must be faced *directly*. We repeat,
it's a cosmic joke that the universally derided Old
Morality—of which the Church (certainly this Pope)
is the last remaining bastion—should suddenly
appear to everybody as the *truth*, however much
they burn to resist it still. Far better to say "We

told you so" than to project the image that the
church has nothing of its *own* to say but "compassion." But then our Shepherds *haven't* been telling
their flocks that kind of thing for decades—they're
out of practice.

Recently I preached and spoke in two dioceses in the
USA on Mother's Day. Never have so many walked out of
Mass—at one Mass about a dozen—as I preached on the
antilife movement. After Mass I always go to the main
entrance to get the flak. My remarks on unmotherhood
(contraception, sterilization and particularly abortion) infuriated one woman. "No topic to discuss with children
present," she blurted, whereupon five women told her they
were glad their children finally heard it from a priest, and
that "it was high time they heard the whole truth from the
pulpit." Undeterred, the protesting mother told me, "You'll
get the message from the collection box." I responded, "I
have never preached for money." (I did not receive one
cent from that parish, but received the largest second
collections ever in two subsequent parishes.) But she
persisted: "No topic for Mother's Day." I finally asked her
where she stood on contraception. No reply, only irrita-
tion.

Contraception is always the worm in the nice apple,
whether for waffling priest or confused and angry contracepting layman. And once you know where either stands
on contraception, you can predict the rest. I for one see
little or no asceticism, spirit of sacrifice or zeal in the
layman or priest who surrenders on the birth control issue.
I do not see these qualities in feminist nuns, either. In
fact, I see a distinct lack of zeal in virtually all of these,
with a good deal of involvement in the peripheral and
nonessential.

Both dioceses I was in are riddled with un-Christian,
dangerous sex education. In both I was assured by reliable persons that practicing Catholic doctors refer mothers
for abortions (a first for me). When this was called to the
bishops' attention, they did nothing, I was told.

One bishop joined Protestant ministers in welcoming
Billy Graham for a rally in his highly Catholic city. Graham, who preaches a safe, middle-class Christianity in
behalf of his $30 million Billy Graham Evangelistic As-
sociation based in Minneapolis, has never spoken out
strongly against abortion. He once returned from Moscow

with only good words for the Communists. Once his wife did lend their home for a meeting of the Christian Action Council, an excellent prolife Protestant group.

ON THE BRIDGE

Thanks to two Catholic lay stalwarts, Niagara University's Dr. Raphael Waters and Canadian lawyer James V. McManamy, every Mother's Day about 3,000 prolifers from Canada and the USA meet in the middle of the bridge spanning the Niagara River to give witness for life with various ceremonies. This year I was privileged to address the group, with the falls roaring in the distant background.

THE KNIGHTS OF COLUMBUS

The Jesuit priest Daniel Lord once described them "as an organization all dressed up with nowhere to go." But one must praise the Knights' national campaign against abortion, as well as their generosity for other good causes. Still, their founder, Fr. Michael McGivney, wanted them to be apostolic, exemplary Catholics. That is why I wish the Knights would be loyal to the whole of Catholic moral teaching.

Above all, I wish they would expel from their ranks U.S. Representatives Edward Roybal and Tony Coelho of California. They, like Jesuit Rep. Fr. Robert Drinan, repeatedly vote to kill the unborn. Last month "Catholic" Loyola-Marymount University of Los Angeles awarded Coelho an honorary doctorate. Last year's LMU commencement speaker was none other than "Catholic" Supreme Court Justice William Brennan, one of the seven who gave us abortion on demand. How tragic that we let so many enemies destroy the Church from within!

PICKETING FOR LIFE

Recently I joined a dedicated group picketing an abortion chamber in Santa Barbara, California. I walked in as self-appointed chaplain to counsel Sara, the collaborating "Catholic" wife (his second wife) of the abortionist, Daniel Joseph. She helps her husband kill thousands of unborn babies. Msgr. Vincent McCabe, pastor of San Roque Church, recently let his deacon baptize her baby. Msgr. McCabe asked no questions and scandalized many. When challenged by prolifers, he defended his actions. He does not seem to mind the Josephs' killing of unborn babies.

SINGAPORE STRUGGLES TO RECOVER

(No. 33—July 1987)

Because Singapore is small—2.6 million people living in 240 square miles— her demographic disaster (stemming from foresight contraception and hindsight abortion) has shown itself quickly.

The government is frantic, seeing the handwriting on the wall (they engineered the fiasco in the '60s and '70s, with the help of Planned Parenthood). Unlike Western countries, Singapore cannot import people to keep itself going. Nor do the sensitive Singaporeans want the ethnic changes now occurring increasingly in wealthy but dying Western countries.

In this island nation, 77 percent of married women aborted their third child because of the earlier Stop-at-Two government pressure. In 1985, 92 percent of women aborted their first pregnancy. The government admits that every year 7,000 married women have "convenience abortions." Last year Singapore was 15,000 babies short of reproduction.

Amazingly, the government now freely publicizes the psychological and physical effects of abortion. The officials even recommend that responsible love and sexual behavior be taught early in adolescence—but sadly, with only a humanistic morality.

Strangely, the authorities also continue to believe the PP lie that biological sex education and wide distribution of contraceptives decrease teen pregnancy. Nor do they understand that the availability of backup, stopgap abortion increases sexual irresponsibility, and that contraception and legal abortion feed each other. This is every country's experience.

Why is it so hard for so many to see this, including Catholics? Is it because they practice sinful contraception themselves, and are therefore blinded? The great British prolife gynecologist Dr. Ian Donald once told me, "As one lives, so one thinks."

Will the Singaporeans succeed in producing a reproductive birth rate? No modern nation ever has. Contraception/abortion creates a point of no return.

BABY FARMS IN SRI LANKA

Colombo's Archbishop Marcus Fernando desperately writes for help, saying "the daily papers" are calling for legalized abortion. The archbishop refers to a "baby farm," where "babies [are] being produced for a fee for export." Tourism has brought in a trail of undesirable values, he laments.

Last Christmas Archbishop Fernando devoted a powerful pastoral to legal abortion and how it totally contradicts the beautiful message of Christ's coming. The archbishop then asked us for "booklets, videotapes and other allied material. We need them now before government and other interested parties begin moving in the matter." We rushed materials by air and sent more by sea mail.

GENOCIDE IN LEBANON

Babies may seem weak and helpless, but they are the only future any nation has. Lebanese Catholics have learned this the hard way.

The wealthier and more educated they became, the fewer children they had. Meanwhile, their Moslems neighbors increased and multiplied. Today the minority Catholics are suffering terribly at the hands of Moslems and Arabs.

According to an eyewitness (a Capuchin priest) Moslems from Iran and Syria persecute Christians devilishly. Christians, mostly Catholics, are not allowed to leave from Beirut airport. Many are murdered indiscriminately. The Moslems perpetrate unspeakable cruelties; they cut a woman open lengthwise and disemboweled her alive.

In the Province of Aleg, Moslems destroyed 58 Christian villages; they bulldozed houses and trees. They gave the same treatment to 62 villages in the Province of Chouf and 24 in the Province of Klim.

Survivors from these 144 villages find themselves in catastrophic, stinking camps north of Beirut where women are routinely raped (and worse). Refugees in Beirut have only one toilet for every 125 persons. The Moslems intercept mail and packages. They have totally cut off these Christians from the rest of the world. Whatever money and provisions the Christians have are taken away. Their only possible escape is by ship to Cyprus.

The Arab states have devalued Lebanese money to destroy the Christian minority. The same Arabs who officially ally themselves with the USA sneak in weapons, money and soldiers to fight the Christians.

As a warning, the Moslems brutally killed a father, his five-year-old son and two grandmothers, while they cut off both of his 16-year-old daughter's legs. The followers of Mohammed have not forgotten their historic cruelties. What will they do when they gain the upper hand in Pill-depopulated "Christian" Europe?

In view of all this, it is mind-boggling that the three-million-member Presbyterian Church, in its nine-day annual meeting, should decide to cuddle up to the more than five million Moslems living in the USA.

The denomination's three-year Islamic study calls on the church to identify, expose and counteract bigotry and prejudice against Moslems and Arabs in a "mutual search for peace and justice."

According to this study (accepted by Presbyterian leaders without discussion or dissent), Islam is in "a phase of vigorous revival, a significant fact in our world today." Ask the Christians in Lebanon, where 150,000 have died in 12 years of civil war, to comment!

There is more: The "pro-choice" Presbyterian assembly also asked federal and state governments to rescind laws governing private sexual behavior between consenting adults. After doing this in 1967, Britain suffered an enormous burgeoning of homosexual groups and crimes. The Presbyterians do not seem to have heard of AIDS; they called upon legislators to pass laws forbidding discrimination based on "sexual orientation."

MOSLEMS IN POLAND

The Moslems are getting stronger every day in Western Europe, where seven million of the 21 million immigrants are Moslems. But now that the Soviets are experiencing a Vietnam of their own in Moslem Afghanistan, they know as never before that the theocratic Moslems (who prop up the still-reproductive Soviet birthrate of 2.3) are not loyal to Communism.

Eventually the Poles may learn this too. In the city of Bialystok, which was heavily Jewish before WWII, the Moslems are raising their fifth mosque with money from Libya's dictator Khaddafi and from other Arab states. The Religious Association of Moslems in Poland, which recently celebrated its 60th anniversary, has only 3,000 members. But they are becoming richer every day. Many young

Libyans are trained in Polish army officer schools. Libyan students, including Palestinians, are sponsored by Khaddafi. In payment, 5,000 Poles work in Libya. "Brother Jaruzelski's" Poland receives Libyan oil as part of the deal.

SUCKING LIFE FROM BRAZIL

In a previous letter I described my first-hand experience in this sleeping giant, her millions of illegal abortions, the intricacies and dangers of liberation theology, and Brazil's economic/political upheaval.

Last year, the government approved "family planning services" in women's health programs. To bring down the 2.4 percent annual birthrate of this resource-rich but underdeveloped country, the government has appointed an inter-ministerial commission to come up with an effective "family planning" policy.

In the middle of it, of course, is BEMFAM (Benefit the Family), Brazil's PP. As always, the latter has been sponsoring propaganda meetings for doctors, nurses and health care workers with your tax money.

BEMFAM has also made the usual "scientific" surveys to prepare the way for its demonic plans, offered under the guise of choice, individual rights, education and health. Of course, they always find "progressive" theologians, priests, Catholic and Marxist university professors, and feminist nuns, to collaborate.

The bishops as a whole have more or less gone along, for fear they would be excluded from all influence in this area and, of course, from all monies. Their own natural family planning programs amount to little more than tokenism. Again, too little, too late.

(Incidentally, the Holy See stopped the Franciscans' second attempt—in Assisi, Italy—to publish their 52-volume series entitled *Theology and Liberation*. Publication was forbidden in Brazil.)

Brazil's statistics are frightening: 27 percent of all women have been sterilized; in northern and western urban areas, the figure rises to 42 percent. PP hypocritically calls these high percentages a sign that modern contraceptive (read abortifacient) methods have been unavailable up to now. BEMFAM (PP) is deeply involved in promoting sterilization.

In the state of Sao Paulo, half of those sterilized were under 30; many had only two children. No one doubts that doctors in private practice commit indiscriminate sterilization. Another factor is Brazil's extraordinarily large number of caesarean births, which makes it easy to snip the mothers' fallopian tubes at the same time.

MASS APOSTASY IN DYING GERMANY

Today only "Catholic" Quebec Province matches West Germany's birthrate: 1.3, the lowest in the world. The cultured Germans have far more theological publications, libraries, books, schools, professors and students than any other nation, proportionally. But theology and theologians are not always a blessing these days: Germany also has one of the world's highest rates of apostasy by Catholics.

In 1985 the number increased fearsomely, according to a report released recently by the German Catholic Bishops' Conference. In 1971, 10.2 million German Catholics attended Mass regularly; in 1985, it was 6.8 million—3.4 million fewer in a stationary Catholic population.

Most German babies are still baptized and most adults are buried with Church rites. But while you could describe Latin American Catholics as "hatched, matched and dispatched," the wealthy, more-or-less-childless, pet-loving German Catholics are just "hatched and dispatched"; they are not getting "matched." Since 1970 there have been 30.9 percent fewer church weddings, a record low, and this at a time when the baby-boomers were of marriageable age.

In 1985, 75,000 Catholics declared they were leaving the Church to avoid the church tax. The Lutherans lost many more. Today, West Germany has more than one million fallen-away adult Catholics. The situation is hardly better in other European countries. For example, 40 percent of the Dutch claim ties to no church.

The Lutheran and Catholic Churches are even worse off in East Germany. Out of 16.6 million people, only 6.9 million belong to the Lutheran Church (about 40 percent), whereas the Catholics number barely a million. Together, they make up less than half of the total population.

West Berlin, where only one out of eight Catholics attends Sunday Mass (compared with one in four in West Germany overall), is a hotbed of homosexuality and AIDS. In East Berlin only seven percent of the Protestants are churchgoers, a smaller percentage of practicing Christians than you find in some large Soviet cities.

Before the recent West German national elections, Josef Cardinal Höffner of Cologne, president of the German

Catholic Bishops' Conference, warned 26.3 million Catholics not to vote for politicians who support abortion "rights." He termed abortion "one of the most brutal forms of domination of human beings over human beings."

Not confused by Cardinal Bernardin's seamless-garment thinking, he rejected the idea that Catholics can vote for pro-abortion politicians who support issues that the Church favors. "The protection of human life," the Cardinal emphasized, "is such a good and inalienable right that any other issue is second." Compare this with the 13 "prolife" issues that an American Catholic bishop equated with abortion some years ago before a presidential election.

Intensive interviews with youth by the prestigious Allensbach Institute found that 60 percent of German young people consider Christianity outmoded and irrelevant. Four out of five have no interest in the Bible; only one out of four who are under 30 says he takes the Ten Commandments seriously.

Meanwhile the Moslems increase and multiply every day, while the affluent Westerners play with sex, despite AIDS. It is interesting that Pill-addicted European young people say the condom is for "old people."

In Latin America, despite the proclaimed glories of liberation theology and base communities, the situation is worse, as far as Mass attendance is concerned. Only in Africa, Oceania, India and South Korea is the Catholic Church growing. In 1966 there were 613 million Catholics worldwide; today, 780 million (the Protestants were 272 million then; now, 326 million). Meanwhile the world's population grew from 3.2 billion to more than five billion.

In the West, the Mormons are the fastest-growing religion, with 6.2 million members. That is why you see the neatly dressed American men walking two by two in the streets of hot Oriental cities, trying to spread Mormonism. The most surprising growth of Christians has been in Red China, with more than 52 million today—mostly Protestants.

DEPOPULATIONISTS CORRUPT MEXICAN YOUTH

On April 25 the government secretly passed a decree (No. 67) declaring that every minor has a right to knowledge of and the means to practice birth control, without parental consent or knowledge. They announced this only on May 5, three days after the conclusion of our international symposium in Mexico City. No nation on earth has

such a wide-open public policy. Minors can even be sterilized without their parents' knowledge.

Mexico has a PP-type sex education program already in
the public school system, a blood supply heavily infected
with AIDS, and an AIDS caseload that increases daily. So
the inevitable explosion of sexual sin will bring unthink-
able problems to this fast-growing Catholic nation.

The new birth-control-to-teens program will be paid for
largely with foreign monies, including your taxes. To
advance this and other deadly plans, the United Nations
Fund for Population Activities (UNFPA) held an International Forum on Population Policies in Mexico in May.
People from 45 developing countries attended.

Also on hand were representatives of the insidious
population controllers: the International PP Federation,
USAID, the Rockefeller Foundation, the World Bank, the
Population Council and others. For public consumption
these neo-fascists recommended respecting local cultural
and religious values, while simultaneously praising Red
China's brutal forced abortion, one-child-only policy! In
practice they do whatever they please, and bring chaos to
the victim nations.

JAPAN FIGHTS TO CONTAIN A.I.D.S.

Our great colleague and prolifer in Tokyo, Fr. Anthony
Zimmerman, insists (as does Dr. Paul Cameron) that
AIDS-spreading homosexuality is public health problem
number one. Japan has 123 million people and a nonreproductive birthrate of only 1.7 children per completed
family. Fr. Zimmerman writes this about the AIDS
plague:

> We hope to control it in Japan, where homosexu-
> als have no status. The condoms are going to take
> their toll in the U.S.A. The *Lancet* (21/28 Decem-
> ber 1985) had a letter signed by five persons stat-
> ing that prostitutes tell that condoms split much
> easier during anal intercourse (up to 50 percent)
> than during vaginal (less than 1 percent). How-
> ever, there are other reasons for failure with con-
> doms; this keeps the pockets of licensed gynecolo-
> gists lined with money in Japan (at least two mil-
> lion abortions yearly, mostly condom failures).

From this we can see the absurdity of PP's and Surgeon General Koop's recommendation of condoms to prevent the spread of AIDS. The Japanese distrusted the Pill and the IUD from the beginning and never approved them, for medical and moral reasons (fearing promiscuity). They have only a few cases of AIDS, contracted from foreigners. Japanese ladies of the night prudently hang out signs reading, "Foreigners not welcome."

BISHOPS AND SCIENTISTS vs. AIDS

In a pastoral letter marking the bicentennial of the U.S. Constitution, Denver's Archbishop Francis Stafford has declared that the declining influence of mainline Protestantism and the divisive character of scandal-ridden evangelicalism has created a "Catholic moment" in the evolution of American democracy. But doesn't the Church, as bearer of the full truth, almost always have such a moment?

Given the AIDS disaster, we now know what a "moment" the bishops had, had they chosen to follow the lead of Pope Paul VI's prophetic *Humanae Vitae* in 1968! And what a "moment" the Church had in the early '60s as the proud Western world embarked on the disastrous sexual revolution ushered in by the Pill—a revolution that has given us the worst plague in history!

Is it "bishop-bashing" to report the truth about the American, Canadian and European bishops' virtually ignoring NFP? At most, they engage in a kind of tokenism even today, despite Pope Pius XII's two urgent pleas for NFP research, development and propagation in 1951. Every day, in every speaking tour and in every country, I become more convinced that contraception is the root cause of and the gateway to the universal sex-mess and mass abortion we have in the West. And if this is true, what are the bishops doing concretely to meet this challenge?

Today the Church has the only solution to AIDS: chastity before marriage and faithful monogamy within. What a "moment" the Church and bishops have now, to clean homosexuality out of their seminaries and radical feminism out of their convents; to foster true love (impossible without sexual control) and a Catholic understanding of marriage and generous parenthood; to stand up fearlessly before the world and proclaim the truth about human sexuality in this most vital area of human and family life.

I am still shocked by Joseph Cardinal Bernardin's telling University of Chicago students that although he "accepts"(!) the papal document on bioethics, "Catholics will make their own decisions." Why did he not tell his listeners that parenthood in the Christian context is a privilege, not a right?

Did any of the Cardinal's advisors remind him that *in vitro* fertilization (IVF) usually involves masturbation, that IVF causes multiple abortions, that the procedure fails 90 percent of the time, and that it occasions all manner of hideous abuses, not least of which are embryo transfer, fetal experimentation and surrogate motherhood?

And surely it is a scandal that so many bishops have at least indirectly given their blessings to homosexuality by allowing special Masses for chapters of the active homosexual group, "Dignity."

The Third International Conference on AIDS was held last month in Washington, DC. Almost 7,000 attended, making it the largest meeting of scientists ever to discuss one disease. It is terrifying that virtually all of the participants were in favor of unbridled sex. They see AIDS as no more than a serious, but hopefully curable, temporary nuisance. As soon as these scientists find a solution (with your tax dollars), people can resume their freewheeling sexual escapades.

Making the most sense of anyone at the conference was Dr. John Seale, the famed British virologist who wrote this in the British *Journal of the Royal Society of Medicine* for April 1987, after saying AIDS "is the ultimate virological nightmare":

> Society's only defence to halt the epidemic is declared to be education—for those engaged in aberrant social behaviour—on how to modify the techniques of their "lifestyle," without actually forsaking it. This, in reality, would merely slightly reduce the high speed with which the deviant behaviour disseminates the virus. Pamphlets on "safe sex" have been showered upon homosexual men, like confetti at a wedding, advising them to use condoms during sodomy. Governments have been lobbied to provide free disposable hypodermics for addicts to inject illicit drugs . . . It matters not one jot to a virus whether the mechanism is an aberrant social custom of primitive or of modern

man, or of 20th-century medical practices. Ethically a virus is neutral. No amount of special pleading by the homosexual or the medical community will alter the laws of biology.

The meeting saw the virtually total surrender of U.S. Surgeon General Koop to the perverts who are so obsessed with the male lower intestine. In the *Village Voice* newspaper, Koop called the heroic Dr. Paul Cameron, who exposes the realities of homosexuality, "one of the most dangerous men in America." Koop went on wildly to accuse Cameron of favoring "genocide of homosexuals."

And has anyone noticed that our prominent progressive theologians have nothing creative to say about the sexual transmission of the AIDS plague? They bear much responsibility for the death toll, given their disloyal teachings.

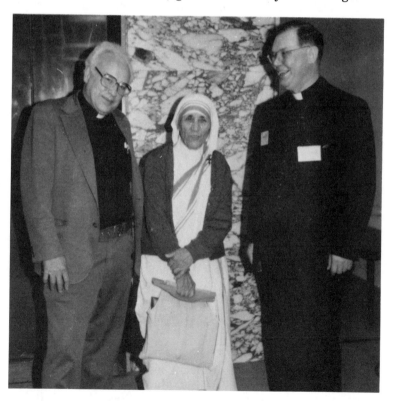

In Japan, with Mother Teresa and Fr. Anthony Zimmerman.

PRO-ABORTION JEWS AND THE NEW HOLOCAUST

(No. 34—August 1987)

There is a most ironic side to the widespread, furious objections of some Jews (and others) to Pope John Paul II's routine diplomatic reception of Austrian President Kurt Waldheim. The same segment of the Jewish community that accuses the Pope of insensitivity to the Jewish Holocaust not only condones but has more or less led the greatest holocaust of all time, the war on unborn babies.

It is obvious to anyone who has studied the abortion movement in the Western world as long as I have (25 years) that a large number of Jews who are disloyal to the teachings of Judaism more or less lead the abortion movement.

It is high time that someone remind these pro-abortionists that there is a holocaust going on that dwarfs even the horrible Jewish one, taking 50 million lives every year, worldwide. It has now engulfed three-quarters of humanity, with no end to the killing in sight. Jews who are pro-abortion must face up to their complicity in the violent deaths of 22 million infant victims (so far) in the USA alone.

They should study the historical links between the Nazis and the birth control–abortion movement in the U.S. They should recall that the Nazis promoted abortion massively among the Eastern peoples and forced Jewish women in concentration camps to undergo abortions—practices condemned by the Nuremberg trials as "crimes against humanity." They should weep for the 40,000 Jewish babies killed every year in Israel. They should recognize—now that abortion is killing off the West—that abortion is Hitler's revenge.

There are various beliefs among Jews across the liberal-conservative spectrum, and many Jews oppose abortion. Some are prolife leaders, such as the great South African Dr. Hymie Gordon of the Mayo Clinic, former abortionist Dr. Bernard Nathanson, New York's Rabbi Yehuda Levin, Rabbi Jacobovitz in Britain, and others.

Even so, I have discovered only one tiny Jewish prolife group—Israel's EFRAT—in the 70 countries I have worked in.

I also know that countless Catholics and Protestants helped to legalize and finance mass abortions in Western countries, from Supreme Court Justice William Brennan to Sen. Ted Kennedy. But I urge pro-abortion Jews to look into their own souls, as we all must do from time to time, to see whether they are not guilty of a monstrous inconsistency.

I urge them to heed the words of the valiant aerospace engineer, Dr. Kenneth Mitzner of California, who founded the League against Neo-Hitlerism around 1970 to fight abortion. Sadly, his fellow Jews gave him virtually no help. After the Supreme Court's Black Monday decision in 1973, Mitzner wrote, "It is tragic but demonstrably true that most of the leaders of the pro-abortion movement are of Jewish extraction."

Again, in a letter to me of 17 July 1987, he declares:

> Jews must decide whether we condemn Hitler and his followers because mass murder is intrinsically evil or whether our quarrel is just with their choice of us as victims. If our concern is only with the killing of Jews, we have no claim on the sympathies of the rest of humanity. Some Jews ask the world to weep with us for the Jewish victims of Nazism, and at the same time they promote the murder of innocent babies by abortion. Such Jews are the most contemptible of hypocrites.

Let me sketch for you the role these hypocrites have played, and are playing, in the abortion holocaust.

If you have my book *The Death Peddlers*, notice how many Jews helped lead the infamous 1971 abortion-planning meeting in Los Angeles, which I exposed; some 40 percent of the speakers were Jewish. Also, note the large number of abortionists (consult the Yellow Pages) and pro-abortion medical professors who are Jewish.

No American doctor did more to promote legalized abortion than the late gynecologist Alan Guttmacher, long-time president of Planned Parenthood (PP) and founder of the Planned Parenthood Physicians. And no antilife group today kills more unborn babies in the USA than PP, with its chain of more than 45 abortion chambers where 95,000

babies die every year. Guttmacher and various Jewish
colleagues also sat on the board of directors of the pioneering American Euthanasia Educational Fund.

Perhaps no one person fostered abortion legalization
worldwide more than the late Dr. Christopher Tietze, a
Jewish refugee who worked for the Rockefeller-founded
Population Institute in New York and who was the darling
of the abortion-promoting International Planned Parenthood Federation (IPPF).

Stanford professor Paul Ehrlich helped condemn millions of babies to death, including his fellow Jews, when he
wrote his best-selling book *The Population Bomb.* Even
though serious demographers have lambasted his scholarship (he wrote the book in two weeks), Ehrlich is the man
most to blame for the hoax of overpopulation.

Another key figure in the American Holocaust was
Anthony Bielenson, the California state senator most responsible for legalizing abortion in that state in 1969. He
is still voting for abortion today in the U.S. Congress.
Bielenson's counterpart in New York was Albert Blumenthal, who led the drive for abortion there in the late '60s;
Blumenthal is still in the New York legislature.

Of the six Jews in the U.S. Senate today, four are
pro-abortion. The great majority of the 27 Jews in the
House of Representatives are for "choice." The chief defender and funder of PP in the House is Henry Waxman of
California (who is also an eloquent defender of the homosexuals).

At the forefront of the abortion-legalization fight in the
USA was the American Civil Liberties Union (ACLU),
which is still staffed and supported largely by pro-abortionists of Jewish descent, although many Jews are hostile to
the ACLU. In state after state the ACLU promoted prena-
tal baby-killing with an almost religious fervor. It has
even gone to court trying to force hospitals to abort babies.

The four chief organizers of NARAL (formerly the
National Association for the Reform of Abortion Laws, now
National Abortion Rights Action League) were Jewish;
NARAL was initially the most potent propaganda organiza-
tion promoting abortion on demand in the USA. One
founder, Bernard Nathanson, is now prolife. Right now a
number of Jewish groups are vigorously opposing the ap-
pointment of Judge Robert Bork to the U.S. Supreme
Court, always mentioning his contention that the *Roe v.
Wade* abortion decision was unconstitutional.

Several prominent Jewish organizations officially support the killing of unborn babies, including the American Jewish Congress, the National Council of Jewish Women, B'nai B'rith Women, the Union of American Hebrew Congregations, the Women's League for Conservative Judaism, and the National Federation of Temple Sisterhoods.

Pro-abortion Jews are prominent among TV/radio/movie executives, authors, columnists (such as the feminist Ellen Goodman), editors, and so on. The famous Lichter-Rothman studies of America's opinion-molders showed that 95 percent of the "movie elite" are pro-abortion, and 62 percent are Jewish. Among the "TV elite," 97 percent favor abortion and 59 percent are Jewish. A mere 90 percent of the "news media elite" are pro-abortion; 23 percent were raised in Jewish households.

At the first World Population Conference in Bucharest in 1974, I was a member of the only prolife group attending a huge pro-abortion assembly sponsored by IPPF as a parallel meeting to the official conclave. The authorities refused to show my prolife films, while showing their own abundant pro-abortion audiovisual propaganda. I stormed into the office of the chairperson. She relented only when I assured her that the world would hear about it if I could not show my films. She was Jewish.

Ironically, my film presentation followed that of Harvey Karman, inventor of the Karman cannula for "menstrual extraction" (early abortion). The often-jailed Karman posed as a Ph.D. in psychology; actually he had a master's degree in theatrical arts.

At this Bucharest meeting I was astonished at how the abortion hierarchy of the whole world was present—especially the Americans. Many of them were Jewish, such as Joseph David, who is very active in advocating and justifying abortion in current historical and legal literature.

Also active and vocal at Bucharest was the king of the abortion propagandists, Lawrence Lader. He wrote the flagrantly untruthful but extremely influential books *Abortion I* and *Abortion II*. (Incredibly, Justice Blackmun quoted Lader 11 times in *Roe v. Wade*; he never cited the world-famous fetologist Dr. A. W. Liley once.)

Lader wrote two other devilishly clever books, the obscene *Breeding Ourselves to Death* and *A Foolproof Method of Birth Control*. The latter praises the Association for Voluntary Sterilization, another gulper of your tax money, now international in its operations. More recently, Lader's

Abortion Rights Mobilization group has taken the U.S. Catholic hierarchy to court, aiming to strip the Church of her tax exemption.

The militantly pro-abortion secular feminist movement was inspired by Betty Friedan. Even today some of its chief "spokespersons" are Jewish, e.g., Gloria Steinem. It was Jewish feminist Simone Weil who, as health minister, treacherously engineered abortion on demand in France in 1974, despite her own great sufferings in Auschwitz. This five-year "experiment" was ratified as permanent law on the last day of 1979, the Year of the Family.

During this incredible experiment in killing, Weil held a news conference in Paris in which she proclaimed, "We are out to destroy the family. The best way to do that is to begin by attacking its weakest member, the unborn child." Someone reminded her that no known society or culture has been without the family, that the family is universal in human experience, and asked her whether she had something better to replace it with. Typically, she ignored the question.

In Canada the leading abortion advocate and chief killer of unborn babies is Henry Morgentaler, who claims to have been in Auschwitz. Morgentaler has set up 11 illegal abortion mills in "Catholic" Quebec province. Now he is challenging the federal law in other provinces.

Currently, prominent Jews are among the chief exponents of euthanasia in Germany, Austria and Holland.

Until recently, the real political power in Austria was in the hands of a fanatically pro-abortion Prime Minister, Bruno Kreisky, an atheist of Jewish descent. Kreisky almost certainly was present when we showed parliament a film of an 11-minute suction abortion. Why was there no Jewish outcry against his extermination of Austrian babies, including Jewish ones?

In 1974–75 I lectured against abortion more than 50 times in Austria, showing films I introduced to that country. In 1975 parliament legalized abortion on demand during the first three months of pregnancy. Although they are supremely sensitive about their own Holocaust, Austria's Jews gave me and my colleagues no help in stopping this new holocaust; on the contrary, they spoke eloquently for killing preborn babies. Today Austria is a dying country, with more abortions than births.

Among the chief crusaders for abortion in England, too, were prominent Jews. And I learned, in Buenos Aires, that leaders of Argentina's two-and-one-half million Jews were pressing for school sex education, which always includes contraception and (subtly) abortion.

American Jews always were the contraceptors in our society, despite their beautiful prolife tradition and culture. Today they average barely one child per completed family. Worldwide, the entire Jewish population is thinning out tragically—only about 15 million have survived Hitler and abortion.

From my research in Israel and my contacts with prolife rabbis there, I think I can prove that Israel's Jews have one of the highest abortion rates in the world, if not the highest, computed as the ratio of killings to births. Strangely, while killing their own offspring, a good number of Israelis adopt Brazilian babies (preferably of German extraction). In the Holy Land I asked a prolife rabbi and a professor about euthanasia also; the professor's wife blurted out, "They don't talk about it—they just do it."

Meanwhile the Knesset (parliament) has actually discussed the very real possibility of Israel's Arabs' voting the Jews out of their own parliament in the foreseeable future, thanks to low Jewish birthrates. To remedy this, HLI's contact Rabbi Mordechai Blanck founded EFRAT (Society for the Advancement of Childbearing), a tiny group of Orthodox Jews trying to raise the Jewish family birthrate.

Jews of all convictions must never forget their Holocaust, and I grieve with them over its victims. But again, Jews who are pro-abortion must face up to their role in the greatest holocaust in all history, the abortion holocaust. They should also reflect on the truth that there have been other and even larger holocausts, e.g., the worst of all (tens of millions) in Red China under Mao; the Soviets' planned starvation of the Ukrainians (nine million); the 20 million Russians and 6.3 million Poles who lost their lives at the hands of Hitler; and others.

Pope John Paul II belonged to the anti-Nazi underground and has prayed at Auschwitz and Maidanek. The protests of pro-abortion Jews over his reception of the Austrian president were political and hypocritical; they had nothing to say about Waldheim's visiting Jordan on his next stop.

The Waldheim affair was really only a subtle attempt to morally coerce the Pope into giving Israel full diplomatic recognition—and this scheme took in even the president of the U.S. hierarchy, who put out a statement sympathetic

to the Pope's critics.   He was rescued by Msgr. Daniel
Hoye, General Secretary of the National Conference of
Catholic Bishops, who issued a clarification.

I urge prolife Jews and Jews who have never thought
much about abortion to form specifically Jewish prolife
organizations, and to take back the leadership of the Jewish community from the pro-abortionists. By doing this
you will not only help save millions of non-Jewish babies,
you may well help save the Jewish nation from the truly
final "solution" of abortion.

PERU: BATTLE FOR LIFE IN THE ANDES

In the mid-1970s the military government closed all of
the centers of the Peruvian Family Planning Association
(PP), destroyed its literature, confiscated its headquarters,
and even jailed its president. (Don't you wish you could
have watched?) But those destroyers of youth and family
crawled out from under their rock when "democracy" returned in 1980.

Last November, President Alan Garcia unleashed PP
and mobilized government health services for "responsible
parenthood" programs, which always mean, "Have intercourse, but don't get pregnant and don't spread venereal
diseases and AIDS." Anyone who criticizes or objects is
resisted or overrun. U.S. tax money pays for huge containers of sterilization equipment and abortifacient IUDs
and Pills.

Peru's population of 20 million is growing by 2.5 percent; the average family has 5.2 children. To reduce fertility, mobile medical units move through poor communities. The deception and lies are familiar: "Even the
Church now says we should have only the children we can
care for," while PP conveniently ignores the Church's insistence on NFP only.

In a June 1987 letter raising U.S. funds for Latin
America, PP claims, "For years medical professionals have
said that family planning improves the health of women
and children." What a gross deception! PP sterilizes
semi-literate women (at times without informed consent or
knowledge), feeds them abortifacient Pills, injects the abortifacient Depo-Provera (banned in the USA) into them, and
embeds Norplant abortifacients under their skin. These
are far more destructive of women's health and fertility,
not to mention the damage they do to youth and the family—not to mention the inevitable legalized abortion, which

kills thousands of babies and many women. Promiscuity, VD and now AIDS are always the aftermath of PP's programs.

With government encouragement, the current 21 small, foreign-financed, mostly PP-operated groups will now burgeon. Dr. Elisen Barron, head of Peruvian PP, remarked, "The private groups are never going to change the demographic profile of Peru because this is something that only governments can handle." This is why PP always infiltrates governments and the media.

MORE ON EUTHANASIA IN HOLLAND

No other medical profession in Europe resisted Hitler's abortion/euthanasia program as did the Dutch. Not one doctor cooperated; some paid the ultimate price. Today, though, no other nation is closer to legalizing active euthanasia than Holland. Legalized assisted suicide is practiced widely. The renowned Belgian Dr. Philippe Schepens has evidence that Dutch doctors kill 20,000 patients annually. He cites an historical first, family doctors' being called in to end the life of an elderly member.

TV and radio openly advocate "mercy" killing in this land of paralyzed Catholicism. About 10 AIDS patients have been killed—so far, voluntarily. The old and very ill are anxious and fearful. A Patients' Union has been formed to help people find trustworthy doctors, as the end of Dutch democracy threatens and the State decides who will live and who will die. The Dutch are fulfilling their old, no-longer-humorous sayings (which refer to their ingenious pushing back of the North Sea for more land): "God created the world, but the Dutch created Holland," and, "God knows everything, but the Dutch know even more."

HONDURAS vs. PLANNED BARRENHOOD

Since 1965, PP of Honduras has been a member of IPPF. IPPF's deadly manual for sex "education" for Latin America includes contraception, sterilization and abortion. The government, the media and the feminists are pushing this program for inclusion in the Honduran education system, first by "educating" the teacher and then by implementing IPPF's "educational" population programs in all Latin American countries, with government help but without parental control.

IPPF gave $385,000 to Honduran PP in 1984, $356,000 in 1985, and $385,000 in 1986. USAID contributed $2.8 million for 1981–85 and more for 1986–87. The American Association for Surgical Contraception (a euphemism for sterilization) contributed $259,285 in 1983 and $313,807 for 1984-85. For this project the Triton Corporation gave Honduran PP $1,161,377 between September 1981 and July 1985. Of course, the result is always promiscuity, increased VD, ever more female sterility, sinking birthrates, fornicating youth and the destruction of the family.

Using prolife materials from HLI, our people in Honduras published a half-page ad exposing the population controllers in the largest newspaper in Tegucigalpa, the capital. Praise God, this ad and lobbying of key government officials (especially the minister of education) have for now stopped this so-called Population Program from being introduced into the schools.

WE TOLD 'EM SO!

A dear supporter wrote, "They are beginning to listen to you!" He was referring to demographer Ben Wattenberg's much-discussed book *The Birth Dearth*, which says what you have been hearing from us for more than a decade: the West is dying because of overcopulation and low birthrates. Wattenberg's book has drawn much media and press attention. He has caught up with us.

Apparently, though, he has not heard of our booklet *Eight Reasons You Should Consider Having One More Child*, because he writes, "In the U.S., everyone is for a family policy, everyone is for taking better care of children—but hardly a soul can be heard endorsing the idea of more children."

In his book, Wattenberg makes a remarkable statement: The demographic disaster threatening to engulf the West can perhaps be remedied—but only by spiritual means. Still, we must correct his assertion that countries in Eastern Europe are reproducing. They are not, except for Poland, which has 2.5 children per completed family.

True, the USSR has a reproductive birthrate (2.3), thanks to her 60 million prolific Moslems. Moslem fertility is of no small concern to the Soviets; Russian women average six abortions in their lifetimes and barely 1.6 children. Romania has a birthrate so low that the government has severely limited abortions and forbidden contraception. (Dear *New York Times*: Why not publish this news, eminently fit to print?) That is why Hungary, Yugoslavia with its multiple languages, and Czechoslovakia welcome HLI's prolife literature, printed by the HLI branch in Yugoslavia.

LIONS CLUB STERILIZES KENYANS

When I was in Nairobi three years ago, I discovered that the Lions Club sponsored sterilization camps in various parts of Kenya. These camps horrified me, especially because they use bribery and coercion to get people to agree to be neutered.

Upon my return I began an investigation, as did a prolife Lion whose help I solicited. We received nothing but put-offs from the Lions. But we persisted. Finally, along comes an incredible letter from the International Association of Lions Clubs' General Counsel admitting that they sponsor these camps. He excused them as "serving the needs of their [Kenyan] communities" and as being "on a strictly voluntary basis." I guess the Lions' motto "We serve" has become "We sterilize."

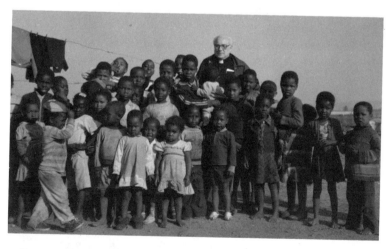

Where prolifers see hope and courage, depopulationists see despair and pain.

RESCUE THE BABIES

(No. 35—September 1987)

[While Fr. Marx was incommunicado on a missionary journey to Eastern Europe, John Cavanaugh-O'Keefe wrote Special Report No. 35.]

En route to Edinburgh for Britain's first international prolife conference, which Fr. Marx and I both addressed, I stopped in London to visit the central offices of International Planned Parenthood Federation. Britain's newspapers were full of stories about Peter Ryan, who killed 16 people on a rampage through Hungersford recently—but they ignored the global slaughter of tens of millions of children orchestrated by PP and her allies.

At the conference in Edinburgh, Fr. Marx gave an overview of what the death lobby has done internationally.

I spoke about peaceful action to protect unborn children from abortion. But before I even opened my mouth, Archbishop Winning of Glasgow had already begun undermining my work verbally. He also imposed an archdiocese-wide news blackout, lest his flock be corrupted by talk of even peaceful picketing.

Rescue missions—peaceful, prayerful sit-ins—have saved the lives of countless babies in America. But there is almost nothing comparable in Europe, and I intended to change that. In response, Archbishop Winning urged people not to be swayed by American rhetoric (mine). Since he did not make the basis for his interference public, it was difficult to answer his objections. He really should explain his position, because my position is based firmly on a century of Magisterial teaching.

I am appalled by people who think that an unjust law alters our duty to protect children. The teaching of the Church is hardly obscure on this point. The great Pope Leo XIII, whose encyclicals laid the groundwork for a century of teaching on social justice, was blunt about unjust laws; he said they are "null." In *Diuturnum* (1881), he taught that "if the will of rulers is opposed to the will and the laws of God, they themselves exceed the bounds of

their own power and pervert justice; nor can their authority then be valid, which, when there is no justice, is null."
Leo XIII was very respectful of civil authority—except
when it contradicted the law of God.

The *Declaration on Procured Abortion* (1974) also states
firmly: "Whatever may be laid down by civil law in this
matter, man can never obey a law which is in itself immoral, and such is the case of a law which would admit in
principle the liceity of abortion."

The American bishops taught the same thing in their
Pastoral Plan for Pro-Life Activities (1985): "Consistent
with our nation's legal tradition, we hold that all human
laws must ultimately be measured against the natural law
engraved in our hearts by the Creator. A human law or
policy contrary to this higher law, especially one which
ignores or violates fundamental rights, surrenders its claim
to the respect and obedience of citizens while in no way
lessening their obligation to uphold the moral law."

Any edict or statute that declares abortion to be legal
is null, and has absolutely no claim to our obedience. The
British Abortion Act is null, and Archbishop Winning
should say so. In the USA, *Roe v. Wade* is null and void,
and the bishops should say so.

Even so, some people hold the opinion that no one is
obliged to protect children. It is a good thing to do, they
say, but is not an obligation. That is nonsense. Proverbs
24:11 commands flatly, "Rescue those being dragged away
to execution. Do not stand back and watch them die" If
you want explicit marching orders from Scripture, there
they are.

The long-suffering prophet Pope Paul VI was impatient
with empty rhetoric. "It is not enough to recall principles,
affirm intentions, underline the strident injustices, and
offer prophetic denunciations: these words will not have
real weight unless in each person they are accompanied by
a more vivid awareness of his responsibility, *and by effective action*," he wrote (in *Octogesima Adveniens*). He insisted that we accept responsibility for the evils around us:
"It is too easy to shift the blame for injustices onto others,
if one is not at the same time convinced that each man
participates in them and that personal conversion is the
first necessity."

Pope John Paul II's pastoral letter on reconciliation
and penance returns forcefully to this theme. In his lit-
tle-read but powerful document, the Holy Father explains a

term that is generally abused by the left and ignored by the right, "social sin." "Some sins . . . constitute a direct attack on one's neighbor, and more exactly, in the language of the Gospel, against one's brother or sister," he writes. "These sins are usually called social sins . . . The term *social* applies to every sin against justice in interpersonal relationships, committed either by the individual against the community or by the community against the individual." Lest anybody miss the significance to the abortion controversy of this profound teaching, the Pope specifies: "Also social is every sin against the rights of the human person, beginning with the right to life and including the life of the unborn." The trendy denunciations of "social sins" that omit abortion are not honest efforts to "think with the mind of the Church."

To hear some theologians, you would think that abortion was the world's first culpritless crime (like prostitution, brazenly labeled a "victimless crime"). But the Pontiff sets that nonsense aside and points out the culprits. Social sins are "the result of the accumulation and concentration of many personal sins."

What are these personal sins, and who commits them? According to the Holy Father, it is not just "those who cause or support evil or who exploit it," but also "those who are in a position to avoid, eliminate or at least limit certain social evil but who fail to do so out of laziness, fear, or the conspiracy of silence, through secret complicity or indifference; of those who take refuge in the supposed impossibility of changing the world, and also of those who sidestep the efforts and sacrifices required, producing specious reasons of a higher order."

The Pope is not talking about hesitations on the lofty road to canonization; he is talking about sins against justice: laziness, fear, silence, indifference, thinking that it is impossible to change the world, avoiding effort and sacrifice. He calls these sin!

The American bishops are even more forceful (at least in theory) in their denunciations of sins of omission. In the pastoral letter on economics, they teach that "the ultimate injustice is for a person or group to be actively treated or passively abandoned as if they were non-members of the human race."

This is a critical proposition. No one has ordered Archbishop Winning to kill a child. Had anyone done so, he would not be all tied in knots over "respect for the law." The problem is that British and U.S. citizens have been ordered to *refrain* from action. That is trickier. But the Pope rejects the proposition that there is a significant difference between action and inaction. If the Supreme Court (or Parliament) commands immoral action you must refuse to obey—and if the Court or Parliament commands immoral inaction, you must still refuse.

Some people buy the bizarre notion that when a child is about to be killed the laws against trespass are still morally binding. Ponder the words of Pope Paul VI in *Populorum Progressio*: "As the Fathers of the Church and other eminent theologians tell us, the right of private property may never be exercised to the detriment of the common good." Never!

It was against this background of teaching that Pope John Paul II made this remark in March 1986, speaking to prolifers in Rome: "In these matters, I take Mahatma Gandhi as my mentor."

And it is this body of thought that lends force to the recent Vatican statement, *The Dignity of Procreation*, which declared that a "movement of passive resistance to the legitimation of practices contrary to human life and dignity is beginning to make an ever sharper impression upon the moral conscience of many," and urging that conscientious objection vis-a-vis laws destructive of human life be "recognized and supported."

I trust that no honest Christian, particularly a Roman Catholic bishop, would take it upon himself to oppose rescue missions without explaining publicly how such opposition can be reconciled with the teaching of the Church. It would be scandalous to abandon a century of teaching on social justice without explanation.

SIT-IN CRITICS IN *FIDELITY* ANSWERED

People who have missed HLI's symposia are likely to be confused about rescue missions, even careful, thoughtful people such as Professor Charles Rice (a member of HLI's Board of Advisers) and E. Michael Jones, editor of *Fidelity*. Jones's magazine devoted an entire issue (July-August 1987) to rescue missions. One of the great things about *Fidelity* is that it has such an excellent letters section. Since readers can respond at length, the writers can explore questions and make mistakes without doing permanent damage. (That is called "dialogue"; it used to be common among leftists.) There was no shortage of mistakes in this issue.

Jones quotes Fr. Richard Roach, SJ, a moral theologian from Marquette University, on rescue missions, asking whether they are persuasion or revolutionary acts. Roach is committed to the Church and opposes the destructive work of Marquette's pro-abortion theologian, Daniel Maguire. But supporting *Humanae Vitae* does not necessarily mean that you understand everything. Roach opines that sidewalk counseling is a better way to persuade, and that if rescues are revolutionary, they must meet just-war criteria, including hope of success. With that analysis, he dismisses them.

Does the moral world contain just two options, persuasion and revolution? Which category does the fire department fall into? Or, to follow the clue placed under Roach's nose by the phrase "rescue mission": are ambulances persuasive or revolutionary? Neither one, obviously. Maybe I should not generalize based on my limited experience, but around here ambulances save people's lives when there is an emergency. I do not understand what is so confusing about that.

In any case, the just-war criteria apply to acts of violence. They are a clarification of the Fifth Commandment, "Thou shalt not kill." It does not make any sense to apply them to nonviolence.

And even if you do apply the standards for apples to my bag of oranges, why does Roach question our chances of success? In the past month, we have closed two abortion clinics in Maryland by nonviolent action. Of course, we have a long way to go (there are more than 40 abortion clinics in the metropolitan area), but we intend to win. I think that Roach's rule would exclude all long-term struggles. The traditional demand for a "reasonable expectation of success" applies to war, not to individual battles, and certainly not to skirmishes—and absolutely not to nonviolence.

Roach and Jones are unhappily locked into the old insidious pattern of thinking of abortion as a political issue. Abortion is a political issue, and a moral issue, and a subject of public debate, and a hallmark of the century of holocausts, and a global catastrophe, and all kinds of other lofty things. But behind all the rhetoric, there are a baby and a mother and a killer with a weapon. The question is: Can we stop this man from killing that child?

That is a practical problem to be answered by action, not a theoretical question to be debated endlessly with ever-spiraling sophistication.

It is a little perplexing (actually insulting, but let that go) that Roach is prepared to offer a moral analysis of rescue missions without reference to *any* of the pertinent Church teachings, some of which have been gathered and published by HLI. (Last October, HLI cooperated with Vince Fitzpatrick at American Life League to publish a collection of excerpts from encyclicals and Church documents relevant to rescue missions.) Amazingly, when Roach discusses how rescue missions "fit into the Church's teaching," he refers to only one document, and that one is irrelevant.

Professor Rice does not do much better. He has been helpful in the legal defense of prolifers all over the country and is a tremendous inspiration to many people. Usually his chief contribution is clear thought based on sound Catholic doctrine. Not this time.

Rice advises caution in picking the right battleground, and warns that prolifers who get arrested and go to jail are out of action. (Could Jesus have accomplished his rescue mission without getting arrested and "put out of action"?) Looking at the limited resources of the prolife movement, Rice wants to maximize the impact of limited dollars and limited hours. He recommends a defensive posture on the firm ground of the First Amendment, which supposedly guarantees our freedom to counsel women and protest at abortion mills.

The problem here is a confusion of metaphor with reality. Abortion is an issue, and we can win or lose a debate about it—and we can get "killed" if our arguments are weak. That is a metaphor. But there is nothing metaphorical about abortion's killing children. The places where millions of children get slaughtered have already been selected. Does it make any sense to debate about where to draw the battle line? If all of us, *including women and children*, could retreat and regroup, then we could argue about proper defense. But right now, only the prolifers can retreat; women and babies cannot. The battle lines are drawn!

To continue the military metaphor: We are allies of pregnant women and unborn children. They are under fire. They are sustaining heavy casualties, including millions of dead babies and millions of abused women. Why are we, the allies, debating about the best way to protect *ourselves*, when our casualties to date include no deaths, a dozen injuries, and only a handful of prisoners taken?

If we encourage people to think of their own safety when children's lives are at stake, where are they going to get the backbone to risk arrest when free speech is at stake?

In Pennsylvania, a woman was arrested praying the Rosary in front of an abortion clinic. She was held in jail over the weekend, and a bladder infection flared up. She filed suit, charging that the arrest was an infringement of her First Amendment rights—and she complained about the damage to her health. In response, a federal judge ordered her to submit to a physical exam by a physician chosen by the abortion clinic. If she thinks she has a right to pray the Rosary on a public sidewalk, she has to let a sex-crazed homicidal maniac paw her!

No, the First Amendment is not a magic shield for our rights. More and more courts and city councils are outlawing prolife speech, leafletting and picketing near abortion mills.

In his critique, Rice carefully makes exceptions for two jailed activists, Joan Andrews and Joe Wall, who have offered their lives to protect children. But he puts them on pedestals, where they are admirable but irrelevant. He pietizes them into the misty distance, where it is possible to praise them without being challenged to imitate their example. By contrast, the real Joan Andrews says that just about everybody should risk arrest to save babies. And the real Joe Wall is a tireless recruiter.

Roach and Jones are solid Catholics, informed and thoughtful. Their problem is that they have not been attending HLI's symposia, where the *whole* prolife/profamily movement is explained and discussed by experts.

THE ABORTION-FREE PAPAL TOUR

Returning to the United States, I flew to Miami, the first city on the Holy Father's tour. Prolife rescuers will work to make Miami safe and peaceful for everybody, including babies, during the papal visit.

My fervent prayer is that the abortionists will agree to a truce and will refrain from bloodshed. But if they are determined to kill somebody, we will intervene. There is no reason to tolerate the publicly advertised, openly scheduled, lethal brutality towards children—especially when we are trying to listen to the world's greatest defender of preborn babies.

Prolife rescuers across America set the goal of making each city an abortion-free zone while the Vicar of Christ is there. By the end of the papal tour, prolife rescuers will have accomplished three things.

First, we will have saved some lives. Many of the killings that are delayed during those special grace-filled days will never be rescheduled. Second, we will get the word out all over the world that determined and courageous people can protect children even if the laws of the land are in disarray. Today, only a few dedicated prolifers are aware that it is *possible* to close down abortion clinics whenever we decide to do so. And third, we will strengthen the impact of the Pope's teaching on whatever topics he addresses. Everyone who hears about us will know that people listen to this great Christian teacher and try to live the gospel he preaches.

ABORTION IN WASHINGTON, DC

In the nation's capital, there are more abortions than births, with approximately 1,500 abortions for every 1,000 births. Forty abortion clinics in the metropolitan area work hard to achieve this incredible death toll.

Last March, HLI and Washington-area prolife activists broke the story about DC's "dumpster babies," the hundreds of bodies found in the trash all over the city. We found the first bodies in back of Alan Ross's Bethesda abortion clinic. Not a single local newspaper reported the bodies in Bethesda (although some reported the larger piles of corpses at other sites). But justice triumphed anyway. On July 31, Ross's neighbors succeeded in forcing him to stop killing babies there. They got a court injunction against killing babies there. They told the judge that our picketing hurt their businesses, and the only remedy was for him to stop killing.

Ross had promised not to run an abortion clinic, and tried to say that advertising abortions and killing children does not necessarily turn his office into an "abortion clinic." The judge's mouth dropped open at that claim!

A few weeks after Ross was closed down, another abortion clinic was in court, fighting eviction. Cygma abortion clinic has a history of deceiving landlords about its business, and this time it looked as if the landlord would toss them out. They defeated their landlord the last time this fight arose.

Cygma is run by Gail Frances, an occasional Catholic (raised Catholic, she kills babies Monday through Saturday and then goes to Mass on Sunday). Frances has been in the abortion industry for years and makes money on both sides of the Potomac.

One of Cygma's more interesting temporary locations was a basement in Chevy Chase. That basement was inaccessible to stretchers and was unsafe as well as illegal. When we publicized their location, they moved out immediately—but Cygma was never prosecuted.

Cygma's next stop was Kensington, where they opened during the weekend of HLI's international symposium in nearby Silver Spring. HLI participants helped picket there, and the picketing shocked the landlord into action. It has taken some time to bring the matter to court, but at long last the events of that weekend are finally paying off, and the abortionist should be out soon.

Cygma's history shows how incredibly gullible people can be. Gail Frances is at the cutting edge (pun intended) of school-based sex clinics in the DC area. She has convinced the people of Alexandria that her new service to teenagers near a high school will offer contraceptives and (abortifacient) Pills but not surgical abortions—and people believe her. Lincoln said that you can't fool all the people all the time, but Gail Frances sure tries.

A.I.D.S. AND AFRICA

Here at HLI, we have been struggling to get people to put together population projections and AIDS projections. So far, no demographer has taken this obvious step. Asked about this curious omission, a researcher at the World Health Organization told me that nobody really has any idea what will happen with AIDS. For example, he said, nobody knows whether AIDS will be transmitted heterosexually in any significant numbers outside Africa, and nobody knows whether AIDS will spread throughout Asia, which is relatively free of the plague right now. But still, in those countries where the extent of AIDS is already known—and is known to be devastating—you would think that governments would call off their programs to abort and sterilize and contracept their children away. The population controllers are blind—or they do not care. In Zambia, where AIDS already affects one person in 10, money for health care is going down and money for population control is going up.

The whole leadership class in some African nations is threatened by AIDS, because they swallowed PP's propaganda about the superiority of modern Western morality. They learned to industrialize and learned at the same time to play with sex. A fatal mistake! New leaders will be forced to put a higher value on chastity.

KOOP'S BALLOONS

While AIDS spreads at an unmeasured rate (even data collection is blocked by politics), the promotion of condoms for "safe sex" continues. Even after the *New England Journal of Medicine* published an article confirming that it is risky to bet your life on a balloon (and recommending masturbation instead—you didn't think they had converted, did you?), the deception spreads. The debate over condoms is nuanced when you listen to all the sexperts, but in the drugstore, when you look for aspirin, the message that you see out of the corner of your eye is blunt: "Condoms are everywhere, because people are fornicating and sodomizing everywhere—so get with it, iceberg! This message is brought to you by local health experts."

Surgeon General Koop's stance on condoms is "I'm personally chaste but . . ." Anyone who doubts that that is bankrupt should take a look at a recent PP analysis of how its abortion clinics and referral services should respond to AIDS. Patricia Donovan, writing in the PP-affiliated Guttmacher Institute's *Family Planning Perspectives* (vol. 19, no. 3) recommends a two-prong response, as does Koop.

But where Koop pushes chastity with condoms as a backup, PP is talking about condoms with *abortion* as the ol' familiar backup. (Abortion will not cure AIDS, but it does prevent the birth of AIDS-infected babies.) PP does not debate Koop's first defense against AIDS, or even mention it. In fact, the words "chastity" and "abstinence" do not even appear in the 5,000-word article.

Despite floods of brave rhetoric about being "the first line of defense in terms of education" about AIDS, these folks abandon the only real solution without a blink. They know, even if Koop is still fooled by his own rhetoric, that chastity-is-best-but-condoms-are-okay means *condoms*.

REBEL ARCHBISHOP vs. VICAR OF CHRIST

(No. 36—October 1987)

Once in a while someone accuses me of bishop-bashing. Will they now accuse the Pope himself of doing a little bishop-bashing during his recent inspection tour of the American Catholic Church?

Imagine the Pope's having to tell 320 American bishops, who are the official teachers and guardians of the deposit of faith in their dioceses, "It is sometimes claimed that dissent from the Magisterium is totally compatible with being a 'good Catholic' and poses no obstacle to the reception of the sacraments. This is a grave error that challenges the teaching office of the bishops of the U.S. and elsewhere. I wish to encourage you in the love of Christ to address this situation courageously . . ." Will they?

The vice president of the American hierarchy, one of four prelates chosen to speak to the Pope for the U.S. bishops, directly contradicted His Holiness in statements to the media. A few years ago, this archbishop approved Jesuit Kenneth R. Overberg's insidious attack on *Humanae Vitae*, distributed nationally in 1983 through the widely used catechetical publication *Update*. When I wrote the archbishop for an explanation, he sent me the usual waffling episcopal response.

The same archbishop, incidentally, staged a kind of liturgical striptease in his cathedral last Holy Thursday, by washing the feet of women who had removed their nylon stockings in the sanctuary. A secular priest from another diocese took the matter to Rome. The reply came swiftly: Washing women's feet is forbidden, and the archdiocese did not consult the proper authorities.

An intelligent Catholic layman wrote this archbishop recently about "girl altar-boys" in the archdiocese. The prelate offered that the issue was being discussed in Rome, that he had broken only a "guideline" (not true), and, strangely, that such matters are best handled "under the principle of subsidiarity" [translation: complain to the pastors, not me]. This is better known as the principle of buck-passing.

The archbishop did not fool the reporters. They spread the message all over the world of "the free-thinking American Catholic Church" and what they termed "the autocratic Vatican." This account by Aileen McCabe of *Southam News* appeared in the Canadian capital's *Ottawa Citizen* (19 September 1987):

> After the showdown between the bishops and the Pope, reporters asked Cincinnati Archbishop Daniel Pilarczyk what he made of it all.
>
> With a straight face and even voice, he replied: "I did not perceive the Pope saying in any way he's displeased with the church in our country."
>
> Surprised, but persistent to the end, a reporter asked what the archbishop would now advise a parishioner who was on birth control and asked if she could still receive communion.
>
> "It's far too simple and easy to say anybody who does this should not receive communion," Pilarczyk replied.
>
> Undaunted, the reporter continued: "Well, the Pope said . . ."
>
> "I don't think the Pope is saying that everyone who practises birth control should leave the church," Pilarczyk interjected.
>
> Heads shook in amazement.

Instead of talk of schisms there were jokes about peasant popes and "grocery store Catholics" who pick and choose which church doctrines they will follow and which they will leave on the shelf.

So disobedient is this archbishop that he proclaimed, "The Bishop of Rome spoke to his brothers and told them how it is, [and] the Bishops will go home and do what they did before." But, he said, "We will do it with more enthusiasm."

Most American bishops have totally tolerated theological rebellion, at least since Pope Paul VI's prophetic 1968 encyclical on birth regulation, *Humanae Vitae.* In doing so, they have surrendered their role as moral guides, especially in the crucial areas of sex, marriage and the transmission of human life itself. As a result, American Catholics now have little sense of sin and go to Confession only rarely. Millions of U.S. Catholics now commit early abortion through abortifacient Pills and IUDs. Even good Catholics do not take their bishops seriously.

Episcopal faces should have been red when the Holy See finally had to order the American bishops to remove rebel Fr. Charles Curran from the faculty of their pontifical Catholic University after he had sowed theological error there for 20 years. They should also have been red when the Pope had to urge them *again* to promote NFP.

Speaking on sexual and conjugal morality, divorce and remarriage, the Pope noted "that there is a tendency on the part of some Catholics to be selective in their choice of the Church's moral teaching." In other words, no pick-and-choose, Greeley/Curran/McCormick/McBrien-type "cafeteria Catholics" for him, please.

But who can deny that the bishops themselves have been selective! For example, approximately 80 percent of all annulments in the Catholic Church are granted to couples in the USA. And within the last four years, four U.S. bishops have had to withdraw *imprimaturs* from books, all of which were notably opposed to certain clear Catholic moral teachings. A fifth U.S. archbishop, a Benedictine, should now withdraw his *imprimatur* from the pornographic New Creation Series on sex education.

But why go on? Suffice it to say that we are obliged to obey bishops and priests (and to support them financially) only when they are loyal to the Pope and the Magisterium, and never when they are obviously disloyal. At the same time, we should aid and defend as never before all of the bishops and priests who do strive to follow the directives of a great and courageous Pope, who called again for a "comprehensive and solid program of catechesis."

Nor must we be afraid to expose (in all charity) error and rebellion in the Church. This is part of our Christian duty, as the Church's great theologians and saints from Paul to Aquinas have taught us. We live in a day and age when the hunger for popularity and the virus of cowardice in the face of opposition immobilize countless bishops, priests and religious. Let us remember always that "cowards hide in crowds while the brave walk in single file."

H.L.I. SHORES UP UNITED KINGDOM

HLI and our Scottish branch co-sponsored the International Symposium on Life and Family, held in Edinburgh in August. Attended by 135 prolife leaders from 12 countries and addressed by experts from five nations, it was a huge success—even though it was boycotted by Archbishop Thomas Winning of Glasgow, who feared the group might actually picket local baby-killing centers. Briefed by our veteran John Cavanaugh-O'Keefe, some 40 participants did stage a peaceful protest in front of a hospital where doctors kill babies daily.

Highlighting the symposium was Miss Monica Pearce, head of one of Britain's 120 hospices, where the terminally ill go to die. "We must oppose euthanasia by making it unnecessary, through a creative handling of all pain by a judicious drug regime, by understanding the process and psychology of dying, and by nursing with a truly Christian kindness," she declared in her magnificent address.

The well-known Dr. Peggy Norris described the hideous nazification of modern medicine, whose only guideline is that what we can do we must be allowed to do. Aberdeen's Bishop Mario Conti gave an encouraging opening address and supported the picketers in front of the abortion center. (He tried to join them but went to the wrong place.) At the Sunday Mass the Archbishop of Edinburgh preached in a friendly way but proved he knows little about the prolife movement.

I gave the final, summary address, urging everyone to have courage, to expect opposition and persecution, not to look for the fruits, and to leave everything to God.

Some months ago, incidentally, the Scottish hierarchy distributed nationally an intelligent brochure which expressed genuine compassion for AIDS sufferers but which was not afraid to condemn the sinful perversion of homosexual acts.

Scotland is very different from England, Wales and Northern Ireland. Whereas some six percent of her Presbyterians go to church regularly, almost 20 percent of Scotland's 800,000 (mostly Irish) Catholics attend Mass weekly. The more conservative and religious Scots contribute far fewer abortions, proportionately, to the UK's annual toll of approximately 150,000 than do the English and the Welsh. In the UK fewer than three percent of Anglicans are churchgoers.

More than 600 citizens of the UK have died of AIDS, and an estimated 100,000 are infected with the virus. In 1986 the government spent 2.5 million pounds on an "AIDS education" campaign that the *British Medical Journal* declared a failure. Now the politicians are spending four million pounds on another "educational" program. It uses shocking, explicit ads aimed at sodomites and drug abusers, under the slogan "Don't Inject AIDS." An 80-second television warning will be combined with an on-slaught in special-interest magazines aimed at the high-risk groups and the 16-to-24 age group. The price of sin has never been higher.

Contributing to more sin is the London Rubber Company, which gave out 21,000 free condoms at a three-day summertime rock festival in London. Meanwhile, virtually all large British insurance companies are moving toward refusing to underwrite policies for AIDS sufferers, the HIV-infected and the promiscuous, even if tests prove negative. (Meanwhile, the USSR has decreed compulsory AIDS testing for high-risk Soviet citizens and all foreigners, and announced jail terms of five to eight years for people who knowingly pass on the deadly virus.)

Our HLI branch in Braemar now has five hard-working staff members under the leadership of Fr. James Morrow, a creative and persecuted parish priest. They are doing heroic work with very little, having sold their furniture to buy necessary equipment! One of their many projects is producing a much-needed prolife/pro-family prayerbook for people all over the world.

UNDER ATTACK IN PILL-HAPPY IRELAND

Because her government borrowed so much capital in the 1970s, this nation of 3.5 million people now has one of the highest per capita foreign debts in the world. And of six European countries I have visited recently, I found Ireland the most expensive, despite having no family al-lowances. Despite the general poverty, the Irish own 200,000 VCRs; observers fear a massive influx of porno-graphic videos imminently from Britain, which recently cracked down on smut. The porn videos would come via Northern Ireland to the Irish Republic's 300 video shops. (These are now a familiar sight in the developed world.)

Out of a work force of one million, some 250,000 Irish men and women are unemployed; in some working-class parishes, 60 percent are out of work. This has led to a worrisome emigration of young people, more than 40,000 of whom left last year. One result of this exodus is that the number of young couples marrying has declined significant-ly, as will the birthrate.

Although Ireland's 17.4 births per 1,000 translates to a completed family size of fewer than three children, the Irish still have the highest birthrate in Europe; Ireland is one of only three countries in the developed world that are still reproducing themselves (the others are Poland and Malta). But contraception/sterilization is fast overtaking Ireland. Doctors sterilize an estimated 800 people annually, mostly women. A national poll showed that 80 percent of the Irish are decidedly against all abortions, but only 15 percent oppose contraception for all, including married couples.

A most perceptive Irish pastor told me that contraception is now the national disease, with virtually no bishops or priests opposing it; the fledgling NFP movement seems to be declining. A change in the law in 1985 allows contraceptives to be sold to anyone over 18, married or single. Last year Ireland had 26,000 teen pregnancies, but 800 of the mothers were married. There were 5,500 illegitimate births.

Because families are smaller, vocations have declined accordingly. Men are still leaving the priesthood, too. Thus, the diocese of Cork recently lost six priests in 18 months; there is already a definite shortage of clergy in that diocese.

A few months ago a homosexual American priest came to Ireland to plead for homosexual "rights" and appeared on the Gay Byrne show, the equivalent of Johnny Carson's show. In response, an Irish bishop made himself part of a new conference pleading for such "rights."

Irish seminaries are riddled with dissenting theologians. The Fr. Charles Curran of Ireland is Fr. Enda McDonagh, who opposed the 1983 anti-abortion amendment (which HLI helped to pass); he is still doing his thing at Maynooth, the national seminary. With more and more contracepting lay teachers replacing fewer and fewer nuns, the Catholic school system seems to be producing graduates who do not know their Faith. As one Irish wit put it, "In the grades they learn nothing; in high school they discuss it." The Catholic school system is bedeviled with "values clarification" courses and cursed by "sex education" that the bishops approved, prematurely but regrettably.

Almost 4,000 Irish girls go to England yearly to have their babies killed. The courts have closed the two organizations referring them for English abortions, the Well Woman Centre and Open Line; both have appealed to the

Irish Supreme Court, where the prolifers hope to win.
Prolifers suspect the Irish Family Planning Association of
referring girls to Britain for abortion.

Denmark has the highest abortion rate in Europe, 142
babies murdered for every 100 born; in the European Economic Community as a whole, doctors kill 38 babies for
every 100 who are born. Compared with those death tolls,
the abortion rate is comparatively low in the Green Isle,
where in 1983 the voters amended their Constitution to
make it impossible for Parliament ever to legalize abortion.
Last year the Irish passed an amendment rejecting divorce,
too. As of September 1, out of 21 cases of full-blown AIDS
in Ireland, 13 have died. Of the 10,000 people who have
requested AIDS tests, 605 were diagnosed as HIV-positive.

The Church's situation in Ireland is much like that of
the Church in the U.S., with little orthodox episcopal leadership and very watered-down seminary training. Everyone is wondering anxiously who will replace the late orthodox Archbishop McNamara of Dublin. Unfortunately,
St. Patrick's land lacks an equivalent of the American
Fellowship of Catholic Scholars, which could help restore
truly Catholic thinking and teaching.

Nevertheless, up to 90 percent of the Irish still attend
weekly Mass. But is it out of conviction or habit? The
nuns are still mostly in religious garb, but there is a decided tinge of secular feminism infiltrating the active convents. According to a May/June newspaper poll of 1,000
people, 54 percent favored ordaining women, 31 percent
opposed it and 15 percent were undecided.

DYING LUXEMBOURG

Abortion was legalized in 1976 in this small, tradition-
ally Catholic country of 356,000 souls. Today an estimated
1,000 women have abortions yearly, but no one knows how
many others go to neighboring countries such as France,
Germany and Switzerland to have their unborn babies
killed. Including the offspring of the 30 percent who are
immigrants, the birthrate is now only 1.6 children per
"completed" family.

Some 15 percent of the "Catholics" in this dying nation
go to church regularly. In the past an average of 18–20
priests were ordained annually, but today the diocese has
only 18 seminarians. The religious orders have virtually
no novices. Good Catholic prolifers told me that priests
roundly reject *Humanae Vitae*, as do virtually all doctors.

A perceptive Franciscan nun remarked that the bishop was "nice to everybody and said yes to all." Few young people go to Mass, never having been taught their Faith or their prayers.

Speaking to the Catholic women of the country, I felt terribly frustrated because the audience was obviously mired in contraception (and because my German is not the best). I slept with strange thoughts in Luxembourg's huge, beautiful Grand Seminary, which the government built for the Church in a better day. (Luxembourg's few seminarians now attend a seminary in France.) The Duchy of Luxembourg has a small prolife group, Pour la Vie Naissante, inspired by a zealous old priest, Canon Chanoine A. Biel.

HOW UNICEF KILLS CHILDREN

Thousands of Catholic and other Christian children will trick-or-treat for UNICEF again this year. This is a crime, because UNICEF is unquestionably involved in global attacks on life and family.

Planned Parenthood let the cat out of the bag in time for Halloween, in a review of its own publication, *The Children of the Nations: The Story of Unicef*, in the International Planned Parenthood Federation's magazine *People*, (vol. 14, no. 3):

As early as 1959, the Swedish delegation to the Unicef Executive Board had brought up the topics of population and family planning, to be met by general embarrassment and hostility from most Catholic countries. In 1966, Harry Bavouisse put forward to the Executive Board meeting at Addis Ababa, the first, cautious suggestion to be presented formally to the governing body of a UN organization, that multilateral funds should be spent on providing poor mothers with access to family planning [translation: contraception, sterilization, abortifacient Pills/IUDs/injections/implants, and surgical abortions]. The result was the most bitter and explosive confrontation in Unicef history.

Slowly, the intransigence of the opposition mellowed, and family planning has found its rightful place in most of Unicef maternal and child health programmes, although the anathema of the Catholic

Church on artificial fertility control has acted as a brake and inhibitor to faster progress.

A few years ago, UNICEF had a meeting in Rome. They asked Pope John Paul II to address them, and he did. Afterwards, whenever I wrote to UNICEF to complain about their involvement in abortion and population control, they only sent me the Pope's speech! Every year thousands of innocent Catholic children trick-or-treat to raise funds for UNICEF. Every year thousands of Catholic adults will buy UNICEF's Christmas cards, already being advertised on TV and radio in free public service announcements. They should read this mail-order appeal by the Nicaragua Medical Aid Advisory Board for money for the Communists: "Each dollar you send buys more than $10 worth of medicines because we purchase our pharmaceuticals from UNICEF." UNICEF medical supplies have been found in the hands of African guerrillas and were also furnished to the Communist government of North Vietnam during its guerrilla war against South Vietnam.

CANADA STILL SINKING

Canada, 80 percent Christian and more than 45 percent Catholic, is the only country in the world where Catholic leaders legalized abortion. How the tricky Prime Minister Trudeau used the bishops is now documented by Anne Roche-Muggeridge in her fascinating book *The Desolate City*. Today Canada is paying the price, particularly in Quebec, its most Catholic province. The average "completed" family in Canada now has 1.67 children (2.2 are needed for national reproduction). This year Canada will accept some 125,000 immigrants. The median age of Canada's population is currently its highest in history.

Between 1981 and 1986, the number of young people 14 to 18 years old in Quebec decreased by 15 percent, whereas young adults 18 to 24 years old experienced an eight percent drop. Meanwhile, the number of people 65 and older has grown from 1.4 million in 1961 to 2.7 million in 1986, a rate of increase more than twice that of Canada's population as a whole. Our neighbors to the north should learn that "God always forgives, man sometimes forgives, nature never forgives."

Like Singapore, Quebec province is dying. The average French-speaking couple there has 1.4 children. English-speaking Quebecers have even fewer children, making the

Anglophone birthrate 23 percent lower than the Francophone rate. Largely because of oppressive French Canadian fanaticism, 293,987 people left Quebec for other provinces in the last 15 years. Of these, 52.4 percent were Anglophones between the ages of 20 and 44, i.e., the age range for starting and raising families. The result for the province: an ever-aging community with ever-fewer children.

Quebec's government is desperate. It needs immigrants badly. The issue is discussed heatedly in the provincial parliament and press. The French-speaking, of course, want immigrants who speak French; there are not many of these, so other immigrants who are accepted will have to learn French. A decade ago the Socialist former Premier René Lévèsque told the English-speaking, "Rely on the power of your loins." But there will be no "revenge of the cradle." The bishops, at whose door you can lay much of the dilemma, do not even seem concerned. They have nothing to say about this unfolding tragedy!

By 1991 Quebec aims to bring in 60,000 immigrants annually. But there is an abiding fear of "terrorist invaders," unkempt, unwashed and not appreciating French culture and language. Will this vast, open, empty, wealthy country succeed in raising its birthrate? No modern, wealthy nation ever has.

Today Quebec is the only province with free-standing abortion chambers. This happened when Henry Morgentaler, Canada's apostle of abortion, challenged the federal law which requires that the killings be done only in a hospital after approval of a three-member doctors' committee. After Morgentaler won three court cases, the provincial government decided to allow him to kill babies freely in separate abortion mills.

Quebec also has 731 daycare centers, which you see in every country in the world with a reduced birthrate. The government recently increased to $90 million the amount set aside for daycare in fiscal 1987–1988; it has nothing to give to the dutiful housewife who stays home to raise her children.

Meanwhile, Canada's hierarchy has much to say about the economy, feminism and a vague "peace and justice." The loudest prelate is the maverick Bishop Remi De Roo of Victoria, British Columbia. Some months ago he gave a notorious major address at a conference in Washington,

DC, on women's ministries within the Church.   Directly
disobeying the Pope, Bishop De Roo pleaded for priestesses.
In 1975 the Canadian hierarchy asked Rome to extend
nonordained ministries to women.   In February 1976,
Toronto's Bishop (now Cardinal) Emmett Carter, in the
name of the bishops' administrative board, asked the Vatican to launch a theological examination of the question of
women's ordination.   In 1977 a Canadian bishops' commission began to assess the extent of women's involvement in
church work.   In 1980, the Bishops' Synod on the Family
in Canada heard Bishop Robert Lebel call for "positive
recognition of the modern feminist movement out of fidelity
to the word of God."   Why is it that today so many bishops
in the Western world trifle with fads while their nations
are dying?

CHURCH, FAMILIES FIGHT BACK IN ARGENTINA

We North Americans no longer live in democracies; we
are manipulated by arrogant governments and the godless
mass media.   That is why you never heard the truth about
Argentine President Raul Alfonsin's recent serious political
setback.   Argentina's newspapers reported that Alfonsin's
massive rejection at the polls was due to the economic
situation of the country.   The truth is, the people were
angry over his attacks on Faith and family.

If economics was the cause of Alfonsin's political debacle, is it not strange that the resignations of the Ministers of Education and Public Welfare were accepted after
the election, but the Minister of Economy was confirmed in
his position?

According to the Argentine constitution, the president
must be a Catholic.   In public, Alfonsin goes through the
motions, but he is actually a Mason, a radical Socialist and
possibly a secret Communist.   And that is how he behaves
behind the scenes.

Thirty days before the elections, the Catholic hierarchy
issued a pastoral letter entitled "The Course of Our Country."   It was a public condemnation of the government's
secular, anti-Catholic laws and its attempts to destroy
Argentina's Christian culture and lifestyle.

Suddenly there appeared a flood of pornography, which
had never been seen or allowed before.   Obscene magazines
at newsstands, X-rated videocassettes and degrading television programs—all were suddenly allowed, in the name
of "freedom of expression."   Then followed a law which

wiped out the legal distinction between legitimacy and illegitimacy, so that "living an alternative lifestyle" (shacking up) became as good as legal marriage. Next the government decreed pensions for concubines.

And then, in a split decision, the Supreme Court decriminalized certain dangerous drugs for personal use. Drug consumption by the young increased alarmingly, as the first AIDS cases became part of the daily news. More recently, after a heated national controversy, the government passed a very liberal divorce law, purportedly to legitimize the irregular situations of more than two million citizens.

Perhaps worst of all, government-promoted "sex education" and "family planning" showed up in schools. (And these in a vast, empty country that is not reproducing itself, and whose people kill some 300,000 unborn babies yearly.) The official public school sex ed books sanction masturbation, oral and anal sex, and much more. Not surprisingly, the government's *Sexual Education Handbook* is in large part the work of the Asociación Argentina de Protección (!) Familiar, the country's branch of IPPF.

Alfonsin has signed a decree authorizing "family planning," with free Pills and the creation of "offices" at public hospitals to "advise" couples on reproduction. The push for offensive "family planning" has been relaxed momentarily, though, because of the national debate over sex education.

In Argentina we see once more the workings of the international game plan of that supragovernmental and paramedical monster, the International Planned Parenthood Federation. Headquartered in London, its brain is in New York's Rockefeller-funded Population Council and its deadly tentacles are everywhere.

POLAND'S ENDLESS MARTYRDOM

(No. 37—November 1987)

After 24 grueling days in Yugoslavia and three countries behind the Iron Curtain, I am still in a state of semi-
shock over the way people are forced to live there. In the
New York Times, Norman Davies, author of *God's Play-
ground: A History of Poland*, remarked recently, "Western
journalists and Sovietologists rarely succeed in conveying
the underlying realities of the Soviet bloc." In this *Special
Report* and the next, I hope I can convey to you some of
the painful realities of Communist society.

This was my fourth missionary journey into the Communist nations.

Before World War II, Poland was an exporter of food.
Thanks to that conflict and four decades of Socialism,
Poland today is a poor and underdeveloped country with a
$30 billion foreign debt; she cannot even furnish clean
drinking water everywhere or, at times, even the unmen-
tionable paper.   I was astonished at Poland's primitive
horse farming.   Poland's industrial cities are severely polluted, as are virtually all such cities in the Red world.

The struggle between Church and Communism was
and is ferocious and unrelenting. The godless Reds have
had to back off again and again, while inflicting more pain
on the Catholics than in any other modern nation.   To
bring the Catholic Church to its knees, the Marxists first
tried to close the churches; from 1953 to 1956, they kept
the great and heroic Stefan Cardinal Wyszynski under
house arrest. These measures did not work.

The desperate atheists eventually realized that they
could maintain order only if they recognized the existence
of the Church, while opposing Her in every possible way.
So, among other tricks, they prohibited the building of
churches for 30 years, excluded the Church from all public
media, and forbade the publication of all Church newspapers and magazines.

It was only in 1981 that the Reds relented on these
three points, as a concession to the Solidarity Movement,
which they tolerated for 16 months. The 34 Catholic publications are now permitted to print about two million

pieces per year—or 1.2 percent of the available paper, which is strictly rationed to keep the Church in line. The government's propaganda output is 38 million pieces.

Inspired by the Pope's first visit, Solidarity was an effort to promote truth, justice and freedom in national affairs, mainly through labor unions. Although Solidarity was short-lived, the benefits it won were many and substantial: (1) the people are free to build Catholic churches; (2) from the original five, Catholic Clubs for Intellectuals have spread throughout Poland; (3) Sunday Mass is now broadcast on radio; and (4) 32 Catholic high schools were given back to the nuns and brothers (in 1963 the Communist government had taken over all Catholic schools, without compensation). During Solidarity days, the Reds were enraged when people demonstrated outside of TV stations at night during the "news" broadcasts, which always amounted to a tissue of lies and Communist propaganda.

I listened to English-language Soviet "news" broadcasts at night. They twist every item of news to serve Communist and atheistic ends, obviously trying to deceive. For example, the Vietnamese "volunteers" are withdrawing from Cambodia, to which they were "invited" to "restore order"; the CIA dictates Persian Gulf military adventures to a naive President Reagan in order to threaten the peace-loving USSR; and so on and on.

It would have been entertaining if I had had the assurance that the listeners did not believe it. But Soviet audiences hear this stuff in their own language day and night, year after year, and little else. The announcers I heard spoke perfect English and copied the famous format of BBC news broadcasts.

At midnight on 12 December 1981, the Communists suddenly inflicted martial law throughout Poland. They arrested 10,000 Solidarity activists and all of the leaders, some for being prolife. Scores of Solidarity supporters died from police beatings, "accidents" and "suicides." That a government could suddenly, without even a hint of its intentions, shut down a whole nation and all its cities shows the satanic ability to deceive which these atheistic leaders possess. They also possess a force of 350,000 policemen (10 times the pre-war figure).

The Communists had hoped that people would strike back violently after the ruthless crackdown; this would have given them the excuse for total suppression, perhaps of the Catholic Church, too. But the Poles were too clever and too disciplined to fall for that trap. I was told on good authority that the Pope had a big hand in this, but was given no details.

The spirit of Solidarity is still very much alive, to my surprise.

P.P. AND REDS vs. CHURCH & N.F.P.

In 1957, one year after allowing virtual abortion on demand for medical and social reasons, the Ministry of Health invited Planned Parenthood into Poland. PP there is known euphemistically as the Polish Association for Conscious Parenthood and, of course, is a member of International Planned Parenthood Federation (IPPF). Together, PP and the Communists promoted contraception and "sexual hygiene" (sex education), "discouraged" abortion with contraception, and gave premarital and marital "counseling." To make their nefarious work look good, they included counseling on infertility.

By 1970 there were two central clinics in Warsaw and Krakow, with branch clinics in all 310 counties and 150 villages, plus 300 counseling centers. Contraception was also promoted in all 1,400 hospitals and in women's outpatient departments. Every new mother had to be indoctrinated in contraception and was given contraceptives. The government bore 70 percent of the costs, and the clients paid the rest.

Some Pills and IUDs were manufactured in Poland; others were imported. IUD production was begun in 1968 by Securitas, a Polish company owned by PP, which always loves filthy lucre. Meanwhile, PP conducted its various familiar "surveys," "polls" and "studies" of things such as students' sex lives. It is highly revealing that PP is so dedicated to killing babies and destroying the family that it does not hesitate to get into bed with bloody-handed Communist police states.

The most common form of birth control in Poland was and still is *coitus interruptus*. Only about two or three percent use the Pill, because women distrust it medically. The IUD is used by perhaps four to six percent. But all the paraphernalia of contraceptives and abortifacients are available. Strangely, sterilization is illegal and is resorted to infrequently, possibly because of its Nazi connotations.

An estimated 30–40 percent of the Poles practice some form of NFP. Part of the credit goes to a two-month, mandatory marriage preparation course introduced by the present Pope when he was Cardinal Archbishop of Krakow. He urged his priests never to marry a couple who had not learned God's built-in means of fertility control, i.e., limited, loving abstinence that expresses concern for the spouse and the children. From the archdiocese of Krakow, NFP became a part of every diocesan marriage preparation course in Poland.

Cardinal Wojtyla's many writings on the theology of the body were meant to aid married couples in their difficult vocation. Thanks to him, Poland today is far ahead of every other nation in the crucial area of NFP. Poland has excellent NFP literature, especially the books and writings of Dr. Professor Wlodzimierz Fijalkowski, which have been published in the USSR, and those of psychiatrist Wanda Poltawska, who escaped a Nazi concentration camp and who is still a close collaborator of the Pope. Poland is only the size of New Mexico, but has 3,000 NFP teaching centers!

The actual number of abortions in Poland is debated fiercely. Government figures are totally unreliable. During my 16 days in 10 Polish cities, I stirred the pot by bringing up the matter again and again. But all agree that abortions are declining. Many women have to undergo treatment for botched abortions.

Ninety percent of all Poles are baptized, and about 70 percent attend Sunday Mass regularly. There are about 90,000 Lutherans and Evangelicals in Poland. Some 25 percent of Catholics are known as "neutrals"; they go to church at Christmas, Easter and perhaps a few other feasts or occasions. The "neutrals" see NFP as "Catholic birth control" and quietly regret "the heavy hand" of the Church. They foolishly seek a kind of middle way between the embattled Church and Communism.

In 1945 the Soviets launched "PAX," an attempt to form a "patriotic Catholic Church" that would undermine loyalty to Rome. Its Polish founder, a layman, had the choice of collaborating or getting shot. Headquartered in Warsaw and supported by the government, PAX runs adult educational centers and bookstores in various cities. They publish enough orthodox Catholic books and literature to seem credible. I lectured at one of their centers and found them very orthodox. Good people do belong to the organization, although the Church never approved it.

Another Red attempt to divide the Church and win Catholics away from the bishops is the Social-Christian Society. They run small discussion groups, have representatives in Poland's rubber-stamp parliament, and publish a magazine called *For/Against*, but they are not very effective. Also, the Church had a huge national charity apparatus before the Communists took it over. The Reds kept the name but have not fooled the fiercely Catholic Poles.

The regime subtly weaves atheism into the school curriculum. It also subverts Poland's nationhood and culture by requiring young people to study Russian from grades four through 12. There are four years of English as well.

Again and again, Poles told me that some Catholic doctors commit illegal abortions in their private offices. These doctors kill by the dilation and curettage ("D and C") method because they cannot afford suction machines. Nor can the hospitals, where the original law requires the little murders to be committed.

The Health Ministry requires doctors to teach contraception to every woman they abort. In 1981, because of falling birthrates and abortion-related health problems, the government urged doctors to discourage women who apply to have their babies killed.

By committing illegal abortions, Polish doctors multiply their official income of only about $25 per month. They often charge this much to kill one baby. So-called Catholic doctors rationalize their baby-killing with such excuses as, "It's not the only thing I do"; "it's only a small part of my work"; "I tell the woman not to"; "I'd get fired and my children would starve, would suffer"; "if I don't do it, she'll go to a quack"; and "if I make her pay, she'll think twice the next time." Before Solidarity was suppressed, members placed lighted candles in front of the homes of doctors who killed babies.

Professional people such as doctors and intellectuals are often paid less than skilled workers. Why? Because the Communists know that doctors will corrupt themselves by getting money in other ways. Intellectuals will be humiliated. They will have to scramble to make a living, so they will have less time and energy to make trouble. Much the same psychology is behind the endless queuing up: it demeans you, humiliates you and wastes your time.

Rarely have I seen so many people waiting for trams and buses. Socialism works nowhere.

One of the many evil effects of legalized abortion in Poland (as everywhere else) is that many truly Catholic doctors leave gynecology altogether and many truly Catholic medical students do not even enter it. Thus the field is abandoned to the worst—who, by making lots of money through abortions, gain control over the medical profession, medical publications, research monies and even admission of medical students. This is why the majority of abortions in Poland are committed in private clinics, even though the health service commits them free of charge.

The Church has private homes for pregnant girls under the name "SOS," but all too few. A spiritual/psychological healing program for suffering, aborted women has yet to begin. This will be one of the ways HLI will help in Poland.

Involved nurses told me that it is not unusual for a girl or a woman to walk into the abortion chamber with rosary in hand, begging for prayers. Poland has virtually no teen fornication and pregnancy problem. But pastors told me that great numbers of women are pregnant at marriage. Many a girl deliberately gets pregnant to force her boyfriend to marry her; the young man knows that if he does not marry her, he must support the child for 18 years, making it impossible for him ever to marry anyone else.

More than 80 percent of abortions are committed on the babies of married women, usually on the third child. Few babies are available for adoption, but there are many babies in foster homes because of marriages wrecked by increasing divorce, alcoholism and drugs. About one of every eight marriages ends in divorce.

Alcoholism is a huge problem. An experienced counselor assured me that at any given moment four million Poles are drunk. Nine-tenths of what they drink is vodka containing 40 percent alcohol; compare this with France, where only 25 percent of alcoholic beverages are hard liquor, and England, whose figure is 12 percent. There are one million alcohol addicts and another million drug addicts.

The government expresses concern but does virtually nothing about alcoholism. In fact, the State abets it by making alcohol easily available, because booze is the regime's chief source of revenue. When some Poles picketed a large liquor store, the authorities put them in jail. One Polish bishop remarked publicly, "We Poles are neither Catholics nor Communists, but alcoholics."

Alcoholism is a problem throughout the eastern European nations, as well as in USSR. No one I talked with knew whether the problem was worse in Gorbachev's land. Beer, wine and soft drinks seemed far less available in Poland than in other lands. But no one could tell me whether this was a government ploy to boost vodka sales.

About eight AIDS deaths have been reported in Poland, despite the Communists' hush-hush policy. Before the Reds took over, the nuns ran many hospitals, schools and other institutions. The Communists confiscated all of these without compensation. They let the nuns run schools for persons with severe handicaps and a few other minor institutions in which the sisters can have little influence.

But because of the shortage of nurses and the general health-care mess, the government has been trying to lure the nuns back to hospital work lately. Hospital beds are very scarce, and health services are abominable. In the whole of Poland there are only three kidney-dialysis machines. Many essential medications are either unavailable or in short supply.

Surgical equipment is so scarce that it is used 'round the clock, with surgeons having to work day and night five times a month. Nurses, afraid of needlessly awakening catnapping doctors, have at times called them too late and had patients die. And in medicine, as in everything else, whether you work hard or not, the Socialist paradise pays you the same wage.

My Polish friends told me that to get good medical care you must have connections. Behind the Iron Curtain is no place to get sick.

Poland's economy is on the critical list. Dull, gray, dilapidated buildings face you at every turn. "Everything is wearing out and getting worse," remarked my interpreter, once a university professor. "The System," as the Poles call the Communist *apparat*, often cannot furnish even ordinary human necessities.

There is supposed to be no unemployment in the People's Paradise, but countless Poles have no work, or only menial tasks; even university graduates find it difficult to secure positions. The average worker makes about $600 a year.

The economy has gone backwards noticeably since martial law was installed in 1981. The U.S. trade boycott was a serious blow. During his second visit to Poland, the Pope referred to the people's helplessness and discouragement, seeing only dull, gray days ahead. He focused particularly on abortion, alcoholism and drug addiction, begging the young not to despair and not to leave the country.

The housing situation could hardly be worse. Even if a young married couple could afford to rent or buy a flat, it is not available. So many live with parents, sometimes waiting 20 years or more to get their own flat. One reason the Reds relaxed the abortion law in 1956 was this severe housing shortage, typical of all Iron Curtain countries.

Meat and other foods are subsidized heavily, because the Reds remember all too well the food riots of 1956, when the police shot some 50 peaceful demonstrators to death and wounded more. Solidarity actually succeeded in putting up a monument to these heroes.

Nowhere in the world have I seen so many people waiting in line. It took me most of an afternoon to buy a pair of shoes ($4); a black suit was not even available. There are mysterious, periodic shortages, such as those of cheese and butter when I was there. Chocolate is rationed and is for children only; parents stand in line to get some. How much of the national product of the satellite countries goes to the Soviet bear, no one knows. For the Communist overlords, human beings are mere barnyard animals to be bred, aborted and worked for the benefit of the fortunate elite on top. It is a horrible, neo-Nazi system, the reality of which you cannot imagine; you have to experience it. If you ever feel sorry for yourself, go spend a week in the Evil Empire.

POLAND'S FLOURISHING CHURCH

Polish Catholicism was founded in Gniezno in 966. The Church truly flourishes despite the hostile, even satanic, environment. "We have in Poland no crazy bishops or wild theologians," a university professor assured me. Some 900 new churches are being built. All 53 seminaries are filled. The largest is in Przemysl, with 426 major seminarians.

Incidentally, Przemysl's Bishop Tokarczyk is Poland's most outspoken prelate, and is building churches all over his diocese. He once said publicly, "You can't compromise

with Satan; all Communists are devils." Needless to say,
the Reds do not like him!

I spoke in four seminaries and addressed three groups
of priests. Seminarians must do two years of military
service. Poland's army is the only Communist army that
has chaplains! I was told that these Catholic soldiers
would not fight without them.

Last year Poland ordained more than 1,000 priests.
She produces more priests and sends out more missionaries
each year (100 priests and nuns) than any other nation.
There are 20,000 priests, 15,000 nuns and 3,000 brothers
in this amazing country.

The diocese of Lublin has one million Catholics, 380
major seminarians and 800 priests; Bishop Pylak ordains
about 75 new priests every year. Fourteen new churches
are going up right now. In the last 10 years the bishop
has erected 300 new churches, catechetical centers and
chapels. Liberation theology is discussed in the seminary,
but rejected.

Polish theological development is far ahead of that in
the West. Poland's devoted nuns are like the ones we used
to know in the USA, all in habit, with not even a hint of
secular feminism or a yen for the priesthood.

At weekday evening Masses which I concelebrated, I
was astonished at the full churches. The congregational
singing was superb, accompanying a beautiful, sensible
liturgy. There was much lay participation, but no women
in the sanctuary. The Polish Catholic Church today is the
Church we used to know in the States, but updated splen-
didly by Vatican II and untouched by liturgical and aes-
thetic vandals. It is what Pope John XXIII envisioned as
the fruit of Vatican II, but which we never really achieved
in the West.

An informed Pole insists that the Communists were
terrified that Cardinal Wojtyla might become the Primate
of Poland. They were convinced that he would never become Pope because he was too tough and uncompromising.
They were dismayed by his election, and now they brace
themselves when the popular Pope visits Poland.

Although blessed with the pontifical Catholic University
of Lublin (where the Pope taught ethics for 25 years) and
two pontifical postgraduate theological academies at Warsaw and Krakow, Poland has only 32 other Catholic
schools, recently given back by the Reds. But through the

genius of Cardinal Wyszynski, the Polish Church has set up catechetical centers in most parishes.

In these centers, priests, religious and some qualified lay people teach children and adolescents the Faith after school. Every parish priest teaches 20 hours per week. And the young do learn their Faith; they also learn to despise Communism. Grade school students receive two hours of instruction weekly. High school students get one hour weekly and feel superior to their few peers who do not attend. After high school there are adult courses.

I did not get a satisfactory answer to my questions of how the Poles get high school students to come so regularly. The many young people's recreational/spiritual activities involving priests may be part of the explanation. In fact, half of all vocations come from the Life and Light youth movement, through which nuns and especially priests engage boys and girls in cultural, spiritual and recreational programs. Virtually every large parish has a priest who devotes himself almost exclusively to the youth, just as every large diocese has a bishop who gives his primary attention to young people.

Another explanation for the regular attendance at religious instruction and for the number of vocations is that there are few distractions in Polish society; sports have never become a form of idolatry as they have in the USA. Little seems to go on in the evenings, as the streets are surprisingly empty.

Virtually all students finish high school; 60 percent of the graduates vie to get into the limited number of university places, and only 30 percent succeed. "Free, competitive education is the only good feature of Socialism," a female professor from Lublin's Catholic University assured me. She gave me a never-to-be-forgotten personal tour of Maidanek, the huge extermination camp near Lublin where the Nazis gassed and cremated many thousands of Soviet prisoners, Jews and Poles. (When the Allies liberated the camp, among their discoveries were thousands of baby shoes.)

Twice in our times the Poles have been brutally overrun, raped and ransacked. First came the Nazis, who treated them as expendable, subhuman slaves. Then came the Soviet "liberators," whose advancing armies promised to help them, then halted and did nothing while the Nazis ruthlessly put down the Warsaw Uprising just across the River Vistula in 1944.

To eliminate future resistance, the Soviets in 1941 had
shot 8,000 Polish army officers in the back of the head and
buried them in mass graves in the Katyn Forest. (Later,
they blamed the Nazis.) Surviving Polish soldiers were
inducted into the Red armies; recalcitrants were sent to
Siberia.

But despite all their sufferings, deprivations and per-
secutions, the Church saved the Poles as a nation. Having
visited them and having seen their flourishing Catholicism,
I feel less sorry for them. They have the Faith and the
finest expression of Catholicism I have found in any of the
72 countries I have visited.

The Church in the USA and the rest of the affluent
West is very sick, from Her too-many spineless bishops on
down to Her soft-living priests and soft-on-abortion, feminist nuns. By contrast, the Church in Poland is alive and
well—and the Polish Pope knows it. Our Western flabbi-
ness must pain him unimaginably.

FR. POPIELUSZKO, A PROLIFE MARTYR

I must tell you something about Poland's newest great
national hero, the martyred Fr. Jerzy Popieluszko, the
37-year-old chaplain to the embattled Catholic workers of
the steel works in Warsaw. A close collaborator of Solidarity leader Lech Walesa, Fr. Jerzy or "Jurek" was an eloquent preacher and fearless defender of religious and human rights, including the rights of the unborn. After
years of threats and two attempted assassinations, the
regime finally found a way to silence the world's second
most beloved Pole on 19 October 1984.

Returning to Warsaw from Mass in a neighboring
town, Fr. Jerzy was stopped by three secret policemen.
They beat him savagely, then tied his feet to his neck from
behind, so the more he struggled the more he choked.
Next they threw him into the trunk of their Fiat and
drove him to an undisclosed place, where they tortured
him beyond recognition.

Meanwhile, the national outcry was so great—expressed in Masses and prayer services day and night—that the
fearful government had to produce the priest. Smiling
security officers pulled what was left of Fr. Popieluszko
from the River Vistula 11 days later. At one point Walesa
was brought to the pulpit to beg people not to retaliate but
to practice forgiveness and charity.

The Reds wanted their victim buried in the remote village where he was born. But the people insisted that he lie near the Church of St. Stanislaw Kostka, where he had served. Poland's Primate, Cardinal Glemp, had abandoned Fr. Jerzy in life and in death but finally gave in.

A huge, beautiful, thick, flat stone cross marks the grave, which is always bedecked with flowers. The cross is surrounded by stones linked by chains to form a giant rosary in the outline of Poland.

The grave has become a center of national pilgrimage; many millions of people have visited it. Hundreds of thousands come every month. (Even hypocritical, pro-abortion "Catholic" Sen. Ted Kennedy recently knelt at Fr. Jerzy's grave.) Fr. Popieluszko's funeral, attended by two million mourners and graced by 350 bouquets, matched that of the heroic Cardinal Wyszynski. Part of the church basement and neighboring building has become a museum of the heroic priest's short life.

I would like to send some naive bishops and other Sandinista admirers to live with the workers of Poland for a few days. They might learn that you cannot dialogue with the atheistic Communists, who have now engulfed 39 percent of the world's people and who have the blood of many bishops on their hands.

TWO H.L.I. CENTERS FOR EMBATTLED POLES

My days in the Evil Empire proved very, very fruitful. We tend to think the Church is dead behind the Iron Wall, but She is flourishing. Her heroic Catholics pray for *us*.

While I was in Poland the government issued an incredible handbook for "marital education." Intended for grade school and high school students, it has very explicit illustrations of adult sex acts. Obviously PP had a part in its production. It is the worst! Its message is: You must learn to become properly erotic and sexually active; then you must choose your contraceptive. Later on you can give thought to marriage.

It is one more piece of evidence of how PP and its cohorts want pornographic "sex education" in every school in the world. As the vice-rector of Lublin's Catholic University told me, "The Communists could not destroy the Catholic Church by closing churches and fostering alcoholism. So now they'll try to do it with sex—hitting the youngest where they are weakest."

The wonderful Bishop Damian Zmion of the Diocese of Katowice (two million souls) was astonished to learn of PP's role in Poland's sex ed and in the world. He promised to call the attention of all the bishops to this at their next national meeting. I gave him all the anti-PP literature I had with me and promised him more. What an opportunity to expose PP!

I have never made so many promises on a trip, promises of help of every kind. They cannot organize openly, but the Polish prolife movement is active in subtle ways in most parts of Poland. I keynoted their unofficial second national prolife convention at Niepokalanow, "the City of the Immaculate," founded by St. Maximilian Kolbe. They need at least $25,000 worth of our films, videocassettes and literature of all kinds.

HLI now has two new branch offices in Poland. One is in the Baltic seaport of Szczecin (Stettin), and the other is in the industrial city of Katowice in the south. They desperately need films, videos, books, literature—the works.

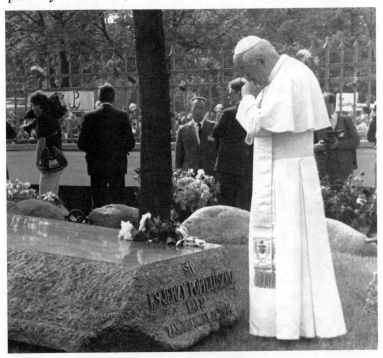

The Pope prays at a martyr's grave.

INSIDE THE PEOPLE'S PARADISE

(No. 38—December 1987)

To pass through the Iron Curtain is to enter the mysterious world of the devil. Communism is truly a satanic "religion," complete with gods (Marx and Lenin), bible (their writings), hierarchy (the Communist Party), a vicious, anti-human philosophy and theology, and a rigid structure of dogmas, rules and regulations.

But the reality—inhumanity and the godless mystique of the Evil Empire—are hard to convey in words. You have to go there to see and experience this nihilistic, totally anti-Christian culture—if culture it be, for the Reds fear and suppress freedom and creativity with a vengeance. And as Mao Tse-tung said, "Political power grows out of the barrel of a gun."

Lenin, who died of syphilis, wrote, "Destroy a nation's morality, and it will fall in your lap like ripe fruit from a tree." The Communists are masters at softening up target nations through drugs and pornography, which they strictly deny to their conquered peoples.

When the Reds take over, they always go after Church leaders first, jailing, torturing and murdering defiant bishops, clergy and religious. Marxists understand well the words of Christ, "I will strike the shepherd and the sheep will be scattered." (Mt. 26:31) They curtail or forbid the activities of all religious organizations as soon as possible, and subject young people to atheistic indoctrination immediately.

All opposition must be eliminated. Potentially troublesome intellectuals and professionals are harassed constantly, neutralized, imprisoned or even shot. Labor unions, civic groups and social clubs are dissolved or taken over.

Like the Nazis, the Communists are masters at "disinformation" and media manipulation. As Stalin said, "Words are one thing; actions, another." Propaganda, lies and deceit of every kind—anything goes if it helps the Party to seize power and keep it.

In Poland, university professors told me the rationalizations, tortured logic and ridiculous word games the Reds use to explain and justify their unjustifiable, Socialist dogma.   There are three kinds of people in the Communist world, they said: (1) the Communist elite, who live like kings;   (2) those who were duped into embracing Marxism but who cannot turn back;   and (3) the silent, suffering majority, who are powerless and without hope, kept in constant fear and distress by the network of informers (before the Hungarian Uprising of 1956, it is estimated that 10 percent of the population were informers).

The Reds are devilishly tricky, knowing when to strike, when to wait, when to compromise, when to retreat (e.g., the Cuban missile crisis); how to use nuns, priests and the Church (e.g., Nicaragua); how to brainwash the young; how to exploit the opposition's weaknesses and gullibility; how to blackmail uncooperative individuals; how to plant rumors and stir up gossip; and how to play chess for the future.

The USSR and its satellite countries are indoctrinating flocks of foreign students in Marxism and revolutionary warfare, new Fidel Castros and Daniel Ortegas being prepared for positions of leadership.   Also under indoctrination are thousands of children kidnapped from Afghanistan and other "liberated zones."

One of the big industries in every Warsaw Pact nation is the manufacture of weapons of all kinds.   The Reds are not only arming themselves to the teeth, but are selling arms to all comers to make money and to influence "nonaligned" nations—while flooding the world with pleas for peace.

The overall leveling of people in the Socialist world has ruined initiative and creativity, except in arms production and military research.   Gorbachev's gigantic problem is how to stir thoroughly cowed people out of their lethargy and away from the alcoholism in which they drown the hopelessness, meaninglessness and dullness of their lives.

The Communists' industrial plant is totally outmoded; their economies are collapsing; and the Reds trail far behind the West in technology and science.   But thanks to the sins, stupidities and spinelessness of the West, the disciples of Lenin have conquered 39 percent of the world's people.   In the process the Communists have murdered 143 million men, women and children, according to the calculations of *Causa Ireland*.

To my surprise, the people of the USSR's satellites know very little about the USSR itself.   They also know very little about each other.   This is no accident.   The

Soviet regime lives in constant fear of disloyalty and collusion among its captive peoples. The State keeps your passport, and when Big Brother lets you travel abroad, you have to surrender your personal papers—to be returned when you give back your passport. Soviet citizens may not visit another city without permission. When citizens from one satellite country visit a neighboring nation or the USSR itself, their movements are strictly controlled. An American or Western European traveling in the USSR is more free than someone from a satellite country.

I talked to Poles who had suffered through the joint German-Soviet invasion of 1939 and the Soviet "liberation" of 1944-45. The Soviets were far worse than the Germans when it came to rapes and other brutalities, especially the Red soldiers who came from the more uncivilized areas of Siberia.

Every literate American should read *In Cold Blood* by Abdul Shams to see the indescribable destruction that Gorbachev's armies are inflicting on the people of Afghanistan. (Is this what some of our unthinking bishops and liberals want in Central America?) No wonder some 100 Poles are escaping via the tourist route into Italy every day. Many of them are the "disenchanted Polish elite." The influx of Poles has become one of Italy's major preoccupations. Even the Pope called it a "sad business."

A CHURCH IN THE CATACOMBS

Formerly a part of the Austro-Hungarian Empire, Czechoslovakia began its national existence after World War I, in 1918. A republic made up of the three provinces of Moravia, Bohemia and Slovakia, it was a functioning democracy until Hitler's brutal invasion in 1938. The Communists took over in 1947 and violently suppressed all opposition.

Of all the Red regimes in Europe, Czechoslovakia's persecutes the Church worst. One reason for this is that Czechoslovakia never experienced a separation of Church and State. Until the Nazi and Communist takeovers, the State properly respected the legitimate role of the Church.

Last September the Catholic hierarchy published a 16-point "Charter for Believers" that calls on the country's Marxist government to end religious discrimination, allow new churches to be built, and agree to the naming of bishops to the country's mostly empty sees. The document

even calls on the world's Catholics to support the Charter
by pressuring Czech diplomats in their countries.

The charter appeals for the release of priests and religious arrested for carrying out their ministries; for permission to form lay parish councils; for State recognition of
deacons; for the legalization of religious orders; and for free
distribution of foreign religious publications, along with
Czech-produced Catholic radio and television programs.

In addition, it insists on an end to "intolerable" government pressure against parents who send their children to
religious instruction and against university students who
continue their religious education; an end to discrimination
against believers seeking professional jobs; and permission
to establish a second faculty of theology in the province of
Moravia.

The 87-year-old Frantisek Cardinal Tomasek is in
charge of six of Czechoslovakia's 13 dioceses, and another
bishop governs a seventh. The rest have only apostolic
administrators, because the Communists resist new nomin-
ations. The Reds have already hinted that they want to
decide on Tomasek's successor. One diocese, by the way, is
Byzantine.

More than 1,100 of the 4,336 parishes are without
priests. The hostile State licenses priests. If any priest is
"too successful," especially with the youth, he loses his
license and must find a job. Also, the government might
remove him to an obscure parish in the country, where
there are few Catholics because of post–World War II mi-
grations.

About 150 Czech priests work underground. I spent a
most interesting evening with two of them. As I looked at
their old, patched shirts and overalls, I thought of our
well-dressed American priests, their nice cars, their monthly paid vacations, comfortable and electronically equipped
rectories, and (in too many cases) well-stocked liquor cabi-
nets. An unknown number of Czech priests are in jail.

Last year the Reds allowed 67 priests to be ordained,
from two seminaries having a combined enrollment of
about 500. Many more would enter the seminaries, but
Gustav Husak's atheistic regime limits the number. Officially, religious orders do not exist. But there are still
some 2,500 sisters and brothers doing what they can to
serve God and His children, some working incognito in
hospitals and other institutions. Gorbachev's ruling pup-

pets want them to die out, so they may not operate novitiates (at least not openly).

Lately, Catholic youth have demonstrated extraordinary courage by making religious pilgrimages openly and in large numbers. This proves the Church is still very much alive, although some priests told me the processions were also a kind of youth protest against an oppressive government, which virtually all Czechs resent.

In Slovakia 100,000 people, mainly young Catholics, made a great pilgrimage to a Marian shrine. Nearly 400,000 believers, 70 percent of them singing young people, took part in three more huge pilgrimages within a few weeks—to the consternation of the police, a bishop told me gleefully.

Besides the barely 10 million Catholics, there are about 500,000 Protestants in 18 denominations. The pre-Reformation heresies of the Czech Jan Hus wreaked havoc in this land, where there are many atheists and agnostics. But nonbelievers too hate the repressive regime of the aging Husak, who demonstrates his fear and hatred of Catholics and Americans in many ways.

Czech priests divide Catholics into three classes: (1) those who were baptized but do not practice; (2) those who were baptized but who go to church rarely, e.g., Christmas and Easter; and (3) the three million or so who practice their Faith rather fervently. Husak's licensing policy makes it exceedingly difficult to catechize, but heroic priests and nuns have their ways and means. The HLI branch in neighboring Yugoslavia prints Bibles and prolife literature for Czechoslovakia on a four-color printing press.

Because parish priests are spied on constantly, there was some hesitancy about allowing me to concelebrate Mass publicly on Sunday. But in all these Red countries people had great fun with my convenient family name, saying that, after all, I was a Marxist and should feel at home!

In the 1960s a surge for democracy emerged under the Slovakian party chief Alexander Dubček. But in 1968 the Soviets and five other Warsaw Pact nations crushed it with a lightning-fast invasion that killed at least 1,000 unresisting Czechs and wounded more. Unlike the Hungarians in 1956, the Czechs did little to resist beyond changing a few street and road signs.

Nonetheless, the Moscow butchers shot a number of army generals for permitting the drive for democracy.

They also promptly shipped thousands of Czech soldiers to the USSR; most went to the Chinese front, never to be heard of again. A reliable source told me that the Communists have murdered at least 30,000 people in this country since 1968.

Before World War II Czechoslovakia was on a par with Germany and England industrially. Her backwardness today is one more proof that Socialism does not work, even if this Marxist land has the smallest foreign debt of any Soviet satellite. Inflation is 30 percent a year.

As in all Red countries, the medical services are inadequate and abominable, run by a bungling bureaucracy. The government claims it lacks funds for essential equipment and medicines, much of which has to be imported from the "corrupt" West.

Housing is in painfully short supply. So are university admissions, and jobs for the lucky ones when they graduate. African students are accused of bringing AIDS into the country. Fifty cases are in the hospitals and five have died, if you can believe the government.

Contraception came to Czechoslovakia in the 19th century, and the Czechs' low birthrates won them the nickname of "Frenchmen of the East." In 1957 the government legalized abortion, with minor restrictions. Typically, subsequent amendments removed most of these.

Two years ago the government began to treat abortion as just one more medical procedure. Abortion became just another means of birth control, with many women submitting to multiple baby-killings. I asked the first professional who might know, just how many babies are actually aborted. He blurted out, "They are uncountable." For every live birth there are at least two babies killed. In some cases abortions are cheaper than Pills and IUDs.

One thing is certain: When you make abortions easy to get, the motivation to contracept begins to evaporate, because people sense that contraception is unnatural and inhuman. Contraceptives, including abortifacient Pills and IUDs, are freely available in Czechoslovakia. The government did publish an amazingly accurate book on NFP in 1972, with a later edition in 1985. Planned Parenthood seems to have entered the scene only in 1970.

Czechoslovakia's 15.4 million people live in a country the size of the state of New York. To rescue the low birthrate of far fewer than two children per family, the government is thinking about tightening up the abortion law. A new mother receives two years of maternity leave; the government pays for one year and guarantees her old job or its equivalent.

Only gynecologists may abort babies; if they refuse, they lose their jobs. Unscrupulous doctors make a bundle committing black-market abortions. As in every country with legalized abortion, good Catholic medical students avoid gynecology. They cannot make an adequate living in that field, but more important, they refuse to help liquidate their nation's future. Poor Czechoslovakia has NO prolife literature, films, videos or slides.

Starry-eyed Communists are hard to find. As the *Wall Street Journal* put it on 13 July 1987, "The State doesn't ask them to believe, merely to make believe that they do." The rewards: country cottages, cars, color TV sets and 200 pounds of salami and ham per person per year. Like the Italians, the average Czech earns about $8,500 a year, while the economy grows by four percent yearly.

Having escaped World War II almost intact, this industrial nation now has superfluous heavy industry, e.g., steel and machine-tool production, while her markets have shrunk. Badly needed reforms proposed by the government call for more free enterprise—which means that layers of self-satisfied bureaucrats will have to become accountable and risk unemployment, besides having to deal with the end of subsidies for various companies, the election of "leading employees" and much more.

The Czechs have tasted democracy and like it. They were not happy with the coming of Mikhail Gorbachev, who understands the economic, social and technical backwardness of Eastern Europe and who is therefore upending the East Bloc. The proponent of *glasnost* is also known for his outspoken intolerance of all religion.

The carefree Czechs do not trust the man from Moscow any more than they do the 74-year-old Husak, even if Gorbachev did say, "Czechoslovakia is making ever better use of the boundless potential of Socialism." The comfortable Czechs, on their way to weekend cottages in Skoda cars loaded with salami, are more than skeptical.

BRINGING PROLIFE AND N.F.P. TO HUNGARY

This ancient Catholic nation numbers 10.6 million in a land slightly smaller than the state of Indiana. The Hungarians are descended from the Magyars and have a difficult, non-Slavic language. Catholicism began with the acceptance of the Faith by King Keza in 875. One need only think of Sts. Stephen and Elizabeth to be reminded of Hungary's great Catholic past.

In 1944–45 the beasts from the East invaded Hungary. In no country behind the Iron Curtain does the Soviet bear have a tighter grasp, nor has it done more harm.

In the period 1949–52 the Reds legalized abortions committed for medical reasons. In 1953–54 there were an estimated 100,000 abortions; government measures to stem the tide were to no avail. The idea spread that the couple, and above all the woman, should decide the outcome of pregnancy. By 1956 the government had removed all restrictions one by one. Today there are an estimated three abortions for every live birth! (There were 140,000 births last year.)

Abortions may be committed only in hospitals, only by gynecologists, and only in the first three months of pregnancy, but exceptions are easily made here, as everywhere. In 1962, Hungary recorded the lowest birthrate in Europe. In 1969, 78 percent of Hungarian women of childbearing age killed at least one baby. As always, illegal abortion continues, but the bad effects on women's health, especially during pregnancies, are of great concern to the government.

Contraceptives are readily available, including abortifacient Pills and IUDs. But for many women, surgical abortion at government expense has been "more convenient and perhaps even more economical than regular use of pills," reported New York City's pro-abortion Population Council.

The Czech Red Cross was naive enough to involve itself in the futile attempts to reduce the dreadful number of baby-killings by spreading contraceptives.

Of course Planned Parenthood, known in Hungary as the Hungarian Scientific Society for Family and Education of Women, has been a big part of the antilife push in this unfortunate, isolated nation. PP even held its notorious 1969 European Near East Regional Conference in Budapest. PP's willingness to collaborate with Communist police states reveals yet another evil side of this sinister global organization.

For 30 years the Red barbarians forbade all religious instruction. They suppressed all religious orders in 1949, but later permitted three to reactivate—the Benedictines (the largest and most scholarly in Hungary before the

Marxist takeover), the Piarists and the Franciscans, all of whose work was, however, seriously curtailed.

In recent years the Communists have relented somewhat; they now allow the religious orders to conduct two gymnasia (university prep schools) each, with permission to teach religion. A mixed group of surviving nuns from various orders run a high school for girls. (This year Fr. Stanley L. Jaki, a Hungarian Benedictine scholar who teaches at Seton Hall University in New Jersey, won the coveted $365,200 Templeton Prize for Progress in Religion; the money is going to benefit 35 Hungarian Benedictines exiled in five Western countries.)

Hungary's clergy and religious are old; priests are in very short supply and are fast dying out. The relaxed persecution allows one seminary of 225 seminarians for the nation's 11 dioceses. Several dioceses are still vacant, a legacy of the confrontational approach of the postwar Cardinal Mindszenty era. Some Catholics believe the Church's subsequent low political profile and cautious, conciliatory policy only contributed to Her decline; she now lacks a clear profile of independence from Communist authorities.

In any case, the Church today is challenged by a growing movement of Hungarian youth who are returning to religion, and by a certain activism which they favor. A movement of conscientious objection to military service has surfaced; it is one of the most volatile manifestations of the new attitudes among East European young people. The government is also suspicious of the "base communities" that have emerged in a number of parishes, especially in rural areas.

Then there is the Piarist priest, Fr. Gjorgz Bulanji, who leads a movement of Catholic lay communities that embrace conscientious objection and various religious-recreational activities. They were originally an underground movement, cultivating their faith through biblical study.

Today they tend to reject the authority of those bishops whom they consider weak, while ruling out any possibility of cooperation with the Marxists. To the dismay of the powerful Bulanjists, a bishops' conference in October 1986 stated that military service was fully compatible with Catholic practice. The Holy See has so far refused to interfere with the influential Fr. Bulanji, however.

I addressed 30–40 seminarians and showed them a videocassette of Dr. Nathanson's latest abortion film, *Eclipse of Reason.* They were fascinated, like Rip van

Winkle awakening to a world they had not known. They kept me far into the night. In Hungary, resistance to abortion is novel; Catholics there have *nothing* with which to curb the killing of the preborn babies. Most Hungarians take abortion for granted; others have fallen into atheism. The problem now, said a seminary teacher, is how to win back the youth whose parents were deprived of Christianity and could not care less.

The rector of the seminary insisted that abortions had been so common for so long that priests were not even aware of bad psychological effects among aborting women, who talk about abortions as freely as they talk about shopping. I asked, "What is taught in reproductive biology?" I added that I find it hard to believe that abortion leaves Hungarian women undisturbed, because non-Christian Japanese are troubled greatly by their baby-killings. In Communist classrooms, I was told, "the fetus is a nothing"; there is no hint of a human being before birth. The development of animals is taught, but contracepting, aborting teachers neglect human development. There is no God, so what difference does it make?

I was traveling with two prolife young people from Eastern Europe. Fortunately, we were able to give out full-color leaflets showing developing preborn babies. The HLI office and press in Yugoslavia print these and other literature in Hungarian. We hope these materials will soon reach every young Catholic in the Catholic high schools. Once again I promised these prolifers a great deal, banking on the generosity of HLI's supporters.

The seminarians were flabbergasted by what they learned. Obviously, they had never heard of NFP, even though John Kippley's excellent *The Art of Natural Family Planning* appeared in Hungarian last July. The professors were vaguely aware of the "Model T" of NFP, the pioneering Ogino-Knaus calendar rhythm method, but nothing more. I explained the latest methods to the seminarians, who vowed to study any books I would send them.

The latest methods of artificial birth control in Hungary are the IUD, the suppository, the Pill and the condom.

Occasionally I am tempted to think I am not doing what God really wants me to do, but not that evening! What a super experience to be with those intelligent but information-starved future priests! Without HLI, when would Catholic Hungary have discovered the prolife movement? HLI is lighting fires all over the world—often where there was not even a spark before.

I shall never forget an old German-speaking professor's description of the Communists' satanic, systematic persecution. He emphasized that Hungary had suffered three invasions in her history: (1) the Tartars, (2) the Communists, and (3) the Abortionists—the last, introduced by the Marxists with the help of PP, being by far the worst.

In 1956, the beleaguered Hungarians tried to throw off the choking Communist yoke in hopes that the West would help them. We did nothing. Soviet tank armies rumbled in. Tens of thousands died in the fighting or were shipped to Siberia. Perhaps 200,000 fled the country. Today the isolated Hungarians are a dying nation. In name, at least, two-thirds are Catholic; the rest are Protestants (Calvinists and Evangelicals) or atheists. Is it any wonder that Hungary has the highest suicide rate in the world? For the young there is no God, no hope—only the painful nihilism of Communism and Planned Parenthood.

A liberalization program that began in 1968 loosened state planning and centralization of the economy and allowed some private entrepreneurship, so living standards climbed ever higher. Some spoke of Hungary's "economic miracle." But investment, production and exports did not keep pace. With inflation at double-digit levels and with gross foreign debt at $16 billion, the highest per capita in Eastern Europe, Hungary's stagnating economy is in very serious trouble.

Severe austerity measures are in place. A very unpopular government has slapped a value-added tax on most goods and services, as well as a far-reaching income tax, both virtually unknown in Communist countries. By taking 20 to 60 percent of annual incomes over $800, the State hopes to tap funds from second jobs or from the "third economy" of gifts and bribes. (The third economy, with all its dishonesties, is characteristic of Communist countries.) Also, because of the low birthrate, this aging, tired nation is trapped in a kind of socioeconomic paralysis, as are the other satellites.

While her economy worsens, 40 percent of Hungary's people live at the subsistence level or below. Of course, for Communist propagandists, mass unemployment is mere "employment dislocation." But the Hungarians are not fooled.

The stagnating countries of the Communist Comecon lack the integration, competition and free-trade laws of the European Economic Community. With their rigid, top-down central planning, they have fallen far behind. And the master in the Kremlin knows it. Meanwhile, the pessimistic, cynical Hungarians quip, "The situation is hopeless, but it is not yet bad."

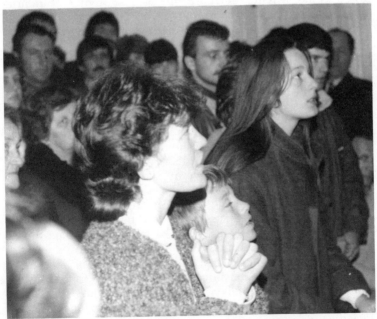

Medjugorje, Yugoslavia: Young people report seeing Mary.

THE SHOWCASE OF COMMUNISM

(No. 39—January 1988)

To cross the border from prison-like Hungary into Yugoslavia at first seems like a fresh breath of air. But soon you breathe in the familiar stench of Marxist inhumanities. Although not behind the Iron Curtain, this fractious, beautiful country of 22.5 million souls is bedeviled by grave socioeconomic ills and many other problems.

According to an old joke, Oregon-sized Yugoslavia is one nation with two alphabets, three religions, four main languages, five principal nationalities, six republics, seven borders and no economy. But you still see pictures of the late dictator, Tito, everywhere.

Yugoslavia has seven million Catholics (mostly Croatians), plus Slovenes, Serbs and some Hungarians, Italians and Albanians (Mother Teresa is an Albanian Yugoslav). The country also has four million indigenous Moslems, thanks to the Ottoman Turkish conquest. The remaining nine million are Greek Orthodox of weak faith and weaker practice; more of Yugoslavia's 50,000 Uniate Catholics go to church on Sunday than do her Orthodox.

Two million Yugoslavs are unemployed, and a million and a half work in foreign countries (including 700,000 in dying West Germany). The country suffers from corruption, mismanagement, a 168 percent inflation rate, a $20 billion foreign debt, increasing strikes, feuding and competing republics that take turns supplying prime ministers, and an inept, struggling national government with no built-in mechanism for improvement. This is the sad legacy of Marshal Tito, who left the economy in potential shambles, having borrowed too heavily in his last years.

The government of Prime Minister Bronko Mikulic has proposed a package of economic belt-tightening measures to renegotiate Yugoslavia's huge foreign debt, but no one seems pleased. The conviction prevails that without a radical switch to a market economy—which assumes a functioning democracy—Yugoslavia cannot solve her problems and defuse her economic, political and social crisis.

Critics say the government should let the economy sort out its problems without outside interference. But how can a divided, demoralized people shake off the thick, strangling web of laws, bylaws, rules, regulations and disincentives? For example, every business employing 10 or more must be State-owned. And how can severely disgruntled people work harder and become more productive while their real wages and living standards are falling and prices are rising? Communist Socialism is a curse.

As you would expect in this most open of Marxist countries, the youth are the first to give expression to the underlying, hitherto-suppressed national aspirations. Among the "progressive" ideas of the young people's nascent pressure groups, particularly in Slovenia, are support for the peace movement, criticism of the military, alternative service for conscientious objectors, environmental concerns, opposition to nuclear power plants, feminist and homosexual issues, and even a multiparty system in a pluralistic society.

HOW THE MARTYR CHURCH LIVES

But despite all these democratic rumblings, the Church is still watched carefully, although less and less so, thanks to the political confusion and all the socioeconomic problems. In no Red country except for Poland have Catholics suffered more at the hands of the Communists.

For example, when Tito's Partisans came down from the mountains and finally won out against the Croatian and Slovenian anti-Communists, they kicked all the wounded soldiers out of Zagreb's bulging hospitals. They tossed them one by one into trucks, then dumped them into holes, dead or alive. Meanwhile, the Reds reoccupied the hospital beds with their own wounded. Once fully in control, Tito ordered the cemeteries where his anti-Communist enemies (and fellow citizens) had buried their dead soldiers, to be plowed under.

The Croatians have a beautiful custom of placing candles in colored plastic containers on the graves of their dearly departed on the eve of All Souls' Day. In one section of a huge cemetery in Zagreb I saw thousands of candles standing together for those whose graves Tito had desecrated and plowed into anonymity.

Among the 250,000 executed by ex-altar boy Tito were 350 priests, many religious and many Catholic professionals and intellectuals. He confiscated virtually all Catholic schools, institutions and property. Ironically, he relented in his persecution later only under American economic pressure, although the Americans (along with the British) were largely responsible for his brutal conquest.

Today Yugoslavia has 3,000 secular priests and 7,000 women religious. She has 10 major and more minor seminaries. Vocations are ample, except in dioceses in coastal tourist regions, where the omnipresent German tourists can always be seen taking part in nude or topless sunbathing. In the country's second largest city, Zagreb, there are 450 Catholic churches, 500 priests, 1,000 nuns, and a good number of Carmels serving two million Catholics. Zagreb is almost all Catholic. Most reluctantly, the government does allow the building of new churches.

I had a fascinating and revealing two-hour conversation with Zagreb's Franjo Cardinal Kuharic. For one thing, I learned that the Communists allowed only one church for a new suburb of 150,000 people. To circumvent restrictions such as these, he (like other bishops) built large, off-the-street houses to which additions could easily be made. Used at first for priests' living quarters, counseling rooms and sometimes a kindergarten, the buildings eventually became parish churches, with the police often looking the other way as the structures grew.

Bishops will also install pastors in large apartment buildings; here the priests celebrate Mass and care for thousands. The fighting little cardinal, whose features and thinking remind you of the Pope's, remarked that the more problems the government has, the less time it has to bother the Church, "so these are good times for expansion!"

The cardinal groaned over the more than 400,000 abortions that he estimates are committed annually in Yugoslavia; some 200,000 of these are committed on teenagers (without parental knowledge), thanks to the Planned Parenthood-type sex "education" in the schools. Of course, this sex "education" only propels the young into more and more fornication, because PP tells them they have a right to intercourse, contraception and abortion.

PP entered Yugoslavia formally in 1967 and now is active within the health service. (Helping PP is the USA's Pathfinder Fund.) PP told the government that contraception would reduce the number of abortions, so contraception became an integral part of "preventive medicine," as sex training became a part of education from kindergarten on.

But by 1969, the ratio of all abortions to births was reported to be four to one. The cardinal's current estimate of 400,000 abortions seems very conservative. Meanwhile, the country's four million Moslems have large families, whereas the nine million mostly non-practicing Orthodox Serbs commit two abortions for every birth. So abortion in Yugoslavia has become a major method of birth control, with many women aborting nine or 10 babies.

Contraceptives of all kinds are available, including the dangerous abortifacient Depo-Provera, also known as "the Shot." As in all Communist nations, medicine is in a shambles, hospital beds are far too few, and equipment is lacking, worn out or outmoded. In several hours of conversation, two female medical students told me that the whole of Zagreb has only one dialysis machine. They also revealed that the government is investing a great deal of money in ultrasound equipment and an amniocentesis program in order to eliminate "defective" preborn Yugoslavs.

PLANNING A MEETING FOR EASTERN EUROPE

I had a marvelous three-hour chat with the 75-year-old Archbishop Frane Franic of Split. Split is a resort and industrial city on the beautiful Adriatic coast, where the Roman Emperor Diocletian had his famed, huge summer palace, still well preserved.

This gracious and intelligently prolife archbishop has 238,000 Catholics, 50,000 Orthodox, 335 priests, 73 major seminarians, more minor seminarians, and only 50 real Communists. The Franciscans have five provinces in Yugoslavia, and 200 men in their major seminary in Split. Tito killed 30 priests from this archdiocese.

Catholicism in Yugoslavia dates back to the seventh century, when Pope John IV (640–642), a Dalmatian by birth, sent the Benedictines to convert the Slavs in 641. At one time, my confreres had 150 monasteries in this country, only to give way to the Franciscans in the 13th century, when St. Francis of Assisi charmed the Moslem satraps.

I proposed to the archbishop that HLI sponsor the first international symposium for prolife leaders in Eastern Europe. He was delighted. At once, he promised his total cooperation, even offering us the 300-seat auditorium beneath his pro-cathedral, plus five adjoining classrooms, all of which he promptly showed me. This is one of the most beautiful modern churches I have ever seen.

He said he wants all his seminarians there, as well as many priests—using the upper church, too, if necessary.

BACK TO MEDJUGORJE

Archbishop Franic is very positive toward the famous reported apparitions of the Blessed Virgin in the Croatian village of Medjugorje. He admitted that many of his priests are skeptical, but said he himself visits the place often. He said the Franciscans at the parish are sincere and do superb work. At times he invites the young visionaries to lunch.

French theologian Fr. René Laurentin erred when he quoted the archbishop as saying, "The visionaries have done more for the area spiritually than all the priests in 40 years." What he did say, in the early years of the reported apparitions, was that the seers had done more privately to shore up people's faith than all the publicly announced parish missions over the years.

It had been almost four years since I first visited Medjugorje. The changes stunned me. The Communists have finally realized the economic potential of millions of Western pilgrims.

This out-of-the-way village of 3,000 people is now being surrounded by many little hotels, restaurants and other facilities catering to more and more pilgrims, among whom Americans predominate, followed by Italians and then the Irish. The Reds have also set up a mile-long gauntlet of booths selling rosaries, statues and other spiritual goods on both sides of the road leading to the church.

Every day thousands of pilgrims come; 100,000 gathered there on the fifth anniversary of the reported appearances, which began in 1981. It is estimated that 10 million have visited Medjugorje.

The local bishop, Pavao Zanic of Mostar, is more than negative about the whole affair—in part, perhaps, because of a centuries-old episcopal quarrel with the powerful Franciscans, who have many parishes in his diocese and in other parts of Yugoslavia.

Bishop Zanic and the national hierarchy have forbidden any priest to lead an official pilgrimage to Medjugorje and offer Mass there. The ruling is mostly ignored. The bishop knows it and has said he will do nothing about it. He and the national bishops' conference have not discouraged people from coming there to pray, to fast and to be inspired to more fervent Christian living; what they forbid

are Church-organized pilgrimages. Meanwhile, the Holy
See has asked Yugoslavia's bishops to make a new, thorough investigation of the reported apparitions and other
phenomena in Medjugorje.

A doctor on the episcopal investigating team showed
me complete documentation of the miraculous healing of a
Pennsylvania woman crippled by multiple sclerosis. In a
two-hour conversation, he said he knew of five other such
documented cures, and that additional healings remain
uninvestigated because of a lack of funds.

Scientists from the universities of Milan, Montpellier
and Grenoble have examined the visionaries thoroughly
and have proclaimed them to be honest young men and
women, with no pathology, who tell the truth as they see
it. The events, say the scientists, have no human or scientific explanation. A French photographer pointed out 'that
all human eyes blink when cameras flash; not so those of
the visionaries when they converse with the Lady of the
visions.

The message is simple: prayer and penance, faith and
reconciliation, loyalty to Church and Pope—or God will
punish the world. I could not verify the celestial prodigies
and other miracles often reported. I will not be surprised
if the Church finds the apparitions authentic. Meanwhile,
Medjugorje has inspired a great deal of prayer and penance, and we cannot have too much of these. We must
await Rome's final decision, but there is no denying that
Medjugorje is an extraordinary phenomenon.

H.L.I.-YUGOSLAVIA THRIVING

HLI's branch in Slavonski Brod, Yugoslavia, is truly
flourishing under the leadership of a saintly, talented
pastor, Father Marko Majstorovic. He spends endless
hours running the four-color printing press HLI purchased,
producing full-color prolife materials in 11 languages for
Eastern Europe, Bibles for Czechoslovakia and Hungary,
and catechetical tools for Yugoslavia's hard-pressed bishops.

He is also the diocesan family life director, the pastor
of 1,500 families, and the builder and director of a much-
needed retreat house that is used for multiple and varied
programs, including prayer meetings. At my request he
organized a two-day prolife training seminar there for
doctors, midwives, nurses, teachers, lawyers, priests, medical students and others. On hand was Fr. Anto Bakovic,
founder of the One More Child movement, with whom I

had a great chat. It was the most productive weekend during my 24 days in four Communist countries.

The zealous Fr. Majstorovic uses some of the Mass stipends you send to buy paper to print Bibles. He also sends stipends in the form of Bibles and other religious materials to the beleaguered priests and bishops of Hungary and Czechoslovakia.

In the last four years Fr. Majstorovic has also built two parish churches for his bishop and has renovated his own church. At times the authorities hassle him, but they seem befuddled by this balding, unassuming priest who refuses to buy a car and visits his people on bicycle. He is surely the most productive priest I know, and it hurts me terribly not to be able to send him everything he deserves and needs.

In all of these Eastern countries, you also meet heroic lay leaders. One of these is Marijo Zivkovic of Zagreb, who, along with his wife Darka, is a member of the Pontifical Council for the Family in Rome. The Communists took away Marijo's passport at the airport just when he was leaving for our First International Symposium in Washington in 1985. This only made him and his family more active for the Lord.

Marijo's apostolic spirit and intelligence have poured over into his brilliant daughter Jelka, who is studying medicine. I drove from Lublin, Poland, down to Zagreb with Jelka, her brother and another medical student. At the Czechoslovak border the Reds held us up for two hours. They were fascinated by the 1,000 "Precious Feet" lapel pins I had carefully hidden away in the trunk. I reassured the customs officials, my fellow Marxists, that the pins were made of cheap metal and were therefore of little value. Into solemn conference went my four comrades: How to handle this major threat to the Revolution?

Meanwhile, I suggested to Jelka that she give two sets of feet to each guard—one for himself and the other for his wife. Our great generosity seemed to win them over; we were highly amused as they studied these filthy products of the capitalist West, then carefully stuffed them into their pockets while we sped off!

The two Catholic medical students told me how you cope when you are a student in a Yugoslav medical school. Generally, all prolife work must be started and carried out within the parish. For example, when Drs. John and Lyn Billings came, they were not allowed to lecture at the university because they were Catholic and the natural family planning method they propagate is "Catholic"!

So the resourceful Jelka founded a group called "Gynecological Socialist Health Workers of Zagreb," which had only two members at first. They then invited the Billingses to a full hall on campus. The response was enthusiastic.

The growing little group now speaks on the Catholic aspects of love, marriage and sex, but must always do it in disguise. Anything Catholic is strictly taboo. At best, chastity is a Catholic idea and must be avoided; for the Communists, promiscuity is a part of liberation.

These Catholic medical students once approached the head of a secondary school and said they would talk about prophylactics and abortion. The director thought they would recommend condoms, Pills and IUDs, and say that abortion was all right. Instead, they spoke on NFP, chastity, the bad effects of abortions, and child development. They showed abortion slides, and proved that abortions kill.

The Catholic students have lots of fun giving new ideas to foreign students. (There are plenty of the last in satellite countries, future Castros and Ortegas learning the glories of Communism so they can subvert their home countries.) For example, a man from India told them there is no need for a woman to prepare herself for marriage and husband, because she is like a cow at the end of a rope held by the husband!

The greatest mistake one could make, these medical students warned me, is to compromise in any way; Catholic teaching, properly presented, appeals to the young people, who have been lied to so much by the Red media and the Marxist professors. Our Lord described the devil as a liar and murderer from the beginning; Communism is surely of the devil, who is everywhere and who never sleeps, as the Church Fathers warned. God save us from the smiling Gorbachev.

H.L.I.'S WORK IN CALIFORNIA

Recently I conducted weekend retreats for young couples and older couples at Our Lady of Peace Retreat in Portland, Oregon; addressed an HLI fund-raising banquet in Sacramento, California; picketed a gigantic abortion center in that city, under the guidance of the wily Albin Rhomberg; preached at seven Masses at Sacred Heart

parish and spoke to the leaders of four groups of Guadalupanos, in Fresno, California; dialogued with four classes at
Garces Memorial Catholic High School in Bakersfield,
California; spoke to the prolifers in that city and to the
Knights of Columbus and the prolife group in Fresno; and
did an hour-long interview on Fresno's Catholic TV channel.

I had a unique experience while preaching at a Sunday
evening Mass, attended largely by university students, at
Fresno's Sacred Heart parish. As usual, I emphasized
chastity, tried to define true love, and explained the
Church's teaching on birth control. I also pointed out the
horrendous, worldwide consequences of disobedience to the
Church's teachings, the correctness of which, I asserted,
was perhaps never more evident than in this age of rampant sex abuse, shacking up, abortions, VD, low birthrates,
divorce and unhappiness.

Suddenly a hand went up. I ignored it at first, but it
stayed up. Finally, I said to the gentleman that this was
not a classroom, that I would talk with him after Mass for
five hours, if he wished. Without genuflecting, he and his
colleague stomped out.

Later I was astonished to learn that the hand belonged
to Val Rios, head of student affairs and the religion de-
partment at the San Joaquin Memorial Catholic High
School, which I was scheduled to address the next day.
Rios canceled my appearance because I was "too negative,"
adding that "in conscience I could not allow him to speak
to our students." (The local bishop later apologized for
Rios' behavior.) From those who know him, I gather that
Rios' hang-up is contraception, that worm in the apple.
Incidentally, California's maverick, pro-abortion, Catholic/-
Buddhist former governor Jerry Brown has spoken at this
high school, as have other pro-abortion politicians.

Fresno is a very interesting diocese, with its own TV
channel, in California's agricultural Central Valley. The
300,000 Catholics of this far-flung diocese are 65 percent
Hispanic, eight percent Portuguese, 25 percent Anglo, 1.5
percent Southeast Asian, 0.4 percent black and 0.1 percent
other. The diocese also contains 30,000 other Asians, most
of whom it sponsored. Among them are 23,000 Hmongs,
the mountain people of now-Communist-ruled Laos, who
still prize their large families. Two priests (who speak
eight languages) serve the Catholic Asians. Increasingly,

the diocese is becoming Hispanic; Bakersfield is the fastest-growing city in California.

I also met with the leaders of the diocese's 40 groups of Guadalupanos, who grabbed up my Spanish prolife literature. The Guadalupanos educate Hispanics and others in knowledge of and devotion to Our Lady of Guadalupe, Empress of the Americas and Patroness of the Unborn. They ordered me to return for another talk.

For one hour without interruption, Fr. Stephen Barham, an intelligent and experienced Maronite priest, interviewed me on Fresno's diocesan TV about the antilife movement worldwide. I have done many such programs, but this was by far the best.

HE HAS KILLED 700,000 BABIES

While in Fresno, I joined some 30 prolifers in picketing one of Dr. Edward Allred's 27 abortion mills in California. Never in my life had I seen such a spacious, specially built, baby-killing chamber.

I walked into a large reception room of this cavernous building and nonchalantly sat down to watch TV. After about two minutes, one of the killer women told me I had to leave. Why, I asked. "You upset people." I told her that I had not spoken to a single person (yet!). I explained, further, that the killing operation was funded mostly by tax money, so it was a public operation, and therefore I had a right to be there. I took my time leaving, seeing one young man crying, aborted girls staggering, and everyone anxious and tense.

Is there a sadder or more somber place in this world than an abortuary, where money-hungry doctors kill troubled mothers' babies for cash? As everywhere, the local health department refers the minority women—blacks and especially Hispanics—to this abortion center. One just-aborted Hispanic woman weepingly told me her whole story outside.

The killer-owner is a conservative Republican and a Seventh-Day Adventist who boasts of having killed 700,000 babies. He has made an astonishing statement about his purpose: He eliminates, above all, immigrant Hispanics—thus doing his fellow Anglo taxpayers a big favor, he says. (Of course, he never mentions the millions of dollars of California tax money he is paid.) He has even said he would like to open a no-charge abortion mill across the border in Mexico. You may remember this millionaire

Allred in the film *The Silent Scream*, aborting babies and nonchalantly making illogical, incredible remarks to justify his bloody killing business.

I also had a great chat with Fresno's Bishop Joseph Madera, who was born to Mexican refugee parents in the U.S., but later raised in Mexico. The head of this varied and growing diocese speaks three languages. Last June he ordained a record six priests.

(To be continued.)

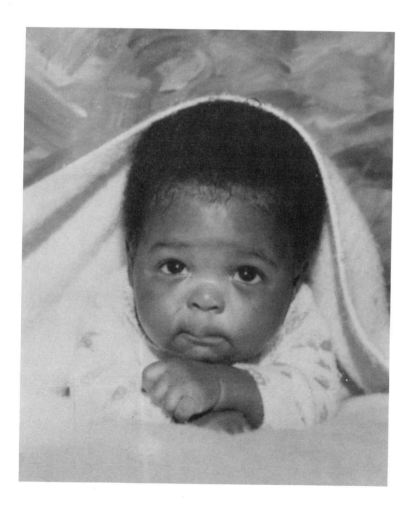

INDEX

Human Life International vs. Planned Parenthood

HLI

- God-centered, totally loyal to the Church and Pope
- *Views people as made in the God's image and having an eternal destiny*
- Believes sexuality is a God-given gift that is good and holy and must be must be used within His laws
- *Recognizes children as gifts of God and the purpose of marriage*
- Affirms the sacredness of every innocent human life from conception onward
- *Insists that chastity and decency must be safeguarded for human happiness and the very survival of society; recognizes that intimate relationships belong within marriage alone*
- Defends the right of married couples to have as many children as they can provide for
- *Opposes sterilization and artificial contraception as attacks upon God's plan and human dignity*
- Founded by Benedictine priest and marriage/family life expert Fr. Paul Marx (called "Public Enemy Number One of Planned Parenthood" at PP meeting)
- *Has 22 offices on five continents helping prolifers in 104 nations*
- Has a budget of less than one percent of PP's budget

PP

- Agnostic, human-centered and totally secularist
- *Views people as mere animals incapable of sexual self-control*
- Believes people can make their own rules and "have sex" with any adult who is willing
- *Sees children as an inconvenient by-product of sex when contraception fails*
- Asserts that "unwanted" preborn children may be killed at will up to birth
- *Teaches that every individual has the right to fornicate, masturbate, use abortifacient "contraceptives," engage in unnatural sex acts, indulge in pornography and kill babies*
- Advocates massive population control programs to force down the birthrates of "undesirable" social groups
- *Sees human fertility as a terrible "problem" to be "solved" by chemical or surgical mutilation*
- Founded by "free love" advocate, avowed racist and anti-Catholic bigot Margaret Sanger, who said Catholics should not be allowed to "breed"
- *Has affiliates in 123 countries; including 45 abortion chambers in the USA that kill 95,000 babies each year*
- Has a budget of $1 million a day, 40 percent from the U.S. taxpayer

Why not share . . .
Confessions of a Prolife Missionary
. . . with others? Give extra copies to friends, pastors, church members, prolife activists, students, reporters, columnists, libraries ($8.95 ppd.; ask for quantity discounts).

Are you receiving Fr. Marx's *Special Reports* regularly? Or HLI's other newsletter, the monthly *HLI Reports?* (Ask about our Spanish quarterly, *Escoge la Vida.*)

Abortion, sexual sins and the war against children and families are a worldwide crisis. If you are not reading HLI's newsletters, you are seeing only a part of the picture. They bring you fascinating and often startling news that you cannot get anywhere else. You will also receive HLI's catalog of the best prolife/pro-family literature, books, films and videos. The suggested donation is $30 (tax-deductible). Please make your check payable to HLI.

[ ] Send me _____ book(s); total, _____.

[ ] Send me HLI's two newsletters. I'm enclosing

my tax-deductible offering of $_____.

TOTAL ENCLOSED: $_____.

name_____tel_____

address_____

city_____state_____ZIP_____

return to:
Human Life International
7845-E Airpark Road
Gaithersburg, Maryland 20879 USA
(301/670-7884)

Why not share . . .
Confessions of a Prolife Missionary
. . . with others? Give extra copies to friends, pastors, church members, prolife activists, students, reporters, columnists, libraries ($8.95 ppd.; ask for quantity discounts).

Are you receiving Fr. Marx's *Special Reports* regularly? Or HLI's other newsletter, the monthly *HLI Reports?* (Ask about our Spanish quarterly, *Escoge la Vida.*)

Abortion, sexual sins and the war against children and families are a worldwide crisis. If you are not reading HLI's newsletters, you are seeing only a part of the picture. They bring you fascinating and often startling news that you cannot get anywhere else. You will also receive HLI's catalog of the best prolife/pro-family literature, books, films and videos. The suggested donation is $30 (tax-deductible). Please make your check payable to HLI.

[ ] Send me _____ book(s); total, _____.

[ ] Send me HLI's two newsletters. I'm enclosing

my tax-deductible offering of $_____.

TOTAL ENCLOSED: $_____.

name_____tel_____

address_____

city_____state_____ZIP_____

return to:
Human Life International
7845-E Airpark Road
Gaithersburg, Maryland 20879 USA
(301/670-7884)

Why not share . . .
Confessions of a Prolife Missionary
. . . with others? Give extra copies to friends, pastors, church members, prolife activists, students, reporters, columnists, libraries ($8.95 ppd.; ask for quantity discounts).

Are you receiving Fr. Marx's *Special Reports* regularly? Or HLI's other newsletter, the monthly *HLI Reports?* (Ask about our Spanish quarterly, *Escoge la Vida.)*

Abortion, sexual sins and the war against children and families are a worldwide crisis. If you are not reading HLI's newsletters, you are seeing only a part of the picture. They bring you fascinating and often startling news that you cannot get anywhere else. You will also receive HLI's catalog of the best prolife/pro-family literature, books, films and videos. The suggested donation is $30 (tax-deductible). Please make your check payable to HLI.

[ ] Send me ＿＿＿ book(s); total, ＿＿＿＿.

[ ] Send me HLI's two newsletters. I'm enclosing

my tax-deductible offering of $＿＿＿＿.

TOTAL ENCLOSED: $＿＿＿＿.

name＿＿＿＿＿＿＿＿＿＿＿＿＿＿＿＿＿＿tel＿＿＿＿＿＿＿

address＿＿＿＿＿＿＿＿＿＿＿＿＿＿＿＿＿＿＿＿＿＿＿＿

city＿＿＿＿＿＿＿＿＿＿＿＿＿＿＿state＿＿＿＿ZIP＿＿＿＿

return to:
Human Life International
7845-E Airpark Road
Gaithersburg, Maryland 20879 USA
(301/670-7884)

Why not share . . .
Confessions of a Prolife Missionary
. . . with others? Give extra copies to friends, pastors, church members, prolife activists, students, reporters, columnists, libraries ($8.95 ppd.; ask for quantity discounts).

Are you receiving Fr. Marx's *Special Reports* regularly? Or HLI's other newsletter, the monthly *HLI Reports?* (Ask about our Spanish quarterly, *Escoge la Vida*.)

Abortion, sexual sins and the war against children and families are a worldwide crisis. If you are not reading HLI's newsletters, you are seeing only a part of the picture. They bring you fascinating and often startling news that you cannot get anywhere else. You will also receive HLI's catalog of the best prolife/pro-family literature, books, films and videos. The suggested donation is $30 (tax-deductible). Please make your check payable to HLI.

[ ] Send me _____ book(s); total, _____.

[ ] Send me HLI's two newsletters. I'm enclosing
   my tax-deductible offering of $_____.
   TOTAL ENCLOSED: $_____.

name_____tel_____

address_____

city_____state_____ZIP____

return to:
Human Life International
7845-E Airpark Road
Gaithersburg, Maryland 20879 USA
(301/670-7884)

Why not share . . .
Confessions of a Prolife Missionary
. . . with others? Give extra copies to friends, pastors, church members, prolife activists, students, reporters, columnists, libraries ($8.95 ppd.; ask for quantity discounts).

Are you receiving Fr. Marx's *Special Reports* regularly? Or HLI's other newsletter, the monthly *HLI Reports?* (Ask about our Spanish quarterly, *Escoge la Vida.*)

Abortion, sexual sins and the war against children and families are a worldwide crisis. If you are not reading HLI's newsletters, you are seeing only a part of the picture. They bring you fascinating and often startling news that you cannot get anywhere else. You will also receive HLI's catalog of the best prolife/pro-family literature, books, films and videos. The suggested donation is $30 (tax-deductible). Please make your check payable to HLI.

[ ] Send me ＿＿＿ book(s); total, ＿＿＿＿.

[ ] Send me HLI's two newsletters. I'm enclosing

my tax-deductible offering of $＿＿＿＿.

TOTAL ENCLOSED: $＿＿＿＿.

name＿＿＿＿＿＿＿＿＿＿＿＿＿＿＿＿＿＿tel＿＿＿＿＿＿

address＿＿＿＿＿＿＿＿＿＿＿＿＿＿＿＿＿＿＿＿＿＿＿

city＿＿＿＿＿＿＿＿＿＿＿＿＿＿＿state＿＿＿ZIP＿＿＿

return to:
Human Life International
7845-E Airpark Road
Gaithersburg, Maryland 20879 USA
(301/670-7884)

Why not share . . .

Confessions of a Prolife Missionary

. . . with others? Give extra copies to friends, pastors, church members, prolife activists, students, reporters, columnists, libraries ($8.95 ppd.; ask for quantity discounts).

Are you receiving Fr. Marx's *Special Reports* regularly? Or HLI's other newsletter, the monthly *HLI Reports?* (Ask about our Spanish quarterly, *Escoge la Vida.*)

Abortion, sexual sins and the war against children and families are a worldwide crisis. If you are not reading HLI's newsletters, you are seeing only a part of the picture. They bring you fascinating and often startling news that you cannot get anywhere else. You will also receive HLI's catalog of the best prolife/pro-family literature, books, films and videos. The suggested donation is $30 (tax-deductible). Please make your check payable to HLI.

[ ] Send me _____ book(s); total, _____.

[ ] Send me HLI's two newsletters. I'm enclosing

my tax-deductible offering of $_____.

TOTAL ENCLOSED: $_____.

name_____tel_____

address_____

city_____state_____ZIP_____

return to:
Human Life International
7845-E Airpark Road
Gaithersburg, Maryland 20879 USA
(301/670-7884)

Marx